Protein Purification
Principles and Trends

Protein Purification
Principles and Trends

Published by iConcept Press

Protein Purification: Principles and Trends

Publisher: iConcept Press Ltd.

ISBN: 978-1-922227-40-9

Printed in the United States of America

Copyright © iConcept Press 2016

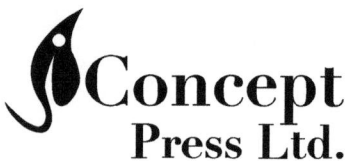

Concept
Press Ltd.

www.iconceptpress.com

Contents

Beste Çalımlıoğlu (*Istanbul Medeniyet University, Turkey*) and Kazim Yalcin Arga (*Marmara University, Turkey*)

Preface

Proteins are biochemical compounds consisting of one or more polypeptides. A polypeptide is a single linear polymer chain of amino acids bonded together by peptide bonds between the carboxyl and amino groups of adjacent amino acid residues. Protein purification is the process of isolating a few proteins from a complex mixture, such as a cell or a tissue. It is an important step for identifying functions, structures or interactions of the protein of interest.

Protein Purification: Principles and Trends discusses several current and important issues related to protein purification. Chapter 1 uses SILAC and TMT quantitative MS methods to identify novel target proteins modulated in the erlotinib (EGFR TKI) resistant lung cancer cells. The use of multiplex quantitative proteomic strategies, such as SILAC and TMT protein labeling are powerful methods for identifying a large number of novel biomarkers. Chapter 2 describes a MALDI-TOF/TOF based proteomic approach to profile HAPE-related proteomic changes in plasma. 25 differential plasma proteins responsible for the discrimination between the two groups from HAPE subjects and healthy controls have been identified and studied based on their biological functions. Furthermore, two of the 25 proteins (Haptoglobin and Apoliprotein A- I) have been considered as putative biomarkers for HAPE. Chapter 3 discusses an important oxidative stress-mediated tyrosine nitration in a protein in tumorigenesis, and addresses the principles of nitroproteomics, isolation and purification of nitroproteins, mass spectrometry characteristics of nitropeptides, methodology used for nitroproteomics in pituitary adenomas, current status of human pituitary nitroproteomics studies, and future trends. Chapter 4 shows the purification of fission yeast Dmc1 and its accessory proteins, and describes a conventional method to monitor DNA strand exchange reaction, which is a powerful tool to understand the biological significance of Dmc1 as well as its accessory proteins.

Chapter 5 introduces the fabrication process of boron nitride nanopores and demonstrates the conductance change in ionic current due to the translocation of both dsDNA and ssDNA through the nanopore. It open a window for DNA sensing with boron nitride nanopores and a potential platform for future DNA sequencing application. Chapter 6 aims to detail with necessary basic methods in protein purification and analysis that leads us to grasp new roles assigned to the $\alpha 1$–$\beta 2$ (and $\alpha 2$–$\beta 1$) interface of the human hemoglobin molecule: one is for stabilizing the HbO2 tetramer against acidic autoxidation, and the other is for controlling the fate (removal) of its own erythrocyte from the blood circulation. Chapter 7 summarizes mouse and human studies that provide mechanisms by which cholesterol could affect inflammation. Apart from the direct effects, its intracellular localization as well as the contribution of different types of cholesterol to the inflammatory response is highlighted – when oxidized, cholesterol is more likely to instigate inflammation. Chapter 8 summarizes major cell sources, important proteins, transcription factors and signaling cascades, which governs mesenchymal stromal cell (MSC) fate towards the osteogenic lineage as well as new trends in the development of scaffold materials with osteoconductive and osteoinductive properties.

Chapter 9 describes features, purification methods and applications of proteins such as membrane bound proteins, enzymes or recombinant proteins produced by halophilic bacteria. Chapter 10 discusses various tau modifications associated with tau aggregation. Tau aggregation is a pathological hallmark of many neurodegenerative diseases including AD. Chapter 11 discusses the properties of the Clostridium difficile toxins, the mechanism of action, and the immunopathogenesis of the toxins. Clostridium difficile toxins will trigger Clostridium difficile infection (CDI) which is the leading cause of hospital-acquired and antibiotic-associated bacterial diarrhea in the United States. Chapter 12 discusses the design of bioseparation strategy for engineering purification of conjugated proteins. The strategy is built on physicochemical properties which include molecular size, surface charge distribution and relative hydrophobicity for size exclusion, ion exchange and hydrophobic interaction chromatography respectively.

Editing and publishing a book is never an easy task. Each chapter in this book has gone through a peer review, a selection and an editing process so as to guarantee its quality. Without the supports and contributions of the authors and reviewers, this book can never be able to complete. We would like to thank all authors and all reviewers who participated in the reviewing process: Anas-Alwogud Abdelmogheth, Shamsozoha Abolmaali, Serefden Ac?kgoz, Minna-Liisa Anko, Glen D. Armstrong, Jean A. Boutin, Stephanie Cabantous, Ben-Kuen Chen, Gianni Ciofani, Aleksandro S. Da Silva, Aaron M. Elliott, Changjian Feng, Frank A. Ferrone, Stephen Florczyk, Peter H. Gilligan, Lan Hu, Paolo Iadarola, Kendall L. Knight, Hans Jörg Kunte, Li Lan, Guang Yu Li, Hung-Wen Li, Jiazheng Lu, Maria D. Mayan, Ayten Nalbant, Karthikeyan Narayanan, Eng-Poh Ng, Nobuaki Okumura, Mana Oloomi, Qi Pang, Spyros Petrakis, Chantal Prévost, Guntars Pupelis, Pablo J. Saez, Songklod Sarapusit, Caroline Schild-Poulter, Alexander Schulte, Hideto Shimahara, Akira Shinohara, Joseph A. Sorg, Erwin Swinnen, Winston Timp, Koji Ueda, Gayatri Vedantam, Chaochao Wu, Wei-Hsiung Yang, Zhen-lin Yang and Qigang Zhou.

Editorial Office, iConcept Press

August 2016

Chapter 1

Discovery of Biomarkers Mediating EGFR Tyrosine Kinase Inhibitor Resistance in Non-small Cell Lung Cancer: A Proteomics Approach

Gregory M. Botting[1], Ichwaku Rastogi[1], Gagan Chhabra[1], Jason T. Fong[1], Ryan J. Jacobs[1], Caleb Shearrow[1], David N. Moravec[1], Joseph Devito[1], Kymberly Harrington[1], Ryan D. Bomgarden[2], John C. Rogers[2] and Neelu Puri[1]

1   Introduction

Lung cancer is the second most prevalent form of cancer in the United States, accounting for more than 224,000, about 14%, of all new cancer cases. In 2016 alone, lung cancer will cause more than 158,080 deaths, accounting for 27% of all cancer-related deaths (Siegel *et al.*, 2016). Lung cancer is subdivided into Non-small cell (NSCLC) and Small cell (SCLC) types, accounting for 85% and 15% of all lung cancer cases in United States, respectively. Epidermal growth factor receptor (EGFR) is a receptor tyrosine kinase (RTK) which is highly expressed on the surface of lung cancer cells and contributes to tumorigenesis through shared signaling pathways (Stella & Comoglio, 1999; Engelman *et al.*, 2007; Puri & Salgia, 2008). Previous research by our group and others suggests that hepatocyte growth factor (HGF) can trans-activate EGFR and that active EGFR can phosphorylate c-Met (Spix *et al.*, 2007; Xu & Yu, 2007; Reznik *et al.*, 2008). These results indicate that EGFR and c-Met have extensive crosstalk, contributing to enhanced tumor

[1] Department of Biomedical Sciences, University of Illinois College of Medicine at Rockford, USA
[2] Thermo Fisher Scientific, Rockford, IL, United States

related signaling in NSCLC. This is also supported by studies which show that EGFR and c-Met inhibitors have a synergistic effect on tumorigenicity in NSCLC (Puri & Salgia, 2008).

There are several driver mutations in tyrosine kinases, which activate signaling in NSCLC to mediate tumorigenesis. Typically, these driver mutations cause constitutive activation of tyrosine kinases through structural alterations of their kinase domains. The most common EGFR mutations are the L858R single-point substitution in exon 21 and the A746-750 exon 19 deletion which constitute 90% of all classical EGFR-activating mutations (Gazdar, 2009). These somatic EGFR-activating mutations in the tyrosine kinase domain are the targets for chemotherapeutic agents, called tyrosine kinase inhibitors (TKIs), which act by inhibiting mutated EGFR signaling. EGFR TKIs competitively bind to the ATP binding pocket of EGFR, thus inhibiting receptor phosphorylation and subsequent activation (Gridellia et al., 2007). Currently, several TKIs and combination therapies are approved for patients who have somatic EGFR-activating mutations. Gefitinib was the first selective EGFR TKI approved for treatment of NSCLC (Cohen et al., 2004). Erlotinib is another effective EGFR TKI which is commonly prescribed following the failure of gefitinib to stop tumor progression (Xu et al., 2010).

Although, EGFR TKIs are effective treatments for NSCLC, their long-term efficacies are limited (Xu et al., 2010) due to the eventual development of resistance (Sierra et al., 2010). The majority of patients who initially respond to TKI treatments usually develop secondary resistance within about 9–14 months, resulting in tumor recurrence (Sequist et al., 2011; Goldman et al., 2012; Spigel et al., 2013). More than 50% of all acquired EGFR TKI resistance is due to the development of the secondary mutation T790M in the EGFR kinase domain (Gazdar, 2009; Dienstmann et al., 2012). The presence of this mutation before TKI treatment has also been shown to result in primary resistance to EGFR TKIs (Kobayashi et al., 2005; Lin & Bivona, 2012). Amplification of c-Met is another mechanism found to be responsible for more than 20% of acquired TKI resistance (Bean et al., 2007; Turke et al., 2010).

Although both EGFR secondary mutations and c-Met amplifications are key mechanisms of resistance to EGFR TKIs, they are not responsible for all forms of EGFR TKI resistance. In order to determine additional mechanisms of resistance to TKIs, it is imperative to identify other proteins which may contribute to TKI resistance and could serve as novel targets for future chemotherapies. Therefore, we developed H358 NSCLC cell lines with acquired resistance to the EGFR TKI erlotinib to elucidate additional proteins involved in TKI resistance. These cell lines were chosen as it expresses high levels of EGFR but did not have pre-existing EGFR mutations which confer resistance. To make these cell lines drug resistant, we exposed cells to step-wise increases of TKIs until cells survived and proliferated at high concentrations of these TKIs (> 10-fold increase in IC$_{50}$ of erlotinib). Following the development of TKI resistance, we used two quantitative mass spectrometry (MS) proteomic methods, SILAC and TMT labeling, to identify novel proteins which were up- or down-regulated in resistant cells.

Stable isotope labeling with amino acids in cell culture (SILAC) is a quantitative method that enables researchers to compare differences in protein expression between two unique cell populations (Mann, 2006). This protein labeling method involves growing one cell population in media containing the light isotope of a particular amino acid (e.g. ^{12}C L-lysine) and growing the other cell population in media containing the corresponding heavy isotope (e.g. ^{13}C L-lysine). Over a number of cell passages, these amino acids become fully incorporated into the proteome of the cultured cells. Since the labeled amino acids differ only in mass and not chemical composition, they can then be detected simultaneously by MS to compare differences in protein levels among the labeled samples. After isotope incorporation, cells can be treated with EGF, erlotinib or a combination of both EGF and erlotinib to alter the expression of proteins which are important in the EGFR tumorigenesis signaling and erlotinib TKI resistance. Following EGF ligand and inhibitor treatments, proteins from parental and resistant cell lines are extracted, combined and prepared for duplex MS analysis to determine levels of target proteins.

Another quantitative proteomic method for differential protein expression analysis is tandem mass tag (TMT) technology (Altelaar *et al.*, 2013). This chemical labeling method utilizes isobaric tags which have the same nominal mass during MS but produce a unique reporter ion upon MS/MS fragmentation. Unlike the SILAC method, TMT labeling does not require the metabolic incorporation for labeling so the tags can be used to label any protein sample including human plasma and tissue samples. Instead, an amine-reactive group is used to label peptides after protein digestion for heavy isotope incorporation. By altering the distribution of heavy isotopes such as ^{13}C and ^{15}N in the structure of the mass reporter, a number of tags can be generated that differ in mass by about one Dalton. This allows TMT reagents to be used to compare differences in protein expression in up to 10 different cell treatment conditions (2–10 plex) in a single MS analysis (McAlister *et al.*, 2012), giving it a distinct advantage over the SILAC method.

We used both SILAC and TMT quantitative MS methods to identify novel target proteins and pathways which may be involved in the EGFR TKI resistance mechanisms. Proteins found to be significantly up- or down-regulated in resistant cells before or after ligand/TKI treatment were considered as potential target proteins. Results from this global proteomic profiling study could provide clinicians with new target options for drug inhibition to overcome TKI resistance in NSCLC patients, potentially increasing progression-free and overall survival rates.

2   Materials and Methods

2.1   Reagents

Erlotinib (N-(3-ethynylphenyl)-6,7-bis(2-methoxyethoxy)-quinazolin-4-amine) was obtained from LC Laboratories (Woburn, MA) and was suspended in DMSO and stored in 50 µL aliquots at –20 °C. EGF was obtained from Cell Signaling Technology (Beverly, MA) and was suspended in PBS and stored in 0.1mL aliquots at –20 °C.

2.2   Cell Culture and Establishment of TKI Resistance

H358 NSCLC cell lines were obtained from the American Type Culture Collection (Rockville, MD, CRL-5807) and were cultured as per ATCC instructions in 6-well plates. Cells were incubated at 37 °C with 7% CO_2 and maintained in Roswell Park Memorial Institute (RPMI) medium (Thermo Fisher Scientific, Pittsburg, PA, Cat No: SH3002701) supplemented with 10% (v/v) fetal bovine serum (Atlanta Biologicals, Lawrenceville, GA) and 1% (v/v) antibiotic/ antimycotic (Invitrogen, Cat No: 15240). For identifying the appropriate concentrations of erlotinib for developing resistance, cells were treated for several months with progressively increasing concentrations of erlotinib (0.5–14 µM) until they were proliferating and surviving at high concentrations. The final IC_{50} was found out to be 11fold greater for erlotinib. Cells were then deprived of drug for 12 passages (12 weeks), but still retained resistance to high concentrations of erlotinib.

2.3   Cell Treatment for Differential Analysis

H358 parental and erlotinib-resistant cells were plated at 4×10^6 cells per dish on 150mm plastic petri dishes and were allowed to adhere and grow for 24 hours. Cells were then incubated in serum-free RPMI medium with 0.5% BSA for an additional 24 hours. Parental and resistant cells were then treated for 24 hours with 10µM erlotinib in serum-free medium containing 0.5% BSA. Following 24 hours of drug treatment, cells were stimulated with 15ng/mL EGF for 2.5 minutes in serum-free medium containing 0.5% BSA. Cells were then rinsed twice with 1× PBS before harvesting by cell scraping. Protein lysates were prepared by drawing cells up with a syringe and expelling them rapidly to disrupt cell components. Lysates were snap frozen in liquid nitrogen and stored at –70 °C until MS analysis.

2.4   SILAC Labeling and MS Quantitation

H358 parental and resistant cells were grown for six passages (30 days) using SILAC RPMI (Thermo Fisher Scientific) containing 0.1 mg/ml "heavy" $^{13}C_6$ L-lysine-2HCl and $^{13}C_6$ $^{15}N_4$ L-Arginine-HCl or "light" L-lysine-2HCl and L-Arginine-HCl with Dialyzed Fetal Bovine Serum. Cells were treated with 5ng/ml EGF for 5 min before harvesting for lysis. For each protein extract sample, 50µg was equally mixed (Parental/Light and Resistant/Heavy) and separated via 4–15% SDS-PAGE. Gels were stained with GelCode Blue Stain (Thermo Fisher Scientific) and protein bands were excised, destained, reduced, alkylated and digested using an In-Gel Tryptic Digest Kit (Thermo Fisher Scientific). Peptides were cleaned up using C18 spin tips (Thermo Fisher Scientific) before MS analysis.

A NanoLC-2D high-pressure liquid chromatography (HPLC) system with a Thermo Scientific PepMap C18 column (75 µm ID × 20 cm) was used to separate peptides using a 5–40% gradient (A: water, 0.1% formic acid; B: acetonitrile, 0.1% formic acid) at a flow rate of 300 nL/min for 120 min. A Thermo Scientific LTQ Orbitrap XL ETD mass spectrometer was used to detect peptides using a top-six experiment consisting of single-stage MS used for quantitation followed by acquisition of six MS/MS spectra with collision-induced dissociation (CID) for peptide identification.

Peptide identification and SILAC quantitation were performed using Thermo Scientific Proteome Discoverer v1.3 software. Identified proteins (2 peptides minimum, FDR < 0.5%) were plotted on semi-log graphs sorted by average SILAC ratios to determine most up- and down-regulated proteins. Mass spectra of heavy peptides containing $^{13}C_6$ L-lysine and $^{13}C_6$ $^{15}N_4$ L-Arginine are shifted to the right of the light peptide spectra by a mass to charge ratio (m/z) of 4 or 5, respectively for +2 charged peptides.

2.5   Tandem Mass Tagging (TMT) and MS Quantitation

Parental and drug-resistant NSCLC cell lines were left untreated or treated with EGF or 10μM erlotinib alone, or treated with both EGF and erlotinib. After reduction and alkylation, proteins from ten different conditions were digested with trypsin, labeled with Thermo Scientific TMT10plex reagents and combined before LC/MS analysis (Figure 2). Magnetic Fe-NTA resin was also used for phosphopeptide enrichment of TMT-labeled samples. Combined peptide samples (unenriched or phospho-enriched) were also fractionated by high pH reverse phase using a novel spin column format containing a polystyrene divinyl benzene resin to generate eight fractions for LC/MS analysis for each sample type.

Samples were separated by RP-HPLC using a Thermo Scientific™ EASY-nLC™ 1000 nano-flow system or a Dionex Ultimate 3000 system connected to a Thermo Scientific™ EASY-Spray™ column, 25 cm × 75 μm or a Thermo Scientific™ Acclaim™ PepMap™ C18 Column over a 5–30% gradient (A: water, 0.1% formic acid; B: acetonitrile, 0.1% formic acid) at a flow rate of 300 nL/min for 210 min.

Spectra were acquired using a Thermo Scientific™ Orbitrap Fusion™ Tribrid™ mass spectrometer using topN FT MS^2 (HCD) at resolution of 60,000 @m/z 200 or using SPS MS^3 quantification was also performed using an FTMS full scan at 120,000 @ m/z 200 resolution followed by IT MS^2 CID and FT MS^3 HCD (resolution 60,000 @ m/z 200) on a total of 10 fragments from the MS^2 spectra. Spectral data files were analyzed using Thermo Scientific™ Proteome Discoverer™ 1.4 software using the SEQUEST®HT search engine, constrained with a precursor mass tolerance of 10 ppm and fragment mass tolerance of 0.02 Da (0.8 Da for CID identification using SPS). Carbamidomethylation (+57.021 Da) for cysteine and TMT isobaric labeling (+229.162 Da) for lysine and N-terminus residues were treated as static modifications while methionine oxidation (+15.996 Da). Data was searched against a Swiss-Prot® complete human database with a 1% FDR criteria using Percolator.

Pathway analysis/protein profiling was performed using Thermo Scientific™ Protein Center™ 3.9 software. The TMT10plex quantification method within Proteome Discoverer 1.4 software was used to calculate the reporter ratios with mass tolerance ±10 ppm without applying the isotopic correction factors. A protein ratio was expressed as a median value of the ratios for all quantifiable spectra of the peptides pertaining to that protein.

3   Results & Discussion

For our initial characterization of differences between parental and erlotinib-resistant cells, we used a duplex SILAC workflow (Figure 1A). After culturing cells in SILAC media containing light (parental cells) or heavy (resistant cells) amino acids, protein extracts from each cell line were equally mixed and separated via SDS-PAGE to fractionate proteins by size prior to in-gel tryptic digests and MS analysis. Overall, we identified and quantified greater than 2800 proteins from the combined LC-MS runs (Figure 1B). Of these, over 500 proteins were found to be up- or down-regulated > 2-fold in resistant cells, compared to parental cells, and considered for a list of target proteins to be further validated (Table 1).

Although we identified a large number of proteins using SILAC that exhibit differential expression between parental and resistant cell lines, this technique is limited to comparing only two to three samples in a single MS analysis. In order to identify proteins which may be changing after treatment with ligand, TKIs or both ligand/TKIs in parental and resistant cell lines, we used multiplex TMT reagents. In the present study, we compared data from SILAC and TMT studies between parental and resistant cell lines only in the presence of EGF, since this was only treatment studied using SILAC. [1]For the TMT workflow, cell lysates from each condition were digested to peptides, labeled with TMT isobaric chemical tags and combined into a single sample before MS analysis (Figure 2). Using this approach, we identified over 4000 unique proteins and measured relative changes in protein levels using TMT reporter ions. Proteins which showed similar changes in expression after each treatment were further grouped using cluster analysis and a heatmap was generated (Figure 3). Proteins which demonstrated significant changes in expression were considered for a list of potential targets to be further validated (Table 1).

SILAC and TMT labeling are two powerful quantitative proteomic methods which enable profiling of relative protein abundance between multiple cell lines and/or cell treatments. Although both methods use stable isotopes for MS-based quantification and sample multiplexing, they have many differences. One important difference between SILAC and TMT is sample compatibility. SILAC is restricted to cultured cells since endogenous protein expression machinery is used for stable isotope amino acid incorporation (Amanchy et al., 2005). In contrast, TMT reagents can label samples derived not only from cultured cells, but also human tissue and serum. Another key difference between these techniques is the time-point at which samples can be combined for multiplexing. Since the SILAC method labels proteins, protein extracts can be mixed immediately after cell lysis. This feature not only reduces errors introduced by parallel sample preparation, but also allows for protein-level separation techniques such as subcellular fractionation, size exclusion chromatography or SDS-PAGE. In contrast, TMT reagents label peptides generated from protein digests, which must be prepared separately. Since samples are mixed much later in the TMT sample preparation workflow, there is opportunity for more error in the quantitative measurements due to sample handling loss, differences in digestion efficiency or pipetting error (Altelaar et al., 2013).

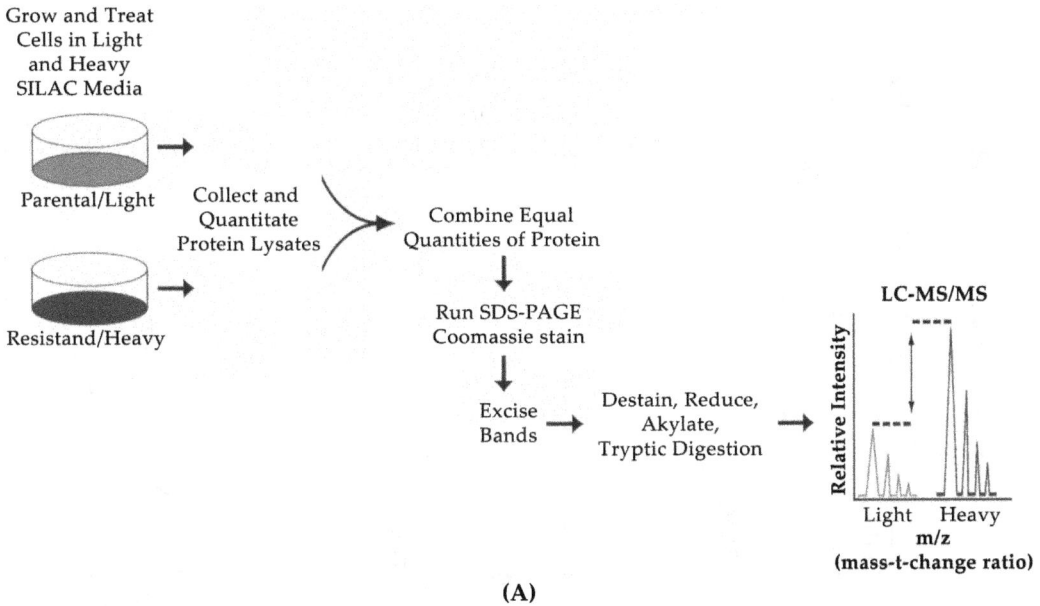

(A)

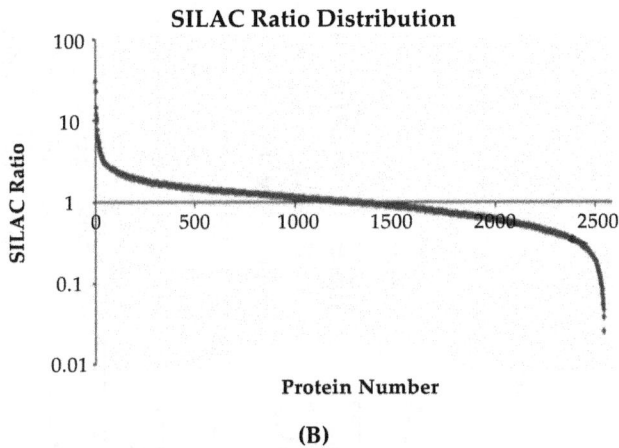

(B)

Figure 1: (A) Schematic of SILAC workflow sample preparation and mass spectrometry analysis. H358 parental and resistant cells were grown for 6 passages using SILAC RPMI with light or heavy amino acids. Cells were treated with/without EGF, lysed and collected. Samples (Parental/Light and Resistant/Heavy) were equally mixed before SDS-PAGE analysis and gel staining. Bands were excised, destained, reduced, alkylated and digested before LC-MS/MS analysis. **(B)** Identified proteins (2 peptides minimum, FDR < 0.5%) were plotted on semi-log graphs sorted by average SILAC ratios to determine proteins which were maximally modulated.

Gene Symbol	Protein Name	UniProtKB Accession Number	Function	Fold-Change by SILAC (resistant/parental)	Fold-Change by TMT (resistant/parental)
CTNNB1	Catenin beta-1	P35222	In presence of Wnt, accumulates in the nucleus activating Wnt responsive genes, which promote tumorigenicity	0.24	0.5
HMGB2	High mobility group protein B2	P26583	DNA binding protein; associated with tumor aggressiveness, growth, and poor prognosis of hepatocellular carcinoma	2.32	1.72
TOMM34	Mitochondrial import receptor subunit TOM34	Q15785	Aids import of cytosolically synthesized pre-proteins into mitochondria	2.51	1.59
MESDC2	LDLR chaperone MESD	Q14696	Assists folding of EGF modules; modulates Wnt pathway through chaperoning the co-receptors of canonical Wnt pathway	0.572	0.792
MCM6	DNA replication licensing factor MCM6	Q14566	Helicase essential for initiation of DNA replication and prevention of re-replication	1.65	ND
AIF1	Allograft inflammatory factor 1	P55008	Actin-binding protein that enhances membrane ruffling and RAC activation. It negatively regulates apoptotic process.	0.56	0.45
GNA1	Glucosamine 6-phosphate N-acetyltransferase	Q96EK6	Catalytic activity: Acetyl-CoA + D-glucosamine 6-phosphate = CoA + N-acetyl-D-glucosamine 6-phosphate	ND	0.57

Continued on next page....

... Continued from previous page

Gene Symbol	Protein Name	UniProtKB Accession Number	Function	Fold-Change by SILAC (resistant/parental)	Fold-Change by TMT (resistant/parental)
BAX	Apoptosis regulator BAX	Q07812	Accelerates programmed cell death by antagonizing apoptosis repressor BCL2 or E1B 19K protein	1.75	1.51
TPR	Nucleoprotein TPR	P12270	Involved in activation of oncogenic kinases	1.57	1.93
SND1	Staphylococcal nuclease domain-containing protein 1	Q7KZF4	Bridging factor between STAT6 and the basal transcription factor	ND	0.76
SDCBP	Syntenin-1	O00560	Adapter protein that couples syndecans to signaling components; may play a role in vesicular trafficking	1.85	ND
MSH6	DNA mismatch repair protein Msh6	P52701	Heterodimerizes with MSH2 to form MutSα, which binds to DNA mismatches, initiating DNA repair	2.69	1.75

Table 1: List of proteins of interest identified and quantified by LC-MS^n from H358 lung cancer cell lines. SILAC and TMT quantitation shows differential protein expression (i.e. fold changes) between parental and erlotinib resistant cells after EGF treatment (n=2 for SILAC and n=3 for TMT). ND is no data acquired for that protein. (*All protein functions are taken from the UniProt Knowledgebase at www.uniprot.org)

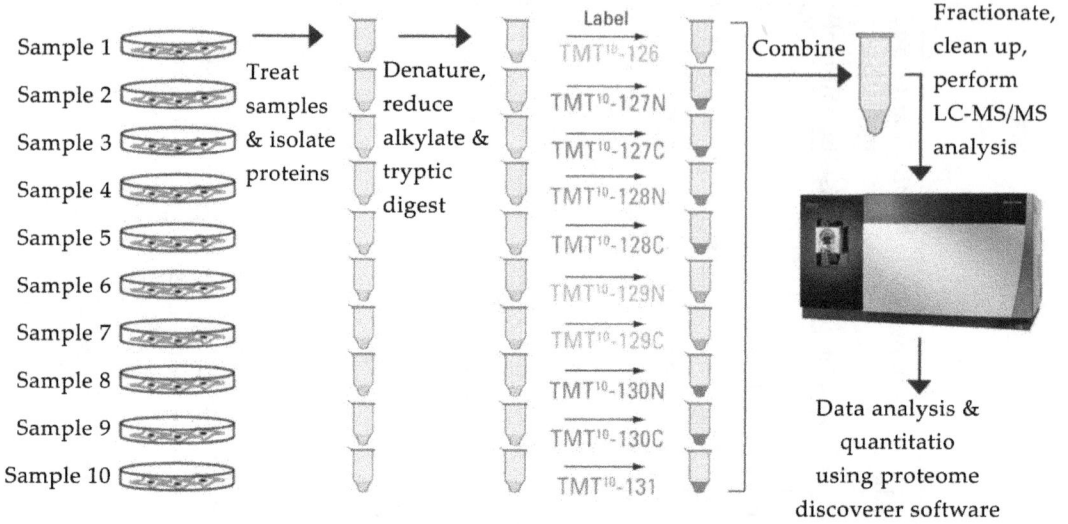

(A)

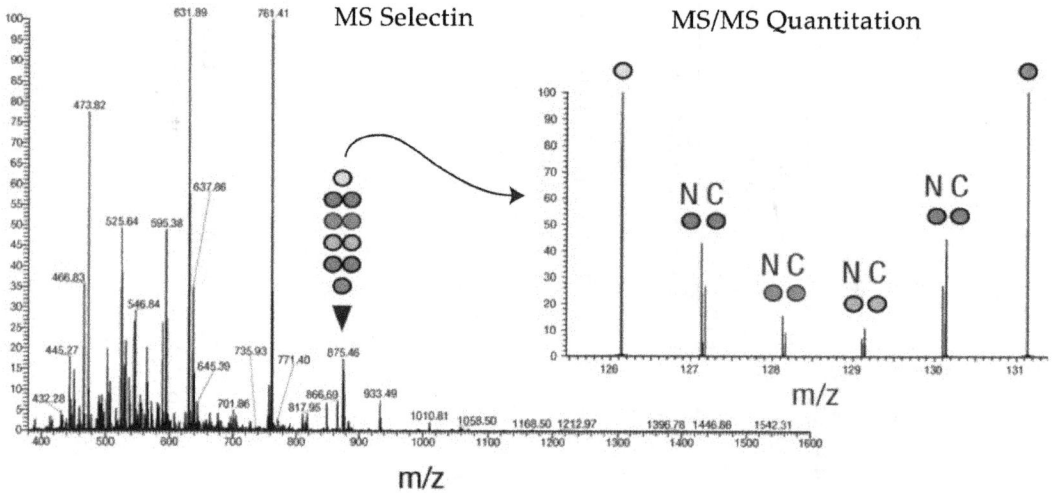

(B)

Figure 2: Schematic of TMT10plex Reagent sample preparation and LC-MS analysis. **A)** Proteins from parental and H358 erlotinib-resistant NSCLC cell lines were treated with diluent, EGF, erlotinib or both EGF/erlotinib were extracted, reduced, alkylated, and digested before being labeled with TMT10plex reagents. Labeled peptides from each treatment condition are combined, enriched for phospho-peptides, fractionated by high pH reverse phase chromatography and analyzed by LC/MS analysis. **B)** TMT10plex-labeled peptides co-elute during MS acquisition but generate 10 unique reporter ion masses during MS^n for relative quantitation.

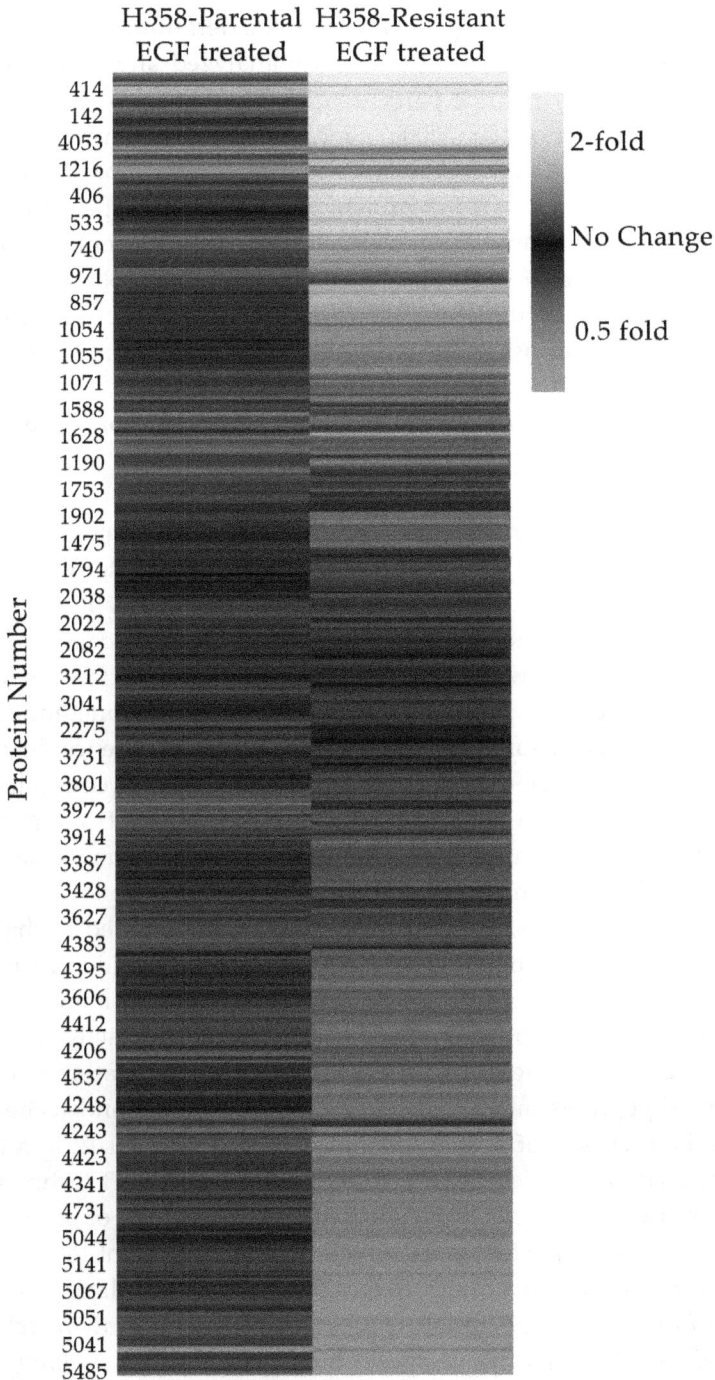

Figure 3: Cluster analysis based on TMT quantitation showing changes in protein expression for 5485 proteins (2 peptides per protein) between H358 parental versus erlotinib-resistant cells for different treatment conditions. Data is normalized to untreated H358 parental cells.

In addition to compatibility and labeling considerations, SILAC and TMT samples have significant differences in how they are analyzed and quantified by MS. For SILAC samples, light/heavy peptide pairs are quantified at the MS-level before peptide identification during MS/MS (Mann, 2006). Since both light and heavy peptides are analyzed simultaneously by MS, SILAC samples are inherently more complex than unlabeled samples. This can result in fewer protein identifications, especially if multiplexing is increased beyond duplex samples. In contrast, TMT-labeled peptides are both identified and quantified during MS/MS. Since TMT reagents are isobaric, labeled peptides have the same nominal mass; therefore, MS complexity is not increased. This allows for higher sample multiplexing using TMT reagents without significant impact to MS acquisition times (McAlister *et al.*, 2012).

Although both techniques require high resolution MS for the best quantitative precision and accuracy, TMT quantitative accuracy can be more affected by interfering ions than SILAC. Since TMT is quantified during MS/MS, interfering ions which are co-isolated during MS acquisition can also contribute to TMT reporter ion signals distorting protein ratios (Altelaar *et al.*, 2013). This background interference can result in suppression of relative differences between samples, potentially leading to more false negatives in the data set. Reducing sample complexity through peptide fractionation is one method that has been shown to reduce background ion interference for isobaric tag quantification. In this study, we used another recently described method, multi-notch or synchronous precursor selection (SPS) MS3, to eliminate interference. In SPS-MS3, multiple precursor ions are selected for a third MS scan to remove co-isolated, interfering ions (Ting *et al.*, 2011). This method dramatically improves TMT quantitative accuracy but can also reduce the total number of quantifiable peptides due to the additional MS scan time on slower MS instruments.

Despite their differences, both SILAC and TMT labeling led to the identification of many novel lung cancer biomarkers. Nearly all of proteins identified using SILAC were also found in TMT experiments which were acquired using a more sensitive, faster scanning MS instrument. Although the fold changes were not exactly identical in SILAC and TMT data, quantified proteins had similar up or down regulation (Table 1). Increasing the number of peptides quantified per protein, biological and technical replicates could improve the accuracy of protein quantitation and may result in a better correlation between the fold differences measured using SILAC and TMT techniques.

Using these two techniques, we have identified a selection of proteins, modulated at least 2-fold in erlotinib-resistant cells, which may be important to EGFR induced tumorigenicity. Our selection of proteins from all acquired MS data sets was based on known protein function and potential relationship with cell growth, cell death, DNA maintenance, EGFR-related pathways and/or lung cancer. A key signaling protein identified using both SILAC and TMT quantitative mass spectrometry was β-catenin which was down-regulated approximately 2-fold in H358 erlotinib-resistant cells (Figure 4). The SILAC method also identified HMGB2, TOM34, MESDC2, AIF1, MCM6, BAX, TPR, Syntenin and Msh6, while the TMT tag approach allowed us to identify GNA1 and SND1 in addition to proteins identified using SILAC as promising targets which may contribute to EGFR/c-Met TKI resistance (Table 1).

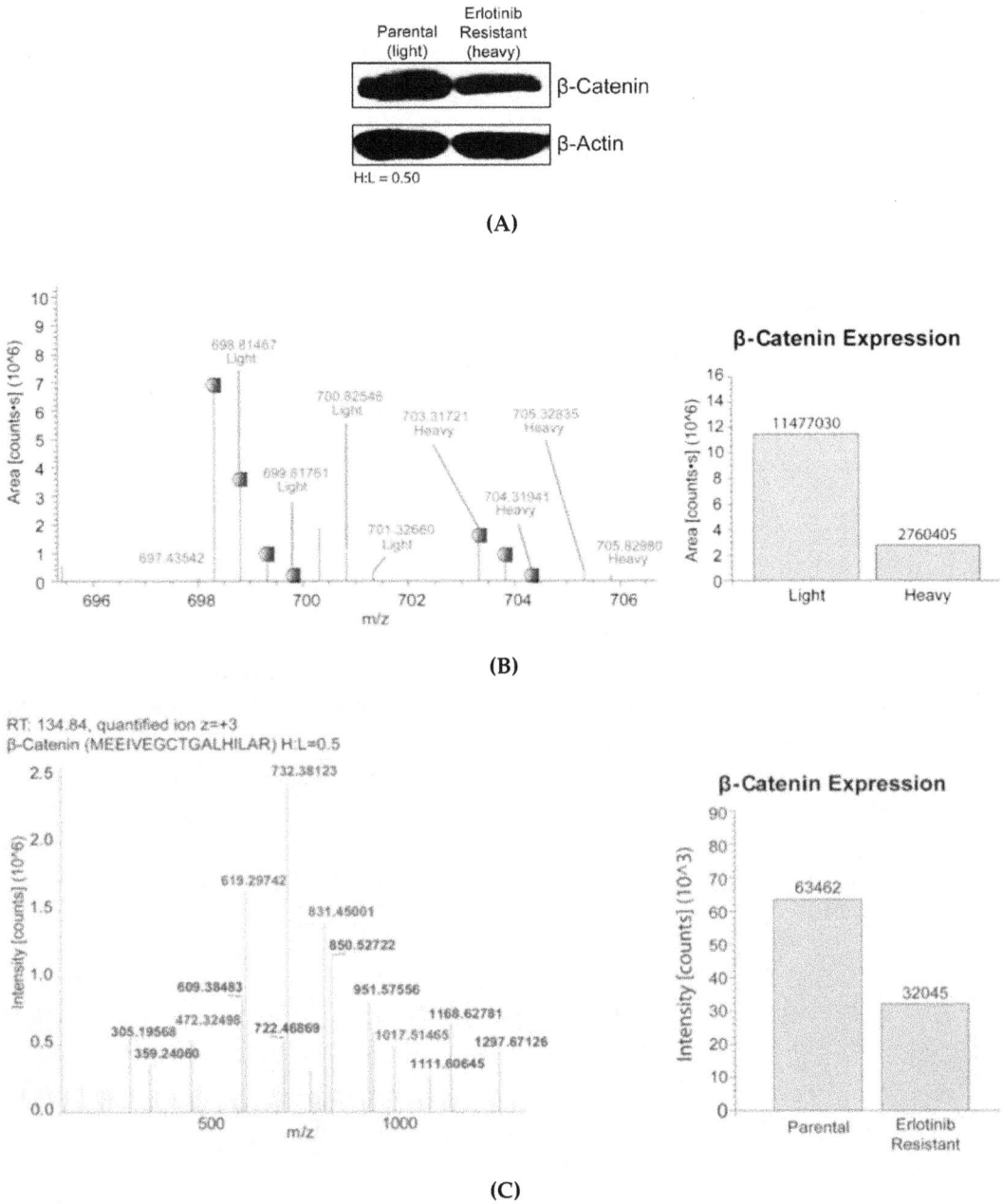

Figure 4: Differential expression of beta-catenin in H358 parental and erlotinib-resistant (ER) cell lines determined by **(A)** Western blot, **(B)** SILAC and **(C)** TMT quantitation. Western blot of protein samples shows comparable beta-catenin levels to those observed by SILAC and TMT analysis. SILAC quantitation is shown for a combined light (parental) and heavy (ER) beta-catenin peptide MS spectrum. TMT quantitation is shown for the reporter ions generated in the low mass region of a beta-catenin MS/MS spectrum which also contains b ions (red) and y ions (blue) used for peptide sequencing.

The use of multiplex quantitative proteomic strategies, such as SILAC and TMT protein labeling are powerful methods for identifying a large number of novel biomarkers. Proteins identified in our experiments using TMT tagging and SILAC suggest that alternative growth/survival signaling such as Wnt and mTOR pathways (Casas-Selves *et al.*, 2012; McAlister *et al.*, 2012; Fong *et al.*, 2013) may play a role in lung cancer resistance. This is further validated by the relative changes in protein abundance identified in our proteomic analysis between parental and erltotinib-resistant H358 cell lines, such as β-catenin, MESDC2 and SND1, which may have roles in mediating Wnt and mTOR signaling (see functions in Table 1) making them candidates for contributing to EGFR TKI resistance. The regulation of these proteins with different cell treatments (e.g. EGF, EGF+erlotinib) using multiplex TMT reagents is an active area of research for future studies. In addition, the actual roles these proteins play in TKI resistance mechanism will need to be further validated in future studies before they are considered as new lung cancer therapeutics.

Acknowledgement

Research reported in this publication was supported by the National Cancer Institute of the National Institutes of Health under award number R21CA158965-01A1 (http://www.nih.gov) to Neelu Puri. The content is solely the responsibility of the authors and does not necessarily represent the official views of the National Institutes of Health. The funders had no role in study design, data collection and analysis, decision to publish, or preparation of the manuscript.

References

Altelaar, A. F., C. K. Frese, C. Preisinger, M. L. Hennrich, A. W. Schram, H. T. Timmers, A. J. Heck and S. Mohammed (2013). *Benchmarking stable isotope labeling based quantitative proteomics. J Proteomics* 88: 14–26.

Amanchy, R., D. E. Kalume and A. Pandey (2005). *Stable isotope labeling with amino acids in cell culture (SILAC) for studying dynamics of protein abundance and posttranslational modifications. Sci STKE* 2005(267): pl2.

Bean, J., C. Brennan, J. Y. Shih, G. Riely, A. Viale, L. Wang, D. Chitale, N. Motoi, J. Szoke, S. Broderick, M. Balak, W. C. Chang, C. J. Yu, A. Gazdar, H. Pass, V. Rusch, W. Gerald, S. F. Huang, P. C. Yang, V. Miller, M. Ladanyi, C. H. Yang and W. Pao (2007). *MET amplification occurs with or without T790M mutations in EGFR mutant lung tumors with acquired resistance to gefitinib or erlotinib. Proc Natl Acad Sci U S A* 104(52): 20932–20937.

Casas-Selves, M., J. Kim, Z. Zhang, B. A. Helfrich, D. Gao, C. C. Porter, H. A. Scarborough, P. A. Bunn, Jr., D. C. Chan, A. C. Tan and J. DeGregori (2012). *Tankyrase and the canonical Wnt pathway protect lung cancer cells from EGFR inhibition. Cancer Res* 72(16): 4154–

4164.

Cohen, M. H., G. A. Williams, R. Sridhara, G. Chen, W. D. McGuinn, Jr., D. Morse, S. Abraham, A. Rahman, C. Liang, R. Lostritto, A. Baird and R. Pazdur (2004). United States Food and Drug Administration Drug Approval summary: Gefitinib (ZD1839; Iressa) tablets. Clin Cancer Res 10(4): 1212–1218.

Dienstmann, R., S. De Dosso, E. Felip and J. Tabernero (2012). Drug development to overcome resistance to EGFR inhibitors in lung and colorectal cancer. Mol Oncol 6(1): 15–26.

Engelman, J. A., K. Zejnullahu, T. Mitsudomi, Y. Song, C. Hyland, J. O. Park, N. Lindeman, C. M. Gale, X. Zhao, J. Christensen, T. Kosaka, A. J. Holmes, A. M. Rogers, F. Cappuzzo, T. Mok, C. Lee, B. E. Johnson, L. C. Cantley and P. A. Janne (2007). MET amplification leads to gefitinib resistance in lung cancer by activating ERBB3 signaling. Science 316(5827): 1039–1043.

Fong, J. T., R. J. Jacobs, D. N. Moravec, S. B. Uppada, G. M. Botting, M. Nlend and N. Puri (2013). Alternative signaling pathways as potential therapeutic targets for overcoming EGFR and c-Met inhibitor resistance in non-small cell lung cancer. PLoS One 8(11): e78398.

Gazdar, A. F. (2009). Activating and resistance mutations of EGFR in non-small-cell lung cancer: role in clinical response to EGFR tyrosine kinase inhibitors. Oncogene 28 Suppl 1: S24–31.

Goldman, J. W., I. Laux, F. Chai, R. E. Savage, D. Ferrari, E. G. Garmey, R. G. Just and L. S. Rosen (2012). Phase 1 dose-escalation trial evaluating the combination of the selective MET (mesenchymal-epithelial transition factor) inhibitor tivantinib (ARQ 197) plus erlotinib. Cancer 118(23): 5903–5911.

Gridellia, C., M. Bareschinob, C. Schettinob, A. Rossia, P. Maionea and F. Ciardiellob (2007). Erlotinib in Non-Small Cell Lung Cancer Treatment: Current Status and Future Development. The Oncologist 12(7): 840–849.

Kobayashi, S., T. J. Boggon, T. Dayaram, P. A. Janne, O. Kocher, M. Meyerson, B. E. Johnson, M. J. Eck, D. G. Tenen and B. Halmos (2005). EGFR mutation and resistance of non-small-cell lung cancer to gefitinib. N Engl J Med 352(8): 786–792.

Lin, L. and T. G. Bivona (2012). Mechanisms of Resistance to Epidermal Growth Factor Receptor Inhibitors and Novel Therapeutic Strategies to Overcome Resistance in NSCLC Patients. Chemother Res Pract 2012: 817297.

Mann, M. (2006). Functional and quantitative proteomics using SILAC. Nat Rev Mol Cell Biol 7(12): 952–958.

McAlister, G. C., E. L. Huttlin, W. Haas, L. Ting, M. P. Jedrychowski, J. C. Rogers, K. Kuhn, I. Pike, R. A. Grothe, J. D. Blethrow and S. P. Gygi (2012). Increasing the multiplexing capacity of TMTs using reporter ion isotopologues with isobaric masses. Anal Chem 84(17): 7469–7478.

Puri, N. and R. Salgia (2008). Synergism of EGFR and c-Met pathways, cross-talk and inhibition, in non-small cell lung cancer. J Carcinog 7: 9.

Reznik, T. E., Y. Sang, Y. Ma, R. Abounader, E. M. Rosen, S. Xia and J. Laterra (2008). *Transcription-dependent epidermal growth factor receptor activation by hepatocyte growth factor. Mol Cancer Res 6(1): 139–150.*

Sequist, L. V., J. von Pawel, E. G. Garmey, W. L. Akerley, W. Brugger, D. Ferrari, Y. Chen, D. B. Costa, D. E. Gerber, S. Orlov, R. Ramlau, S. Arthur, I. Gorbachevsky, B. Schwartz and J. H. Schiller (2011). *Randomized phase II study of erlotinib plus tivantinib versus erlotinib plus placebo in previously treated non-small-cell lung cancer. J Clin Oncol 29(24): 3307– 3315.*

Siegel, R., Miller K. D. and A. Jemal (2016). *Cancer statistics, 2016. CA Cancer J Clin 66(1): 7– 30.*

Sierra, J. R., V. Cepero and S. Giordano (2010). *Molecular mechanisms of acquired resistance to tyrosine kinase targeted therapy. Mol Cancer 9: 75.*

Spigel, D. R., T. J. Ervin, R. A. Ramlau, D. B. Daniel, J. H. Goldschmidt, Jr., G. R. Blumenschein, Jr., M. J. Krzakowski, G. Robinet, B. Godbert, F. Barlesi, R. Govindan, T. Patel, S. V. Orlov, M. S. Wertheim, W. Yu, J. Zha, R. L. Yauch, P. H. Patel, S. C. Phan and A. C. Peterson (2013). *Randomized phase II trial of Onartuzumab in combination with erlotinib in patients with advanced non-small-cell lung cancer. J Clin Oncol 31(32): 4105– 4114.*

Spix, J. K., E. Y. Chay, E. R. Block and J. K. Klarlund (2007). *Hepatocyte growth factor induces epithelial cell motility through transactivation of the epidermal growth factor receptor. Exp Cell Res 313(15): 3319–3325.*

Stella, M. C. and P. M. Comoglio (1999). *HGF: a multifunctional growth factor controlling cell scattering. Int J Biochem Cell Biol 31(12): 1357–1362.*

Ting, L., R. Rad, S. P. Gygi and W. Haas (2011). *MS3 eliminates ratio distortion in isobaric multiplexed quantitative proteomics. Nat Methods 8(11): 937–940.*

Turke, A. B., K. Zejnullahu, Y. L. Wu, Y. Song, D. Dias-Santagata, E. Lifshits, L. Toschi, A. Rogers, T. Mok, L. Sequist, N. I. Lindeman, C. Murphy, S. Akhavanfard, B. Y. Yeap, Y. Xiao, M. Capelletti, A. J. Iafrate, C. Lee, J. G. Christensen, J. A. Engelman and P. A. Janne (2010). *Preexistence and clonal selection of MET amplification in EGFR mutant NSCLC. Cancer Cell 17(1): 77–88.*

Xu, K. P. and F. S. Yu (2007). *Cross talk between c-Met and epidermal growth factor receptor during retinal pigment epithelial wound healing. Invest Ophthalmol Vis Sci 48(5): 2242– 2248.*

Xu, L., M. B. Nilsson, P. Saintigny, T. Cascone, M. H. Herynk, Z. Du, P. G. Nikolinakos, Y. Yang, L. Prudkin, D. Liu, J. J. Lee, F. M. Johnson, K. K. Wong, L. Girard, A. F. Gazdar, J. D. Minna, J. M. Kurie, Wistuba, II and J. V. Heymach (2010). *Epidermal growth factor receptor regulates MET levels and invasiveness through hypoxia-inducible factor-1alpha in non-small cell lung cancer cells. Oncogene 29(18): 2616–2627.*

Xu, Y., H. Liu, J. Chen and Q. Zhou (2010). *Acquired resistance of lung adenocarcinoma to EGFR-tyrosine kinase inhibitors gefitinib and erlotinib. Cancer Biol Ther 9(8): 572–582.*

Chapter 2

Haptoglobin and Apolipoprotein A-I as Biomarkers of High Altitude Pulmonary Edema

Yasmin Ahmad[1], Narendra K. Sharma[1] and Manish Sharma[1]

1 Introduction

Impaired pulmonary gas exchange occurs in high altitude pulmonary edema (HAPE) and in some persons with acute mountain sickness (AMS). HAPE is a form of noncardiogenic pulmonary edema that occurs in persons who ascend to altitudes above 2,500 m and remain there for 24 to 48 hours or longer (Schoene, 1985). Although the pathogenesis of HAPE is unknown, most reports focus on hydrostatic mechanisms leading to capillary leak and pulmonary edema. These mechanisms include hypoxic pulmonary vasoconstriction (Hultgren, 1978; Bartsch, 1991) regional over perfusion (Hultgren, 1978), or capillary rupture from high pulmonary vascular pressure and shear stress (West *et al.*, 1991). Hypoxia, cold, exertion, fluid retention, and pulmonary vasoconstriction have also thought to be contributed (Hultgren, 1978; Houston, 1960). Although pulmonary hypertension has been documented in many HAPE patients, (Hultgren, 1978; Bartsch, 1991) there is also evidence that increased capillary permeability and inflammation may play an important role in the pathogenesis of HAPE. Evidence for the presence of inflammation in people with HAPE has come from several sources. Many patients with HAPE have fever, peripheral leukocytosis and raised erythrocyte sedimentation rates (Schoene *et al.*, 2001). Examination of bronchoalveolar larvage fluid from individuals with established HAPE has high levels of inflammatory cells (Schoene *et al.*, 1996; Schoene *et al.*, 1988; Kubo *et al.*, 1996; Kubo *et al.*, 1998). When brochoalveolar

---

[1] Peptide and Proteomics Division, Defence Institute of Physiological & Allied Science (DIPAS), Delhi, India

lavage was performed in the field, in patients suffering from HAPE for 24 hours or less, there was a marked increase in total cells, with macrophages being predominant, along with elevated levels of cytokines including IL-6, IL-8 and tumor necrosis factor alpha (Kubo *et al.*, 1998). In hospitalized patients later in the course of HAPE, the proportion of neutrophils increase and the observation is an inflammatory process similar in magnitude and pattern due to acute respiratory distress syndrome in the critical care unit (Kubo *et al.*, 1996). Further evidence for an inflammatory component of HAPE is provided by the high rate of preceding respiratory-tract infection in children who develop HAPE (Durmowicz *et al.*, 1997), association between certain major HLA-immunomodulating alleles with susceptibility to HAPE (Hanaoka *et al.*, 1998) and raised plasma E- selectin concentrations in hypoxemic climbers with AMS and HAPE (Grissom *et al.*, 1997). Thus, in addition to pulmonary hypertension, signs of inflammation are present in HAPE.

Plasma proteins are useful targets for diagnostic, prognostic, and or therapeutic development. With proteomic tools available recently, profiling of human plasma proteome becomes more feasible in searching for disease-related markers (Anderson *et al.*, 2002). The presence of a particular protein and/or its isoforms in the plasma represents the likelihood of other biologically active molecules. These in turn may correspond to cellular functions. Since cellular functions often change during different disease states, the measurement of protein expression and modification may lead to the detection and identification of particular disease. To the best of our knowledge, there are no plasma or serum biomarkers with high sensitivity and specificity for the diagnosis and monitoring of HAPE. We therefore aimed to identify the differentially expressed proteins in the plasma of HAPE patients as these have the potential to be developed as biomarker for the detection of disease. These differentially expressed may also play roles in the disease development and manifestation.

To date, some studies have attempted to identify biomarkers of HAPE however; no study has attempted to identify non-invasive, blood-based, diagnostic biomarkers that can discriminate between healthy control subjects and HAPE patients. Using a proteomics approach, we have identified a panel of two blood-based biomarkers which, when used in combination, can discriminate between healthy control subjects, patients with high altitude pulmonary edema and has the potential to be a valuable tool in the clinical diagnosis of high altitude related pulmonary disease. The results showed that most of the plasma proteins found in patients with HAPE are acute phase proteins (APPs), compliment components and apolipoproteins generated by hypoxia-induced inflammation.

2   Materials and Methods

2.1   Materials

Bio-Lyte pH 3–10 Ampholyte, 17 cm Ready Strips™ IPG strips pH 5–8 (Biorad, Hercules, CA, U.S.A), Mineral oil, Urea, Bromophenol blue, CHAPS, agarose, Acrylamide, Bis, Tris, SDS, DTT, Ammonium persulfate, Iodoacetamide, TEMED, sodium thiosulfate, silver nitrate, sodium carbonate, Potassium ferricyanide and Trypsin Singles™ Proteomics Grade were obtained from Sigma (St. Louis, MO, U.S.A). ELISA kits of haptoglobin and apolipoprotein A-I were purchased from AssayPro (Triad South Drive, St. Charles, MO, U.S.A). The primary antibodies to haptoglobin (mouse monoclonal, IgG₁) and apolipoprotein A-I (rabbit polyclonal, IgG) were both from Santa Cruz Biotechnology, Inc. (Santa Cruz, California, USA). Other analytical-grade chemicals used in this study were from domestic sources. All buffers were prepared with Milli-Q deionized water.

2.2   Subject Characteristic and Selection

Blood plasma of stringently selected HAPE patients (n = 20) and compared with matched healthy male sea level control (n = 10) were studied. The plasma from HAPE patients (ages 25 to 30 yrs) were collected at high altitude medical research centre (HAMRC, Leh, India). The plasma from the healthy sea level controls were collected in Defence Institute of Physiology and Allied Sciences (Delhi, India). Prior to the present experiment they had not been exposed to altitude. The control groups were non-smokers, ages 25 to 30 yrs. Volunteers were provided details of the study design as approved by the Ethical Committee of Defence Institute of Physiology and Allied Sciences and written consent was obtained. Fasting venous blood samples were collected from an antecubital vein in EDTA – treated vials in the morning (8 a.m. to 9 a.m.) at sea level and kept at 4 °C until preparation to prevent coagulation and minimize protein degradation. Blood samples from HAPE patients were collected only at high altitude following the same procedure. Patients were classified as having HAPE if they presented to the medical clinics complaining of shortness of breath or chest discomfort and had conventional diagnostic features of the HAPE. These included recent ascent to altitude, vigorous exercise, and no other acute or chronic medical condition. The degree of AMS was also determined by the Lake Louise score by the same interviewer. AMS was diagnosed when the Lake Louise score was > 5. Chest radiogram was performed when the clinical assessment and/or the analysis of blood gas indicated HAPE by X ray unit (TRS, Siemens) at HAMRC (Leh, India) with a fixed target to film distance of 140 cm at 95 kV and 3 to 6 mA/s. HAPE was diagnosed if the X ray film showed interstitial and/or alveolar edema compared with the chest radiograph taken at lower altitude. Subjects presenting with pneumonia or other factors explaining room air hypoxemia were excluded. To prepare plasma, anticoagulants either EDTA, heparin or sodium citrate, were added to the blood specimens immediately after the blood was drawn to prevent clotting (EDTA plasma: 10 mL containing approximately 1.7 mg potassium EDTA; heparin plasma: 5 mL containing heparin 1 vial ; sodium citrate plasma: 10 mL containing 1 mL of 0.118 mol/L (3.2%) citrate solution). The specimens were then centrifuged at 1500 g for 10 mins/4 °C to avoid hemolysis, decanted and transferred into Eppendorf tubes as aliquots. To each 1.0 mL plasma aliquots, 10 µl of protease inhibitor were added to obtain the reproducible results by 2DE analysis (Hulmes *et al.*, 2004). The plasma samples were stored at –80 °C until further analysis.

2.3   Depletion of High-Abundance Plasma Proteins

Because albumin and immunoglobulin IgG collectively account for ~ 70% of the total plasma protein content (Hulmes *et al.*, 2004), we selectively removed these proteins to enrich for proteins of lower abundance. A dye-based Proteoprep blue albumin and IgG depletion kit (Sigma Aldrich, Germany) was used according to the manufacturer's instructions. Briefly, the provided suspended slurry medium were added to the spin columns, centrifuged and equilibrated at 8000 × g for 10 seconds. The spin columns were collected in fresh collection tube. To each spin column 0.1 mL of plasma sample were added to the packed medium bed, incubated for 10 min, centrifuged at 8000 x g for 60 sec, repeated the same step twice to remove the additional albumin. The two times depleted plasma were remained in the collection tube and pooled for optimal protein recovery. The albumin/IgG depleted plasma samples were stored at –80°C for long-term storage.

2.4   SDS-PAGE Analysis

Sodium dodecylsulfate-polyacrylamide gel electrophoresis (SDS-PAGE) analysis was carried out with the Tris/glycine buffer system according to Laemmli (Laemmli, 1970). Two microlitres (20 μg) albumin and IgG depleted proteins of healthy sea level controls and HAPE patients were separated under reducing conditions on 12% SDS-PAGE mini gels (10 × 10.5 cm) at 250 V, 40 mA, and constant currents for 2h and visualized by colloidal Comassie Blue G-250 or Silver staining according to standard protocols. The gels were scanned in Ultra Lum Omega 16Vs system.

2.5   Acetone/TCA Precipitation

A 100 μl of depleted plasma sample was diluted with 900 μl of 10% TCA in acetone. The mixture was incubated overnight at –20 °C and centrifuged at 15000 g, 4° C for 10 min. The supernatant was removed and 1000 μl of 90% ice-cold acetone were added to wash the pellet. The sample was incubated at –20 °C for 10 min and centrifuged as above. The acetone containing supernatant was removed and the pellet was air dried. For 2D gel electrophoresis, the protein pellet was suspended in 100 μl of lysis buffer containing 8M urea, 2.5 M thiourea, 40 Mm Tris-HCl, 3% w/v CHAPS and 0.5% v/v Igepal CA-630. The protein sample was stored frozen at –20 °C until analysis.

2.6   First-dimension Separation

The protein concentration in plasma was determined by Bradford assay and employed bovine albumin standards. Each sample was analyzed in triplicate. For each sample of plasma, HAPE patients and sea level control, 750 μg of protein were reconstituted in rehydration buffer containing 7 M urea, 2 M thiourea, 1.2%, w/v CHAPS, 0.4% w/v ABS-14, 20 mM dithiothreitol (DTT), 0.25%, v/v, pH 3–10 ampholytes and 0.005% w/v bromophenol blue (BPB) to a final volume of 300 μl. The samples were incubated (RT, 1

h) and then used to rehydrate 17-cm IPG strips (Bio-Rad) with a pH 5–8 linear gradient. The strips were passively rehydrated for 18 h without current in a Protean isoelectric focus (IEF) Cell (Bio Rad). First dimension IEF was carried out at 20 °C in a PROTEAN IEF CELL by the following protocol: 250 V for 1 h (slow ramping), changing the wicks every 30 min (to assist removal of ionic contaminants), 1000V for 1 h, linear ramping 10000 V to over 3 h and a constant of 10000V until approximately 60 kVh was reached. Strips were removed and stored at −80 °C until run on the second dimension.

2.7   Two-dimensional SDS-PAGE

After IEF, strips were equilibrated by agitating for 15 min in 50 mM of Tris-HCl, pH 8.8, 6 M urea, 30% v/v glycerol, 2% w/v sodium dodecyl sulfate (SDS), 1% w/v DTT and 0.01% w/v bromophenol blue (BPB) and then agitating for 15 min in 50 mM of Tris-HCl, pH 8.8, 6 M urea, 30% v/v glycerol, 2% w/v sodium dodecyl sulfate (SDS), and 2.5% (w/v) iodoacetamide and 0.01% w/v bromophenol blue (BPB). The equilibrated IPG strips were slightly rinsed with milli-Q water, blotted to remove excess equilibration buffer and then applied to SDS-PAGE gels (20cm × 20cm × 1mm 8–19% polyacrylamide (30% (w/v) acrylamide: 0.8% (w/v) bis-acrylamide, 37.5:1 stock) using a PROTEAN II XL system (Bio Rad) at 4 °C at constant 10 mA per gel for 30 min followed by 35 mA per gel for 12 h in a running buffer containing 25 mM Tris, 192 mM glycine, and 0.1 % (w/v) SDS until the dye front had run off the edge of the 2-D gel.

2.8   Staining and Imaging

After electrophoresis, proteins were visualized by modified silver staining procedure compatible with MS (Yan *et al.*, 2000). The gels were fixed in 50% v/v methanol, 12% v/v acetic acid and 0.05% v/v formaldehyde for at least 2 h. The fixed gels were rinsed with 50% v/v ethanol three times for 20 min each, then again sensitized with 0.02% w/v sodium thiosulfate followed by three washings with milli-Q water each for 20 sec. The gels were immersed in 0.1% w/v silver nitrate and 0.075% v/v formaldehyde for 20 min and rinsed with milli-Q water twice for 20 sec each. It was developed with 6% sodium carbonate and 0.05% v/v formaldehyde. Finally, the reaction was terminated by fixing with 50% v/v methanol and 12% v/v acetic acid. The stained gels were imaged using an Investigator™ ProPic II Genomics Solutions and the analysis of digitized images with Image Master 2D Platinum v.6 software (GE Healthcare). Automatic spot detection and matching of the gels was done, followed by manual rechecking of the matched and unmatched protein spots. The intensity volumes of the individual spots were normal-ized with the total intensity volume of all the spots present in each gel (%V). Differences of ≥ 1.5 in expression (ratio %V) between matched spots were considered significant whenever a spot group passed statistical analysis (t test, P ≤ 0.05) and a second manual verification of the spots on the gel images. For those proteins with multiple spots in gel, such as haptoglobin, the sum of pixel volumes of individual spots from isoforms was used for analysis.

3   MS Analysis

3.1   In-gel Digestion with Trypsin and Extraction of Peptides

The procedure for in-gel digestion of protein spots from silver stained gels was performed. In brief, protein spots were excised from stained gels and cut into pieces. The gel pieces were destained and incubated for 30 min with 30 mM Potassium ferricyanide and 100 mM sodium thiosulfate at room temperature. The gel pieces were rinsed several times with water to remove destaining solution. The gel pieces were washed for 15 min at room temperature with water and 50 mM NH_4HCO3/Acetonitrile. Enough acetonitrile were added to cover gel pieces for shrinking the gel pieces. The gel pieces were rehydrated in 10 mM NH_4HCO3 for 5 min, equal volume of acetonitrile were added and removed after 15 min of incubation.The gel pieces were again covered with acetonitrile and removed. The gel pieces were dried in a vacuum centrifuge. The dried gel pieces were digested with 20 μl of trypsin (20 ng/ul, Trypsin Singles™ Proteomics Grade, Sigma) and incubated the sample at 37 °C overnight, the tryptic peptide were sonicated for 10 min and dried in a speed Vac. The dried peptides were extracted with 5 μl of 0.1% TFA.

3.2   MALDI-TOF/TOF

Prior to mass spectromeric analysis, α-cyano-4-hydroxy cinnamic acid (CHCA) matrix 10 mg/ml was made in 70% acetonitrile and 0.03% TFA. 0.5 μl of the peptide extracts mixed with the 0.5 μl of the matrix were manually spotted onto a 600 μm/384 well AnchorChip™ sample target (Bruker Daltonics) and dried at ambient temperature. Peptide mass spectra were recorded in the reflectron mode using an Ultraflex III Tof/Tof mass spectrometer (Bruker Daltonics) equipped with a 384-sample scout source. The ion acceleration voltage after pulsed extraction was 29000 V. The instrument was calibrated by using external standard calibration Peptide Mixture for the m/z range of 700 Da to 4500 Da by using the peptide peak of Bradykinin (757.39 Da) Angiotensin II (1046.54 Da), Angiotensin I (1296.68 Da) Substance P (1347.73 Da), Bombesin (1619.82 Da), ACTH fragment 1–17 (2093.08 Da), ACTH fragment 18–39 (2465.19 Da), Somatostatin 28 (3147.47 Da). The monoisotopic peak list was generated in Post Processing s/w and True peptide mass list was generated by Bruker Flex Analysis software version 3.0 and Biotools ver 3.1 without using the smoothing function and the peak filter was applied to exclude the masses lower than 700 Da and the signal to noise ratio of 20. The generated peptide mass list was sent for the online data base search to find and match the Protein Identity. The search engine "MASCOT Server" (www.matrixscience.com) was used to obtain the protein identity by undertaking the Peptide Mass Fingerprinting approach. Search was performed in NCBInr, MSDB and SwissProt database with the following search parameter: Mass Tolerance: 50 ppm to 100 ppm; species, Homo sapience; maximum number of missed cleavages was set to 1 for all samples. Once the protein was identified, the identity was confirmed by using Tandem Mass spectrometry. For each identified Protein, at least one Peptide was selected for MS/MS (Tof/Tof) to validate the Protein Identity. Instrument was used in the Lift mode (Tof/Tof) to obtain the MS/MS spectra. Again the Flex Analysis3.0 and Biotools 3.1 s/w were used to generate the fragments mass list and the sequence Tag of peptide. The mass list was sent to database in same way as was done in case of above PMF approach. The mass tolerance error of 0.5 Da to 1 Da was used for MS/MS ion search. The MS/MS ion search confirmed the protein identity and provided the amino acid sequence of particular peptide.

3.3   Quantitative Validation by Enzyme-linked Immunosorbent Assay

To determine the correlation of haptoglobin and apolipoprotein A-I with HAPE, 30 plasma samples, including 20 HAPE patients and 10 from normal control groups were used for quantitative validation. The total haptoglobin and apolipoprotein A-I were quantified by using competitive ELISA kit with the purified polyclonal antibody against haptoglobin and apolipoprotein A-I (Assaypro, USA) according to the manufacturer's instructions. Briefly individual plasma samples (1 µl) were diluted with mix diluent (2000 µl for haptoglobin and 800 µl for apolipoprotein A-I). The diluted mixtures of 25 µl were added onto 96-well plate and immediately 25 µl of Biotinylated haptoglobin and apolipoprotein A-I were added, mixed and incubated for 1 h. After five washes with buffer, 50 µl of streptavidin-peroxidase conjugate were added and incubated for 30 min. After five washes, 50 µl of chromogen substrate were added and incubated for 10 min till the optimal blue color density developed. A 50 µl of stop solution were added to each well and yellow color developed and measured absorbance on a microplate reader at a wavelength of 450 nm immediately.

3.4   Quantitative Validation by Western Blot Analysis

The protein quantification of haptoglobin and apolipoprotein A-I were selected to be validated by western-blot analysis because the expression changes of these proteins were more obvious than that of the other proteins and the obtaining of their antibodies was convenient. Briefly, plasma samples were first diluted 10 times by 1 × PBS, and then total proteins (40 µg) were separated by SDS-PAGE and electro-blotted to nitrocellulose membrane. After being blotted with 5% nonfat-dried milk in 1 × TBST (25 mM Tris, pH 7.5, 150 mM NaCl, 0.1% Tween 20) overnight, membranes were incubated with primary antibodies for 2 h, followed by secondary antibody for another hour. All these experiments were conducted at room temperature. The immunocomplexes were visualized by chemiluminescence using the chemiluminescent peroxidase substrate kit (Sigma-Aldrich, St. Louis Mo 63103, USA). The film signals were digitally scanned and then quantified using image J software.

4   Results

4.1   Removal of High Abundance Proteins from Plasma and Acetone/TCA Precipitation

Albumin and IgG collectively account for ~70% of the total plasma proteins therefore mask the presence of low abundance proteins. In order to maximize the coverage of disease specific proteins low abundance proteins depletion of albumin and IgG was performed. Figure 1 demonstrates representative one dimensional gel profile human plasma from control and HAPE patient. Depletion of human plasma resulted in significant removal of albumin and IgG at 64 kDa and IgG bands at 50 kDa and 25 kDa (Lane 4, 8) with no apparent loss of other proteins (Lane 2, 3, 6, 7) in both the groups compared to undepleted plasma (Lane 1, 5). Concomitant with the removal of albumin there was a significant enhancement of the staining of several protein spots as observed in two dimensional gel profiles in control and HAPE group. We carried out acetone/TCA precipitation for the removal of protease activity, biological contaminants and enrichment of proteins.

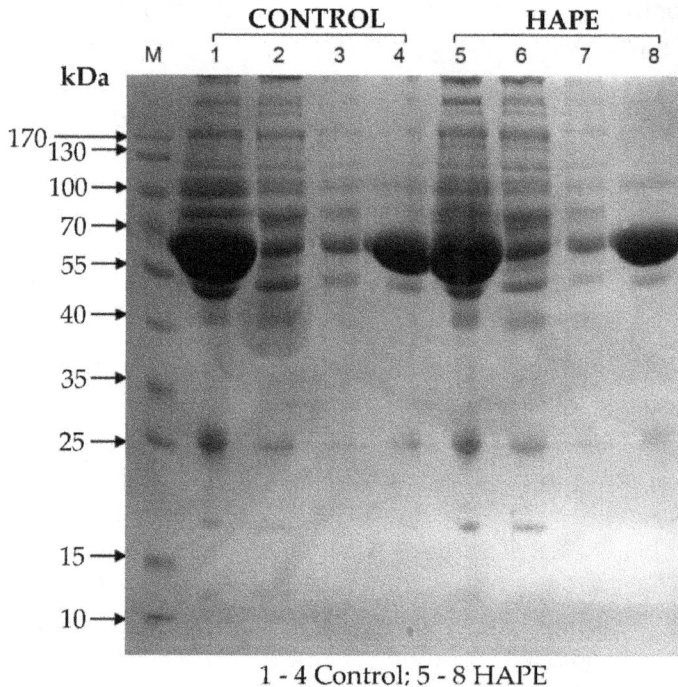

1 - 4 Control; 5 - 8 HAPE

Figure 1: Removal of high ab-undance proteins from plasma: Depletion of human plasma of control and HAPE resulted in significant removal of albumin band at 64 kDa and IgG bands at 50 kDa and 25 kDa (Lane 4, 8) with no apparent loss of other proteins (Lane 2, 3, 6, 7) in both the groups compared to undepleted plasma (Lane 1, Lane 5).

4.2   Proteome Profiles of Plasma Patients with HAPE

The difference of protein profiles between HAPE patients and healthy controls were examined using 2DE with linear IPG strips of 17 cm ranging from pH 5–8. Each plasma samples were run on duplicate gels and proteins were visualized by silver staining. Figure 2 shows the representative proteome profiles for HAPE patients. The relative intensities of the protein spots (normalized spot volume) were compared and analyzed between patients and healthy samples using 2DE gel analysis software. More than 300 protein spots in each silver stained gel can be visualized by 2D ImageMaster software. The quantitative evaluation of the differentially expressed plasma proteins in normal vs HAPE patients was performed by using Student's t-test. In comparison with 2DE from the patients with healthy controls, many chains of spots that may represent different degrees of protein modification and/or degradation products were significantly varied. We compared 25 clear plasma protein spots in 2DE gel maps, which were analyzed by MALDI-MS and MS/MS (Figure 2). Identification was based on NCBInr, MSDB and SwissProt database entries with the mascot search engine. In HAPE patients and healthy control, 25 common proteins were identified (Table 1). Table 1 lists the Swiss port accession numbers as well as the full names of the 25 protein spots, molecular mass and pI values, and the number of matching peptides and protein amino acid sequence coverage by matching peptides. A comparison of 2DE gels from patients with those of healthy controls indicated that 14 spots were significantly upregulated. Among these upregulated protein spots, 11 protein spots clearly showed several fold increases in quantitative protein expression for HAPE patients and were selected for further analysis. The close-up images of up-regulated proteins in the HAPE patients are presented in Figure 3. Among these proteins, haptoglobin Hp-β chain expression was significantly increased in HAPE patients as compared to sea level healthy controls ($p <$ 0.001). Only a marginal increase was observed in Hp-α2 chain in HAPE patients ($p <$ 0.034) compared to healthy controls. Comparison of Hp-β spots from patients with those of healthy control indicated that some chains of Hp-β spots were representing different degree of modification or degradation products. In addition, the HAPE patients exhibited a significantly high content of ApoA-I ($p < 0.001$) when compared to sea level healthy controls (Table 2). We can see the representative gels of HAPE patients and controls in Figure 2. Especially, the expression of Hp-β chain and ApoA-I ($p < 0.001$) displayed remarkably significant differences between the patients and control subjects.

4.3   Validation of Hp and ApoA-I with ELISA and Western Blot Analysis

To validate the result of proteomic analysis, 2 proteins were selected for ELISA and western blotting analysis. We verified whether the expression patterns of selected proteins of haptoglobin and apolipoprotein A-I observed in 2-DE gels paralleled those validated by ELISA and western blot analysis. ELISA analysis of 20 patients with HAPE and 10 healthy controls confirmed that concentrations of haptoglobin and apolipoprotein A-I were significantly increased in the plasma of patients with HAPE (Figure 4).

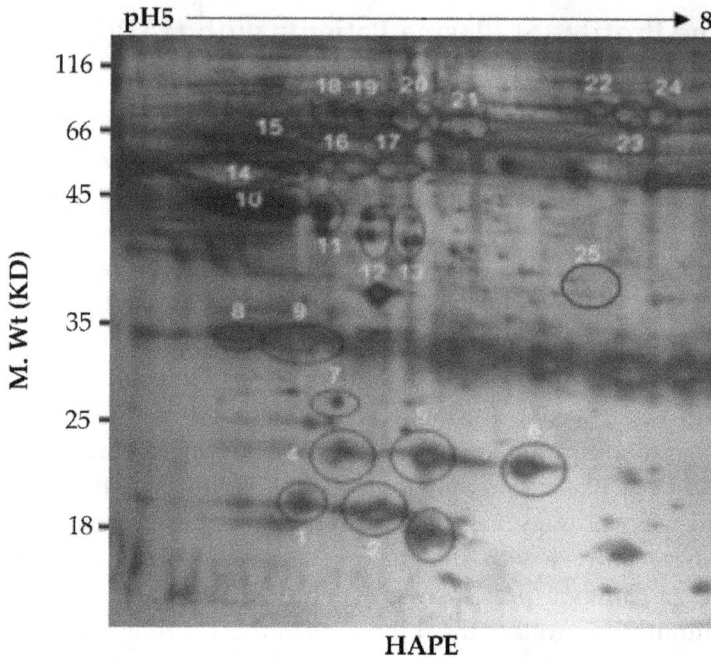

Figure 2: A representative 2D gel of plasma from one HAPE patient with a pH range from 5-8. Distribution of differentially expressed protein spots (marked by circle) and each spot number relates to data shown in Table 1.

The mean plasma Hp concentration was 3800 ± 754.24 µg/ml (mean ± SD) in HAPE patients versus 340 ± 67.987 µg/ml in sea level controls ($p < 0.01$); the mean APO A-I concentration was 5088.9 ± 807.59 µg/ml in HAPE patients versus 688 ± 102.54 µg/ml in sea level controls ($p < 0.01$). The expression patterns of both proteins haptoglobin and apolipoprotein A-I were up-regulated in plasma of HAPE patients (Figure 5) and in agreement with 2-DE results, so the results of ELISA analysis and western blot analysis confirmed the reliability of the proteomic analysis.

5   Discussion

The present study demonstrated the use of proteomic analysis to study the nature of the identified proteins and their significance in disease pathogenesis. Our studies demonstrate that plasma analysis is not only more feasible but safer. In addition, because of the close communication between the alveolar space and blood circulation during lung inflammation, the pathological events occurring in the inflamed lung may be attainable by simply analyzing the patient's plasma. This study has identified a number of overexpressed plasma proteins with different functions in patients with HAPE. Selected description of these proteins that may play a role in HAPE pathogenesis is discussed below.

1	Transthyretin precursor (validated)	VBHU	47	1	20	5.26	15.59
2	Haptoglobin α2 chain	HPHU2	98	10	22	6.13	45.86
3	Haptoglobin α2 chain	HPHU2	98	10	22	6.13	45.86
4	Haptoglobin α2 chain	HPHU2	77	10	22	6.13	45.86
5	Haptoglobin α2 chain	HPHU2	94	10	22	6.13	45.86
6	Haptoglobin α2 chain	HPHU2	97	11	22	6.13	45.86
7	Plasma retinol binding protein precursor (validated)	VAHU	61	7	61	5.48	23.19
8	APOA1 protein	APOA1_HUMAN	80	12	40	5.56	30.75
9	APOA1 protein	APOA1_HUMAN	172	20	59	5.56	30.75
10	Haptoglobin β chain	HPT_HUMAN	59	11	24	6.13	45.86
11	Haptoglobin β chain	HPT_HUMAN	59	11	24	6.13	45.86
12	Haptoglobin β chain	HPT_HUMAN	59	11	24	6.13	45.86
13	Haptoglobin β chain	HPT_HUMAN	59	11	24	6.13	45.86
14	Alpha-1-antitrypsin-precursor	ITHU	117	1	3	5.3	46.87
15	Vitamin D –binding protein precursor	VYHUD	62	5	21.5	5.3	54.49
16	Vitamin D –binding protein precursor	VYHUD	62	5	21.5	5.3	54.49
17	Vitamin D –binding protein precursor	VYHUD	62	5	21.5	5.3	54.49
18	Hemopexin precursor (validated)	OQHU	97	9	26	6.55	52.38
19	Hemopexin precursor (validated)	OQHU	97	9	26	6.55	52.38
20	Hemopexin precursor (validated)	OQHU	101	8	24	6.55	52.38
21	Hemopexin precursor (validated)	OQHU	93	8	24	6.55	52.38
22	Hemopexin precursor (validated)	OQHU	93	8	24	6.55	52.38
23	Hemopexin precursor (validated)	OQHU	93	8	24	6.55	52.38
24	Transferrin precursor (validated)	TFHUP	144	17	31	6.81	79.28
25	Transferrin precursor (validated)	TFHUP	103	8	15	6.81	79.28
26	Transferrin precursor (validated)	TFHUP	103	8	15	6.81	79.28
27	Compliment Component 4A	Q5JNXO_HUMAN	90	10	25	6.27	30.22

Table 1: List of proteins identified in plasma from patients with HAPE.

Protein name	Patients ($n = 20$)	Control ($n = 10$)	p-value[a]
Haptoglobin-β chain	1.328 ± 0.147	0.623± 0.401	< 0.001
Apolipoprotein A-I	2.125 ± 0.412	1.236 ± 0.259	< 0.001
Transthyretin	0.722 ± 0.118	0.231 ± 0.056	< 0.001
Haptoglobin-α2 chain	1.795 ± 1.102	0.958 ± 0.865	0.034
Compliment Component 4A	1.112 ± 0.221	0.466 ± 0.085	< 0.001
Plasma Retinol Binding Protein	0.393 ± 0.043	0.191 ± 0.030	< 0.001

Table 2: List of Differentially Expressed Proteins ($p < 0.05$) [Protein Expression (% Vol)].

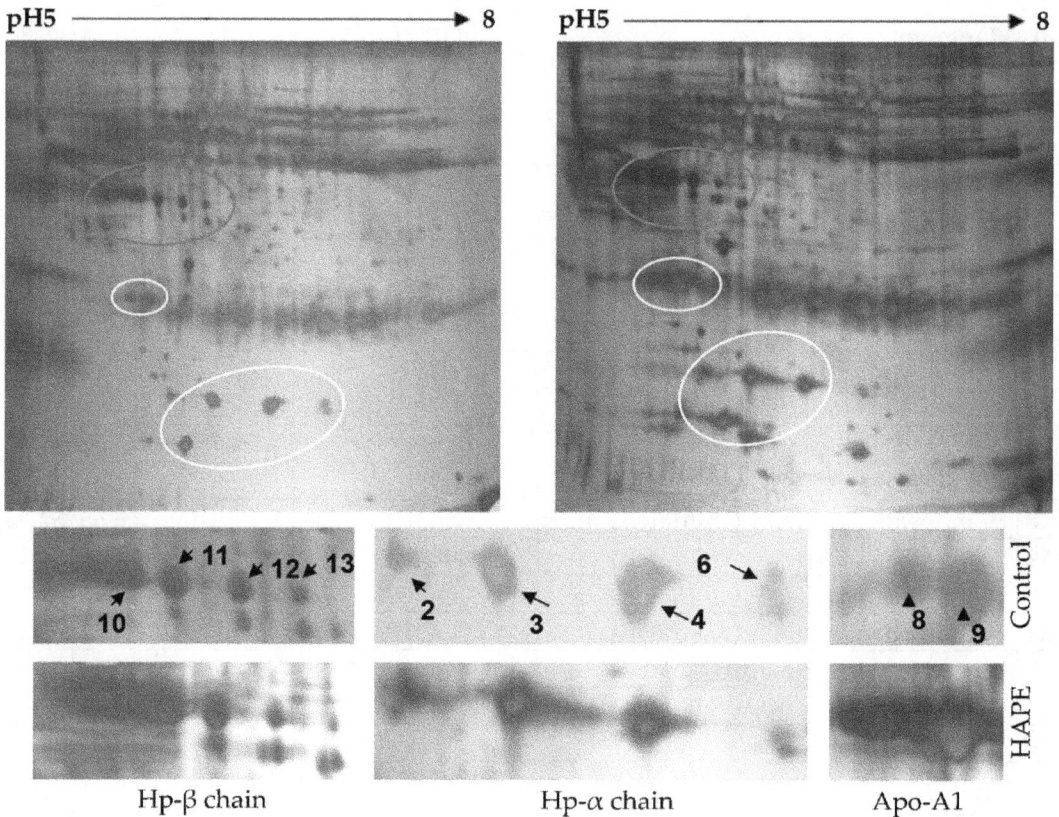

Figure 3: The representative gels of HAPE (A) and controls (B): Two dimensional gels of human plasma from a subject with HAPE and a healthy comparison subject, displaying proteins with isoelectric points (pI) between 5 and 6 and molecular weights between 200 and 10 KDa. **(C)** The expression of haptoglobin-β (10–13) chain and Apo A-I (8, 9) displayed remarkably significant differences ($p < 0.001$) between HAPE patients and control subjects. The expression of haptoglobin-α chain (2–6) showed only a marginal increase in HAPE patients ($p = 0.034$) as compared to healthy control subjects.

Plasma Haptoglobin

Plasma Apo A-I

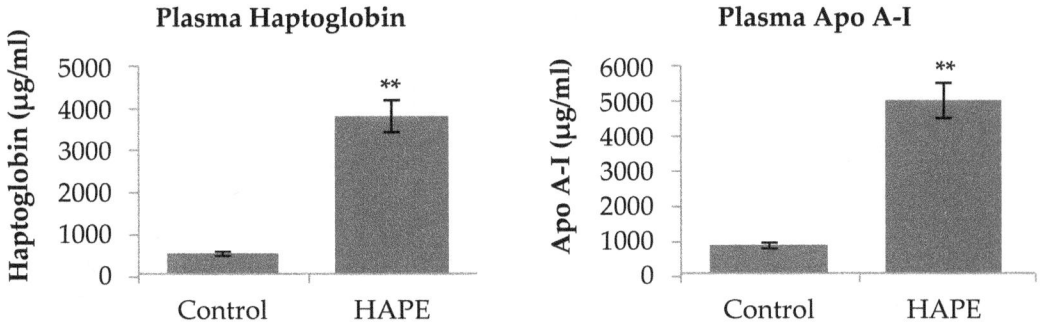

(A) Quantitation of Haptoglobin in Patients against Controls ($P < 0.01$).

(B) Quantitation of Apolipoprotein A-I in Patients against Controls ($P < 0.01$).

Figure 4. ELISA analysis of patients with HAPE and healthy controls: ELISA confirmed that concentrations of haptoglobin (A) and apolipoprotein A-I (B) were significantly increased in the plasma of patients with HAPE. The mean plasma Hp concentration was 3800 ± 754.24 µg/ml (mean $\pm$ SD) in HAPE patients versus 340 ± 67.987 µg/ml in sea level controls ($p < 0.01$); the mean Apo A-I concentration was 5088.9 ± 807.59 µg/ml in HAPE patients versus 688 ± 102.54 µg/ml in sea level controls ($p < 0.01$).

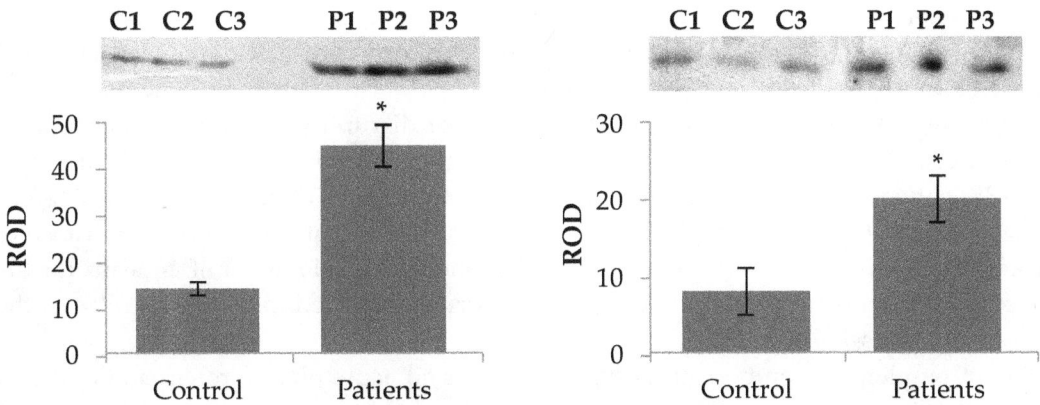

(A) Western blotting of Haptoglobin in Patients against Controls ($P < 0.05$).

(B) Western blotting of Apo A-I in Patients against Controls ($P < 0.05$).

Figure 5. Western blot analysis of haptoglobin and Apo A-I from plasma of three healthy controls and three patients with HAPE. Blots of haptoglobin (A) and apolipoprotein A-I (B) were represented along with their respective relative optical densities (ROD). Data represents the mean $\pm$ SD of three independent experiments. Densitometry analysis of results from western blot, indicating significant change between the two groups compared by student t test. *Significantly different ($p < 0.05$) vs. control.

In this study, we have found that many APPs in plasma of patients with HAPE. These proteins may provide a fast and effective control of inflammatory damage until the subsequent defensive mechanisms can begin to operate (Moshage, 1997). Our findings are in agreement with previous reports.

Along with inflammation caused by injury, trauma, autoimmunity or infection, acute phase proteins (APP) are massively synthesized and released systemically (Gabay & Kushner, 1999). This process is called the "acute phase response", and it is supposedly induced in order to minimize and repair tissue damage. In general, concentration of various positive and negative regulators of acute phase proteins (APP) increase and decrease in response to inflammation (Cecilliani *et al.*, 2002). Among the acute phase proteins found in HAPE patients, transthyretin, haptoglobin β chain, Compliment Component 4A, haptoglobin α2 chain and plasma retinol binding protein showed an increase in the plasma concentration during acute inflammation. Transthyretin (spot no.1) has been shown to be a valuable prognostic factor of nutritional and inflammatory indices in patient's acute respiratory failure (Schlossmacher *et al.*, 2002). Because it is known as a negative APP (Doherty et al, 1998), i.e., an increase in the plasma concentration during acute inflammation, it indicates that the multimeric form of plasma transthyretin showed upregulation in HAPE. A persistent low level of serum transthyretin is predictive of lethality, whereas increased levels were associated with improved ventilatory performances. Additionally, transthyretin interacts with retinol binding protein (spot no.7), thus enabling retinol transportation. Lower levels of transthyretin coincide with lower levels of retinol and retinol binding protein, as reported for ovarian cancer (Zhang *et al.*, 2004). A decrease in transthyretin plasma levels is also seen in negative acute phase regulation during inflammation; correspondingly its increased expression might be utilized as a biomarker for cancer. The transthyretin monomer may also serve as a marker to cerebrospinal fluid barrier disruption and lung cancer (Maciel *et al.*, 2005). We also observed up regulation of transthyretin by 3.0-fold in plasma of HAPE patients, alongside an overexpression of retinol binding protein by 2.0-fold respectively. Our findings in 2DE analysis suggested the conformational significance of transthyretin in patients with HAPE condition and the development of a means for the detection of transthyretin in its conformation forms is needed to clarify its roles in the disease progression.

Complement component C4 (spot no. 25) is an acute phase protein and essential component of the effector arm of the humoral immune response. Compliment C4 exists as two isotypes, C4A and C4B. Although sharing >99 % sequence identities, they have different hemolytic activities, covalent affinities to antigens and immune complexes, and serological reactivities (Schifferli et al, 1986). C4A may be functionally advantageous for ensuring the solubilization of antibody- antigen aggregates (or inhibition of immune complexes (IC), and clearance of IC through binding to complement receptor CR1. In this study, we found that C4A was up-regulated in blood plasma during inflammation.

Haptoglobin (Hp) (Spot no. 10–13) is a positive acute-phase plasma glycoprotein. It is synthesised by hepatocytes, but is also found in adipose tissue and in lung, and is normally released in the blood during acute and chronic inflammation (Gabay *et al.*,

1999; Cecilliani *et al.*, 2002; Wang *et al.*, 2001; Quaye *et al.*, 2008). Haptoglobin is considered to have significant antioxidant and anti-inflammatory properties because of its ability to bind hemoglobin, and haptoglobin depletion could add to vascular dysfunction in the hypertensive lung (Belcher *et al.*, 2009). This might also affect the expression of other proteins because in silico analysis has been used to identify a group of genes that are coexpressed with haptoglobin and hemopexin and modulated in their absence (Fagoonee *et al.*, 2006). Hemoglobin in plasma is instantly bound with high affinity to Hp- an interaction leading to the recognition of the complex by HbSR/CD 163 and endocytosis in macrophages (Madsen et al, 2001). Hp also acts as an antioxidant, has antibacterial activity and plays a role in modulating many aspects of acute phase response. Hp is expressed at high levels in specific cells, including alveolar macrophages and eosinophils in diseased or inflamed human lung tissues, but not in the normal lung. Because the Hp-hemoglobin complex can be removed efficiently by alveolar macrophages, Hp synthesised by alveolar macrophages at the site of inflammation could contribute significantly to the clearance of hemoglobin and thus protect the lower respiratory tract against hemoglobin-mediated oxidative damage (Funmei *et al.*, 2000). Hp has been identified as one of the serum angiogenic factors required for the proliferation and differentiation of endothelial cells (Cid *et al.*, 1993; Cockerill *et al.*, 1995). Increased serum concentration in chronic inflammatory and (or) ischemic conditions are important for tissue repair and promoting the growth of collateral vessels (Padma & Valli, 1989). In this study, we found that Hp was up- regulated in HAPE plasma patients. The concentration of plasma Hp increased to 3800 ± 754.24 µg/ml (mean $\pm$ SD) whereas that of controls was 340 ± 67.987 µg/ml ($p < 0.01$). We might conclude that overexpression of Hp might attenuate hypoxia-induced inflammation in HAPE patients.

Apolipoprotein A-I (Apo A-I) (spot no. 8, 9) is the major protein of high-density lipoprotein (HDL), comprising about 70% of total HDL protein. The best characterized functions of Apo A-I are related to its role in reverse cholesterol transport and include lipid and cholesterol binding, lecithin: cholesterol acyl transferase (LCAT) activation, and receptor binding (Rodriguiza *et al.*, 1997). Beyond its role in cholesterol metabolism, there are many other disparate activities attributed to apo A-I (and HDL) that may be physiologically relevant, some of which may also contribute to apo A-I's anti-atherogenic properties, such as its anti-inflammatory and antioxidant activities (Cockerill *et al.*, 1995). Plasma HDL, quantified by either its cholesterol or Apo A-I content, is the best single predictor of coronary artery disease (CAD), with high HDL levels being correlated with low CAD (Calabresi *et al.*, 1997). In terms of the mechanism of ApoA-I, previous researchers showed that ApoA-I could bind LPS to interrupt activation of macrophage (Ma *et al.*, 2004), inhibit LPS-activated macrophage to release inflammatory cytokines (Yan *et al.*, 2006), and inhibit activation of neutrophils (Liao et al, 2005). Recently, a study examined the effect of ApoA-I overexpression on LPS-induced systemic inflammation and multiple organ injury in mice and concluded that ApoA-I overexpression has a protective effect on LPS- induced multiple organ injury (Li *et al.*, 2008). Increasingly studies provide new evidence supporting the notion that HDL plays a protective role in the lung. ABCA1, which interacts with lipid-poor Apo A-I, was earlier shown to be essential for maintaining normal lipid composition and architecture of the lung as well as respiratory physiology (Bates *et al.*, 2005). More recently, proteomic studies revealed that homozygous sickle cell anemia patients with pulmonary arterial hypertension (PAH) consistently had lower Apo A-I levels than sickle patients without PAH (Yudiskaya *et al.*, 2009). Interestingly, genetic deletion of endothelial lipase resulted in a nearly 2- fold increase in HDL, which was credited with decreasing airway hyperresponsiveness and pulmonary inflammation in ovalbumin-sensitized BALB/c mice (Otera *et al.*, 2009). There is emerging evidence that, Apo A-I plays a critical role in protecting pulmonary artery and airway function as well as preventing inflammation and collagen deposition in the lung (Wang *et al.*, 2010). In this study, Apo A-I was found to be up regulated in HAPE patients as confirmed by ELISA and western blotting, suggesting the anti-inflammatory role of Apo A-I in HAPE.

Considering that the expression of Hp and Apo A-I show roughly 2-fold variances in HAPE, which were acceptable criteria for disease biomarkers in differential display techniques, we suggest that these two proteins might become biomarkers for HAPE diagnosis and prognosis. Furthermore, changes in the proteome observed in the analysis require validation over a much larger sample size for sensitivity and specificity. While it is unlikely that the change in expression of a single protein will be specific indicator for a particular disease, an understanding of different proteins behave in combination may provide an indication of the occurrence of disease. Ongoing investigation into the roles of these differentially expressed proteins will determine their possible use and specificity in the diagnosis and monitoring of HAPE.

5.1   Study Limitations

One important limitation of our study is that the protein quantification is based on only 2D-gels. Most of the proteins have multiple isoforms that differ in electrophorectic mobility. We could not estimate all the isoforms of the identical protein in 2D- gel, and this may affect the accuracy of the single protein quantification. Second limitation of the 2D gel-based proteomic approach is the variable validity of the protein identification. Some gel spots may contain more than one protein. The identification of proteins from peptide sequence is calculated as a high probability. Therefore, the validity of the approach has to be confirmed by different methods. However, since only a few of the respective antibodies against the observed proteins are currently available, it remains necessary to confirm the validity of our gel-based protein expression data by antibody-based techniques. (e.g.Western blotting) whenever antibodies become available.

Acknowledgements

Financial support for this study is provided by a grant from TC/321/Task – 145 (YA)/ DIPAS/2008, Defence Research Development Organization (DRDO), Ministry of Defence, Government of India. We gratefully acknowledge the staff of High Altitude Medical Research, Leh for helping with the sample collection.

References

Anderson, N. L., & Anderson, N. G. (2002). The human plasma proteome: history, character, and diagnostic prospects. Molecular Cellular Proteomics, 1, 845–867.

Bartsch, P., Maggiorini, M., Ritter, M., Noti, C., Vock, P., & Oelz, O. (1991). Prevention of high-altitude pulmonary edema by nifedipine. The New England. Journal of Medicine, 325, 1284–89.

Bates, S. R., Tao, J. Q., Collins, H. L., Francone, O. L., & Rothblat, G. H. (2005). Pulmonary abnormalities due to ABCA1 deficiency in mice. American Journal of Physiology Lung Cell. Molecular Physiology, 289, L980–L989.

Belcher, J. D., Beckman, J. D., Balla, G., Balla, J., & Vercellotti, G. (2009). Heme degradation and vascular injury. Antioxidant Redox Signal 12, 233–248.

Calabresi, L., & Franceschini, G. (1997). High density lipoprotein and coronary heart disease: insights from mutations leading to low high density lipoprotein. Current Opinion. Lipidology. 8, 219–224.

Cecilliani, F., Giordano, A., & Spagnolo, V. (2002). The systemic reaction during inflammation: The acute phase proteins. Protein Peptide Letter 9, 211–223.

Cecilliani, F., Giordano, A., &Spagnolo, V. (2002). The systemic reaction during inflammation: The acute phase proteins. Protein Peptide Letter. 9, 211–223.

Cid M. C., Grant, D. S., Hoffman, G. S., Auerbach, R., Fauci, A. S., & Kleinman, H. K.. (1993). Identification of haptoglobin as an angiogenic factor in sera from patients with systemic vasculatis. Journal Clinical. Investigation, 91, 977–85.

Cockerill, G. W., Gamble, J. R., & Vadas, M. A. (1995). Angiogenesis: Model and modulators. International Review of Cytology. 159, 113–60.

Cockerill, G. W., Rye, K. A., Gamble, J. R., Vadas, M. A., & Barter, P. I. (1995). High-density lipoproteins inhibit cytokine-induced expression of endothelial cell adhesion molecules. Arteriosclerosis Thrombosis and Vascular Biology Biol. 15, 1987–1994.

Doherty, N. S., Littman, B. H., Reilly, K.., Swindell, A. C., & Buss, J. M. (1998). Analysis of changes in acute-phase plasma proteins in acute inflammatory response and in rheumatoid arthritis using two-dimensional gel electrophoresis. Electrophoresis, 19, 355–363.

Durmowicz, A. G., Noordeweir, E., Nicholas, R., & Reeves, J. (1997). T. Inflammatory processes may predispose children to high-altitude pulmonary edema. Journal of Pediatrics. 130, 830–840.

Fagoonee, S., Di. Cunto. F., Vozzi, D., Volinia, S., Pellegrino, M., Gasparini, P., Silengo, L., Altruda, F., & Tolosano, E. (2006). Microarray and large-scale in silico-based identification of genes functionally related to Haptoglobin and/ or Hemopexin. DNA Cell Biology, 25, 323–330.

Funmei, Y., Andrew, J. G., Damon, C. H., Frank, J. W., Christi. A. W., & Jacqueline, J. Pulmonary expression of the human haptoglobin gene. American. Journal of Respiratory

Cell Mol.ecular Biology, 23, 277–282.

Gabay, C., & Kushner, I. (1999). *Acute-phase proteins and other systemic responses to inflammation. The New England. Journal of Medicine, 340, 448–454.*

Gabay, C., & Kushner, I. (1999). *Acute-phase proteins and other systemic responses to inflammation. The New England. Journal of Medicine, 340, 448–454.*

Grissom, C. K., Zimmerman, G. A., & Whatley, R. E. (1997). *Endothelial selectins in acute mountain sickness and high-altitude pulmonary edema. Chest, 112, 1572–78.*

Hanaoka, M., Kubo, K.., Yamazaki, Y., Miyahara, T., Matsuzawa, Y., Kobayashi, T., Sekiguchi, M., Ota, M., & Watanabe, H. (1998). *Association of high-altitude pulmonary edema with major histocompatibility complex. Circulation, 97, 1124–28.*

Houston, C. S. (1960). *Acute pulmonary edema of high altitude. The New England. Journal of Medicine, 263, 478–80.*

Hulmes, J. D., Betheab, D., Ho, K.., Huang, S.-P., Ricci, D. L., Opiteck, G. J., & Hefta, S. A. (2004). *An investigation of plasma collection, stabilization, and storage procedures for proteomic analysis of clinical samples. Clinical. Proteomics Jounal, 1, 17–31.*

Hultgren, H. N. (1978). *High-altitude pulmonary edema. In: Staub N, ed. Lung water and solute exchange. New York: Marcel Dekker.pp. 437–49.*

Kubo, K., Hanaoka, M., Hayano, T., Miyahara, T., Hachiya, T., Hayasaka, M., Koizumi, T., Fujimoto, K.., Kobayashi, T., & Honda, T. (1998). *Inflammatory cytokines in BAL fluid and pulmonary hemodynamics in high-altitude pulmonary edema. Respiratory Physiology, 111, 301–10*

Kubo, K.., Hanaoka, M., Hayano, T., Yamaguchi, T., Hayano, M., Hayasaka, M., Koizumi, T., Fujimoto, K.., Kobayashi, T., & Honda, T. (1996). *Cytokines in bronchoalveolar lavage fluid in patients with high altitude pulmonary edema at moderate altitude in Japan. Thorax, 51, 739–42*

Laemmli, U. K. (1970). *Cleavage of Structural Proteins during the Assembly of the Head of Bacteriophage T4. Nature, 227, 680–685.*

Li, Y., Dong, Ji. B., & Wu, M. P. (2008). *Human ApoA-I overexpression diminishes LPS-induced systemic inflammation and multiple organ damage in mice. European Journal of Pharmaceutical, 590, 417–422.*

Liao, X. L., Lou, B., Ma, J., Wu, M. P. (2005). *Neutrophils activation can be diminished by apolipoprotein A-I. Life Sci.ence, 77, 325–335.*

Ma, J., Liao, X. L., Lou, B., Wu, M. P. (2004). *Role of apolipoprotein A-I in protecting against endotoxin toxicity. Acta Biochimica Biophysica. Sin. (Shanghai), 36, 419–424.*

Maciel, C. M., Junqueira, M., Paschoal, M.E., Kawarmura, M.T., Carvalho, M. G., & Domont G. B. (2005). *Differential proteomic serum pattern of low molecular weight proteins expressed by adenocarcinoma lug cancer patients. Journal of Experimental and Therapeutic Oncology. 5, 31–38.*

Madsen, M., Graversen, J. H., & Moestrup, S. K. (2001). *Haptoglobin and CD 163: Captor and* receptor gating hemoglobin to macrophages lysosomes. *Redox Report, 6, 386–388.*

Moshage, H. *Journal of. Pathology. (1997). Cytokines and the hepatic acute phase response. 181, 257–266.*

Otera, H., Ishida, T., Nishiuma, T., Kobayashi, K.., Kotani, Y., Yasuda, T., Kundu, R. K., Quertermous, T., Hirata, K., & Nishimura Y. (2009). Targeted inactivation of endothelial lipase attenuates lung allergic inflammation through raising plasma HDL level and inhibiting eosinophil infiltration. American Journal of Physiology Lung Cell. Molecular Physiology, 296, L594–L602.

Padma, T., Valli, W. (1989). ABO blood groups, intestinal phosphatase and haptoglobin types in patient with serum hepatitis. Human Heredity 39, 345–50.

Quaye, I. K. (2008). Haptoglobin, inflammation and disease. Transactions of the Royal Society of Tropical Medicine and Hygiene, 102, 735–742.

Rodrigueza, W. V., Williams K. J., Rothblat, G. H., Philips, M. C. (1997). Remodeling and shutting: Mechanisms for the synergistic effects between different acceptor particles in the mobilization of cellular cholesterol. Arteriosclerosis Thrombosis and Vascular Biology, 17, 383–393.

Schifferli, J. A., Steiger, G., Paccaud J. P., & Sjoholm, A. G. Differences between C4A and C4B in the handling of immune complexes: the enhancement of CR1 binding is more important than the inhibition of immunoprecipitation. Clin. Exp. Immunol. 1986, 63, 473–477.

Schlossmacher, P., Wassermann, M., Meyer, N., Kara, F., Delabranche, X., Kummerlen, C., & Ingenbleek Y. (2002). The prognostic value of nutritional and inflammatory indices in critically ill patients with acute respiratory failure. Clinical. Chemistry and Laboratory Medicine, 40, 1339–1343.

Schoene, R. B. (1985). Pulmonary edema at high altitude: review, pathophysiology, and update. pp. Clinics in Chest Medicine, (6) 491–507.

Schoene, R. B., Hackett. P. H., Henderson, W. R., Sage, E. H., Chou, M., Roach, R. C., Mills, W. J., & Martin, T. R. (1986). High-altitude pulmonary edema: characteristics of lung lavage fluid. JAMA, 256, 63–69.

Schoene, R. B., Hultgren, H. N., & Swenson, E. R. High-altitude pulmonary edema. In: Hornbein T., F, Schoene RB, eds. High altitude: an exploration of human adaptation. New York: Mercel Dekker. (2001) 777–814.

Schoene, R. B., Swenson, E. R., Pizzo, C. J., Hackett, P. H., Roach, R. C., Mills, W. J. Jr. Henderson, W. R. Jr.; & Martin, T. R. (1998). The lung at high altitude: bronchoalveolar lavage in acute mountain sickness and pulmonary edema. J of Applied Physiol.ogy, 64, 2605–13.

Wang, W., Xu, H., Shi, Y., Nandedkar, S., Zhang, H., Gao, H., Feroah, T., Weihrauch, D., Schult, M. L., Jones, D.W., Jarzembowski, J., Sorci-Thomas, M., & Pritchard, K. A. (2010). Genetic deletion of apolipoprotein A-I increases airway hyperresponsiveness, inflammation, and collagen deposition in the lung. Journal of Lipid Research, 51, 2560–2570.

Wang, Y., Kinzie, E., Berger F. G., Lim, S. K.., & Baumann, H. (2001). Haptoglobin, an inflammation-inducible plasma protein. Redox Report, 6, 379–385.

West, J. B. Tsukimoto, K., Mathieu-Costello, O., & Prediletto, R. (1991). Stress failure in pulmonary capillaries. Journal of Applied Physiology,70, 1731–42.

Yan, Y. J., Li, Y., Lou, B., Wu, M. P. (2006). Beneficial effects of ApoA-I on LPS-induced acute lung injury and endotoxemia in mice. Life Science, 79, 210–215.

Yan, Y. X., Wait, R., Berkelman, T., Harry, R. A., Westbrook, J. A., Wheeler, C. H., & Dunn, M. J. (2000). A modified silver staning protocol for visualization of proteins compatible with matrix-assisted laser desorption/ionization and electrospray ionization-mass spectrometry. Electrophoresis, 21, 3666–3672.

Yuditskaya, S., Tumblin, A., Hoehn, G. T., Wang, G., Drake, S. K.., Xu, X., Ying, S. A., Chi, H., Remaley, A. T., Shen, R. F., Munson, P. J., Suffredini, A. F., & Kato, G. J. (2009). Proteomic identification of altered apolipoprotein patterns in pulmonaryhypertension and vasculopathy of sickle cell disease. Blood, 113, 1122–1128.

Zhang, Z, Bast, R. C. Jr., Yu, Y., Li, J., Sokoll L. J., Rai, A. J., Rosenzweig, J. M., Cameron, B., Wang, Y. Y., Meng, X. Y., Berchuck, A., Van, Haaften-Day, C., Hacker, N. F. de Bruijn.; H. W., van der Zee., A. G., Jacobs, I. J., Fung, E. T., & Chan, D. W. (2004). Three biomarkers identified from serum proteomic analysis for the detection of early stage ovarian cancer. Cancer Research, 64, 5882–5890.

Chapter 3

Analysis of Nitroproteome in Human Pituitary Adenomas

Xianquan Zhan[1] and Dominic M. Desiderio[2]

1 Introduction

Protein tyrosine nitration is an important reactive oxygen species/reactive nitrogen species (ROS/RNS)-related modification that is derived from the main *in vivo* peroxynitrite pathway and the secondary myeloperoxidase reaction pathway (Scaloni, 2006, Khan *et al.*, 1998, Zhan & Desiderio, 2009a, 2009b, and 2009c, Dalle-Donne *et al.*, 2005, Zhan, Wang, & Desiderio, 2013). Tyrosine nitration adds an electron-withdrawing nitro group ($-NO_2$) to the tyrosine phenolic ring (Zhan & Desiderio, 2006). Addition of this nitro group will decrease the electron density of the tyrosine phenolic ring, change the phenolic pKa value (from ~10 for tyrosine) into the physiological pH range (~7.1 for 3-nitrotyrosine), and affect chemical properties of the tyrosine residue (Zhan & Desiderio, 2006, Yee *et al.*, 2003, Irie *et al.*, 2003). Thus, the decreased electron density will negatively affect the interaction intensity between enzyme-substrate, receptor-ligand, or antigen-antibody when the nitration occurred within those interacting regions, and impact on functions of that protein (Zhan & Desiderio, 2006). Moreover, *in vivo* protein tyrosine nitration might be denitrated with a putative denitrase to result in a dynamically reversible process between nitration and denitration (Irie *et al.*, 2003, Aulak *et al.*, 2004, Koeck *et al.*, 2004). Thus, protein nitration would have a biological function such as neurotransmission and redox signaling besides its pathological consequences. Tyrosine ni-

[1] Key Laboratory of Cancer Proteomics of Chinese Ministry of Health, Hunan Engineering Laboratory for Structural Biology and Drug Design, National Local Joint Engineering Laboratory for Anticancer Drugs, Xiangya Hospital, Central South University, China

[2] The Charles B. Stout Neuroscience Mass Spectrometry Laboratory, Department of Neurology, University of Tennessee Health Science Center, USA

tration also occurs within a tyrosine phosphorylation motif ([R or K]-x2(3)-[D or E]-x3(2)-[Y]), which might compete with the tyrosine phosphorylation to affect cellular signaling (Zhan & Desiderio, 2011, Zhan *et al.*, 2007, Mallozzi *et al.*, 2012). Therefore, protein tyrosine nitration can alter protein functions, and is extensively associated with multiple pathophysiological processes including tumors, neurodegenerative diseases, and inflammatory diseases (Zhan & Desiderio, 2004, 2006 and 2009a, Haddad *et al.*, 1994, Miyagi *et al.*, 2002, Yeo *et al.*, 2008, Halliwell *et al.*, 1999).

A global nitroproteomics method, namely the use of proteomics to investigate protein tyrosine nitration, was used to analyze protein tyrosine nitration in human tissues. The challenging issue in nitroproteomic analysis of endogenous nitroproteins is its very low abundance (one nitrotyrosine per $\sim 10^6$ tyrosine residues) in a proteome (Haddad *et al.*, 1994, Shigenaga *et al.*, 1997) and limited sensitivity of a mass spectrometry (MS). Therefore, it is necessary to preferentially enrich endogenous nitroproteins or nitropeptides prior to MS analysis (Zhan & Desiderio, 2009a). The effective approaches that detect and preferentially enrich endogenous nitroproteins are anti-nitrotyrosine antibody-based enzyme-linked immunosorbent assay (ELISA) (Khan *et al.*, 1998, Torreilles & Romestand, 2001), immunoprecipitation (Zhan & Desiderio, 2006), and one/two-dimensional gel electrophoresis (1DGE/2DGE)-based Western blot analyses (Zhan & Desiderio, 2004 and 2007, Aulak *et al.*, 2001, Miyagi *et al.*, 2002). The commercially available ELISA assay kit (Upstate Catalog No. 17–136) can measure nitrotyrosine content. 1DGE/2DGE-based Western blots can separate and preferentially enrich endogenous nitroproteins and also determine the relative level of nitrotyrosine. Immunoprecipitation can preferentially enrich endogenous nitroproteins from a complex proteome before MS analysis. Tandem mass spectrometry (MS/MS) can characterize a nitrotyrosine site in a nitroprotein (Zhan & Desiderio, 2004, 2006, 2007 and 2009a).

As a potential marker of oxidative/nitrative injuries, protein tyrosine nitration might be an important molecular event in human hypothalamic–pituitary–target organ axis systems (Zhan & Desiderio, 2004 and 2006). The up-stream molecules that promote formation of tyrosine nitration, nitric oxide (NO) and nitric oxide synthase (NOS), participate in those pituitary-mediated axis systems (Zhan & Desiderio, 2004, Lloyd *et al.*, 1995, Ueta *et al.*, 1998, Ceccatelli *et al.*, 1993): luteinizing hormone (LH) (Ceccatelli *et al.*, 1993, McCann *et al.*, 2001, McCann *et al.*, 2003, Pinilla *et al.*, 2001), follicle-stimulating hormone (FSH) (McCann *et al.*, 2001), adrenocorticotropin (ACTH) (Riedel, 2000), prolactin (PRL) (Duvilanski *et al.*, 1995), and growth hormone (GH) (Bocca *et al.*, 2000, Cuttica *et al.*, 1997, Pinilla *et al.*, 1999). The nitrotyrosine level was elevated in a pituitary adenoma. For human pituitary nitroproteomics studies, 2DGE-based nitrotyrosine Western blot analysis (Zhan & Desiderio, 2004 and 2007) and nitrotyrosine immunoaffinity enrichment (Zhan & Desiderio, 2006) were used to separate and preferentially enrich endogenous nitroproteins from a complex human pituitary control and adenoma tissue. Enriched nitroproteins were subjected to trypsin digestion, followed by MS/MS analysis to identify nitroproteins and nitrotyrosine sites. Bioinformatics was used to determine structural/functional domains and motifs of a nitroprotein, and to locate the nitrotyrosine site within a protein domain/motif to clarify roles of tyrosine nitration in a protein (Zhan & Desiderio, 2006). Pathway analysis-based systems biology was used to discover pathway networks that involved endogenous nitroproteins from a systematical and comprehensive angle (Zhan & Desiderio, 2010). In addition, MS characteristics of standard nitropeptides (Zhan & Desiderio, 2009c) were analyzed to obtain the fragmentation to assist interpretation of a MS spectrum of a tryptic peptide derived from an endogenous nitroprotein in a proteome. A total of eight nitrotyrosine-containing proteins (nitroproteins) in a human pituitary post-mortem tissue, and nine nitroproteins and three nitroprotein-interacting proteins in a human nonfunctional pituitary adenoma tissue (Zhan & Desiderio, 2004, 2006 and 2007), were identified with MS/MS. Nitrotyrosine sites located within important protein domains or motifs (Zhan & Desiderio, 2006) were involved in the tumor biological characteristics (Zhan & Desiderio, 2006) and important pathway network systems (Zhan & Desiderio, 2010).

2   Materials and Methods

2.1   Synthetic Standard Peptides

MS analysis of synthetic standard nitropeptide was described to assist interpretation of the MS spectrum of endogenous nitropeptide (Zhan & Desiderio, 2009c). Briefly, three synthetic standard peptides (leucine enkephalin acetate hydrate, LE1, Y-G-G-F-L, 555.1818 Da; nitro-Tyr-leucine enkephalin, LE2, $(3-NO_2)$Y-G-G-F-L, 600.0909 Da; and d_5-Phe-nitro-Tyr-leucine enkephalin, LE3, $(3-NO_2)$Y-G-G-(d_5)F-L, 605.1818 Da) were prepared as a series of dilutions including 5000, 1000, 500, 100, 50, 10, 5, and 1 fmol/μl, respectively. Each prepared peptide solution (4 μl) was mixed with 4 μl of the 5 mg/mlα-cyano-4-hydroxycinnamic acid (CHCA) matrix solution, and was loaded onto a vMALDI 96-well plate for MS characterization of each standard peptide with a vacuum matrix-assisted laser desorption/ionization-linear ion-trap mass spectrometer (vMALDI-LTQ). MS and MS/MS spectra were obtained for each synthetic standard peptide. Laser fluence and the normalized collision energy (NCE) were optimized. The spectrum (MS; MS^2) of each scan ($n = 30$ scans) in each file was processed and accumulated ($n = 30$) to obtain a synthetic spectrum. The m/z value and peak intensity in the synthetic spectrum were used for data analysis and graph construction. Each experiment was carried out in triplicate.

2.2   Detection and Identification of Pituitary Nitroproteins with 2D-Western Blot and MS/MS

A 2D-Western blot-based MS/MS method was described to identify nitroproteins from a pituitary post-mortem control tissue (Zhan & Desiderio, 2004 and 2007). The brief experimental procedure includes: (1) 2DGE and Western blot. A human control pituitary post-mortem tissue (male, 45 year-old, drowning) was used for extraction of proteins. Extracted pituitary proteins (70 μg) were arrayed with isoelectric focusing (IEF; an 18-cm IPGstrip pH 3–10 NL) with an Amersham Multiphor II instrument, following by equilibration with the solution that contained dithiothreitol (DTT) or iodoacetamide, and sodium dodecyl sulfate-polyacrylamide gel electrophoresis (SDS–PAGE) with a home-made 12% PAGE resolving gel (190 × 205 × 1 mm) on a vertical PROTEAN-plus Dodeca Cell (Zhan & Desiderio, 2003a). 2DGE-separated proteins were transferred onto a PVDF membrane (0.8 mA/cm^2; 1 h, 40 min), incubated (1 h) with a primary antibody (rabbit anti-human nitrotyrosine antibody; Millipore product), and incubated (1 h, room temperature) with secondary antibody (goat anti-rabbit alkaline phosphase-conjugated IgG). The membrane was visualized with 5-bromo-4-chloro-3-indolyl phosphate/nitro blue tetrazolium (BCIP/NBT) (Pierce, Rockford, IL, USA). A parallel negative-control experiment (only incubated with the secondary antibody but not primary antibody) was performed to observe any cross-reactivity of the secondary antibody. The 2DGE gel, after transfer of proteins to PVDF membrane, was silver-stained to determine efficiency of the protein transfer. Images of 2D gel and Western blot membrane were analyzed with PDQuest 2D gel image software. Detailed gel image analysis was described (Zhan & Desiderio, 2003b). (2) MS characterization of nitroprotein. Silver-stained 2D gel-spots that corresponded to positive Western blot spots were excised, and proteins were subjected to in-gel trypsin digestion (Zhan & Desiderio, 2003a). The tryptic peptide mixture was purified with a ZipTipC18 micro-column, and analyzed with a capillary liquid chromatography-electrospray ionization-LCQ^{Deca} mass spectrometer (LC-ESI-Q-IT) to obtain MS/MS spectrum of each peptide. *De novo* sequencing was also used to independently and accurately determine each amino acid sequence. MS/MS data were used for protein database analysis with SEQUEST software with mass modifications [+45 kDa (+NO$_2$–H) at Tyr and of +57 kDa (+NH$_2$COCH$_2$–H) at Cys].

2.3   Identification of Pituitary Adenoma Nitroproteins with NTAC and MS/MS

A non-gel method, nitrotyrosine affinity column (NTAC)-based MS/MS approach (Figure 1) was described to identify nitroproteins from a pituitary adenoma tissue (Zhan & Desiderio, 2006). Briefly, The NTAC was prepared with a Pierce Seize X mammalian immunoprecipitation kit with a detailed procedure (Zhan & Desiderio, 2006). A portion (62 mg wet weight) of a nonfunctional human pituitary adenoma tissue (white male, 39 years old, negative expression of FSH, LH, GH, PRL, TSH, and ACTH) was used to extract the protein into a volume (600 μl) of protein extraction buffer (Pierce, Rockford, IL, USA), and was diluted (1:1, v/v) with binding/washing buffer. A volume (500 μl) of diluted sample was incubated (overnight, gently rocking, > 19 h, 4 °C) with the prepared NTAC to bind nitroproteins and nitroprotein–protein complexes. The bound nitroproteins and nitroprotein–protein complexes were eluted with 200 μl elution buffer (pH 2.8) that contained a primary amine (gently mix well, centrifuge 3,000 g, 1 min, 3×). The eluates that contained nitroproteins and nitroprotein–protein complexes were collected for trypsin treatment and MS/MS analysis. Moreover, another volume (500 μl) of diluted sample was added to the control column, followed by the same experiment steps listed above. MS/MS data were used to identify the protein and nitrotyrosine sites by searching the Swiss–Prot and NCBInr databases with Bioworks 3.2 software with mass modifications of +45 Da (+NO$_2$ –H) at Tyr and of +57Da (+NH$_2$COCH$_2$ – H) at Cys. Moreover,

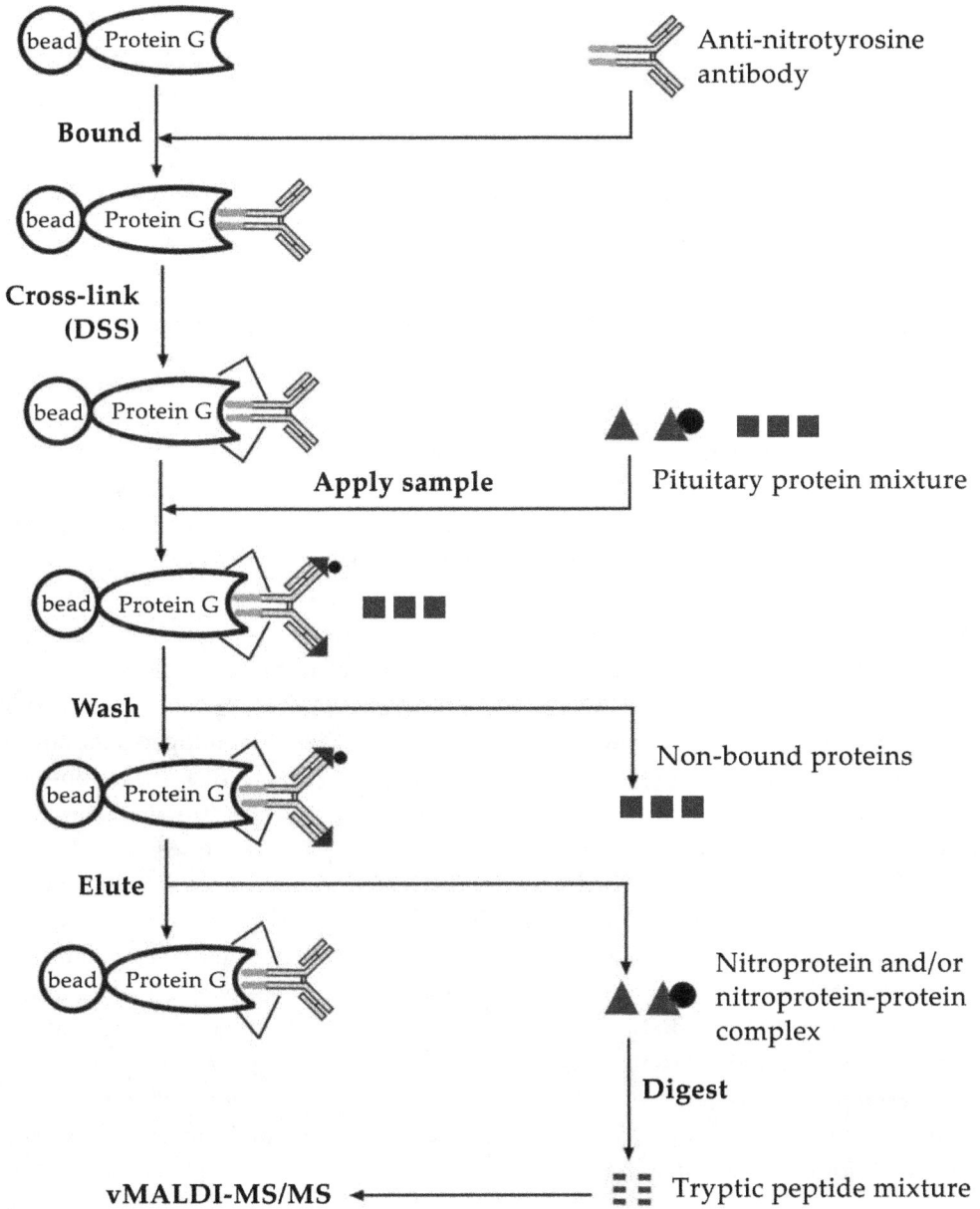

Figure 1: NTAC-based experimental flow chart that was used to identify nitroprotein and its complexes. The control experiment without any anti-3-nitrotyrosine antibody was performed in parallel with the NTAC-based experiments. Reproduced from Zhan and Desiderio (2006), with permission from Elsevier Science, copyright 2006

results derived from NTAC were compared to results derived from the control column to remove any nonspecific binding proteins. Protein domains and motifs analysis with ScanProsite software (http://us.expasy.org/tools/scanprosite) and MotifScan software (http://myhits.isb-sib.ch/cgi-bin/motif _scan) were used to locate the nitrotyrosine sites within protein domain/motif. An experimental data-based model of nitroproteins and their functions was proposed on the basis of the functional information of those nitro-proteins on the Swiss-Prot annotation page and the related literature data.

2.4   Pathway Network Analysis of Identified Nitroproteins

Ingenuity pathway analysis (IPA) system (http://www.ingenuity.com) was used to mine the signal pathway networks that involved the nitroproteins from human pituitary control and pituitary adenoma tissues (Zhan & Desiderio, 2010). Briefly, the Swiss-Prot accession numbers of all nitroproteins were input to the IPA data upload workflow. The IPA system automatically searched the matched Gene/molecules, and generated a two-dimensional table-style format to show the matched proteins and the unmapped proteins. The Swiss-Prot accession number of unmapped protein was converted to the corresponding gene name by searching the ExPASY proteomics server. All Swiss-Prot accession numbers of matched proteins and gene names of unmatched proteins were input to the IPA data upload workflow to generate the final mapped list for next-step analysis. Five subdatasets were generated including All IDs, Unmapped IDs, Mapped IDs, Network-eligible IDs, and Functions/Pathways/List-eligible IDs. Each sub-dataset contained ID, notes, molecules, description, location, type of biofunction, and drugs. The name of each molecule appeared in the pathway network nodes. The Network-eligible IDs were used as the pathway network analysis by comparing the network-eligible molecules with the IPA Knowledge Base (IPAKB) with a Fisher's exact test. The level of statistical significance was set to $p < 0.05$. Each Pathway analysis generated the top networks, biofunctions/Tox functions, and top canonical pathways with a statistical significance ($p < 0.05$). A toxicity pathway is defined as a canonical pathway that is significantly associated with toxicity lists that are functional gene groupings based on critical biological processes and key toxicological responses; and those toxicity lists describe adaptive, defensive, or reparative responses to xenobiotic insult, and could be used to understand biological responses.

3   Results and Discussion

3.1   Mass Spectrometric Behavior and Characteristics of a Synthetic Nitropeptide

The MS behavior of a nitropeptide is much different between MALDI and ESI (Zhan & Desiderio, 2009c, Petersson *et al.*, 2001, Sarver *et al.*, 2001). The MALDI UV laser commonly induces photochemical decompositions of the nitro group ($-NO_2$) to decrease the precursor-ion intensity of a nitropeptide and to complicate the MS spectrum (Zhan &

Desiderio, 2009c, Petersson *et al.*, 2001, Sarver *et al.*, 2001). ESI does not induce those decompositions (Zhan & Desiderio, 2009c, Yeo *et al.*, 2008, Petersson *et al.*, 2001, Sarver *et al.*, 2001, Lee *et al.*, 2007, Kim *et al.*, 2011, Lee *et al.*, 2009). In our experiments, MALDI MS and MS/MS were used to study the fragmentation pattern of *in vitro* nitropeptides (Zhan & Desiderio, 2009c) through analysis of synthetic LE1 (Y-G-G-F-L, 555.1818 Da), LE2 [(3-NO$_2$)Y-G-G-F-L, 600.0909 Da], and LE3[(3-NO$_2$)Y-G-G-(d5)F-L, 605.1818 Da] with a vMALDI-LTQ mass spectrometer.

The results showed that UV laser-induced photochemical decomposition (loss of one or two oxygen atoms of the nitro group to form the unique decomposition pattern of ions ([M+H]$^+$ - 16 and [M+H]$^+$ - 32) in LE2 and LE3 relative to LE1 (Figure 2) (Zhan & Desiderio, 2009c). A similar decomposition pattern ([M+H]$^+$ + Na - 16 and [M+H]$^+$ + Na - 32) occurred for the sodium adduct ([M+H]$^+$ + Na) of LE2 and LE3 relative to the sodium adduct of LE1. A product ion ([M+H]$^+$ - 30) was also observed in the LE2 and LE3 spectra, which could result from the reduction of the nitro group (-NO$_2$) to an amino group (-NH$_2$) (Sarver et al., 2001). Meanwhile, the base-peak intensity of the [M+H]$^+$ ion of LE1 (NL = 1.01E5) was much higher than that of LE2 (NL = 3.25E4) and LE3 (NL = 9.09E4) because photochemical decomposition decreased ion intensity and complicated the MS spectrum. However, recognition of this unique decomposition pattern can unambiguously identify a nitrotyrosine.

For a vMALDI-MS/MS analysis, b- and a-ions were the most-intense fragment ions relative to y-ions (Figure 3) (Zhan & Desiderio, 2009c). Compared to unmodified LE1, more collision energy optimized fragmentation of the nitropeptides LE2 and LE3 (Figure 4A). However, higher collision energy increased the intensity of the a$_4$-ion and decreased the intensity of the b$_4$-ion (a-ion = the loss of CO from a b-ion) (Figure 4B). Also, the optimized laser fluence maximized fragmentation of the nitropeptides LE2 and LE3. Although MS^3 analysis confirmed the MS^2-derived amino acid sequence, MS^3 analysis requires a higher amount of peptides relative to MS^2 (Zhan & Desiderio, 2009c). Thus, MS^3 analysis might not be suitable for routine analysis of endogenous low-abundance nitroproteins. To detect an endogenous nitropeptide, the amount of peptide must reach the sensitivity of a mass spectrometer; for our synthetic nitropeptides, the sensitivity of vMALDI-LTQ was 1 fmol for MS detection and 10 fmol for MS^2 detection (Zhan & Desiderio, 2009c). The detailed results were described (Zhan & Desiderio, 2009c). Those MS data of synthetic nitropeptides would be useful to assist the interpretation of MS spectrum of an endogenous nitropeptides.

3.2   Enrichment of Endogenous Nitroproteins in Human Pituitary and Adenoma Tissues

Nitrotyrosine is formed from the reaction of free or protein-bound tyrosine with RNS including peroxynitrite (Beckman, 1996) and free-radical nitrogen dioxide (Squadrito & Pryor, 1998) and has a very low abundance (1 in ~10^6 tyrosines) in an *in vivo* proteome (Haddad *et al.*, 1994, Shigenaga *et al.*, 1997). MS is the essential technique for identification of a nitroprotein/nitropeptide and nitrated site (Zhan & Desiderio, 2004, 2006 and 2007). However, MS is limited by it's certain sensitivity (Zhan & Desiderio, 2009a).

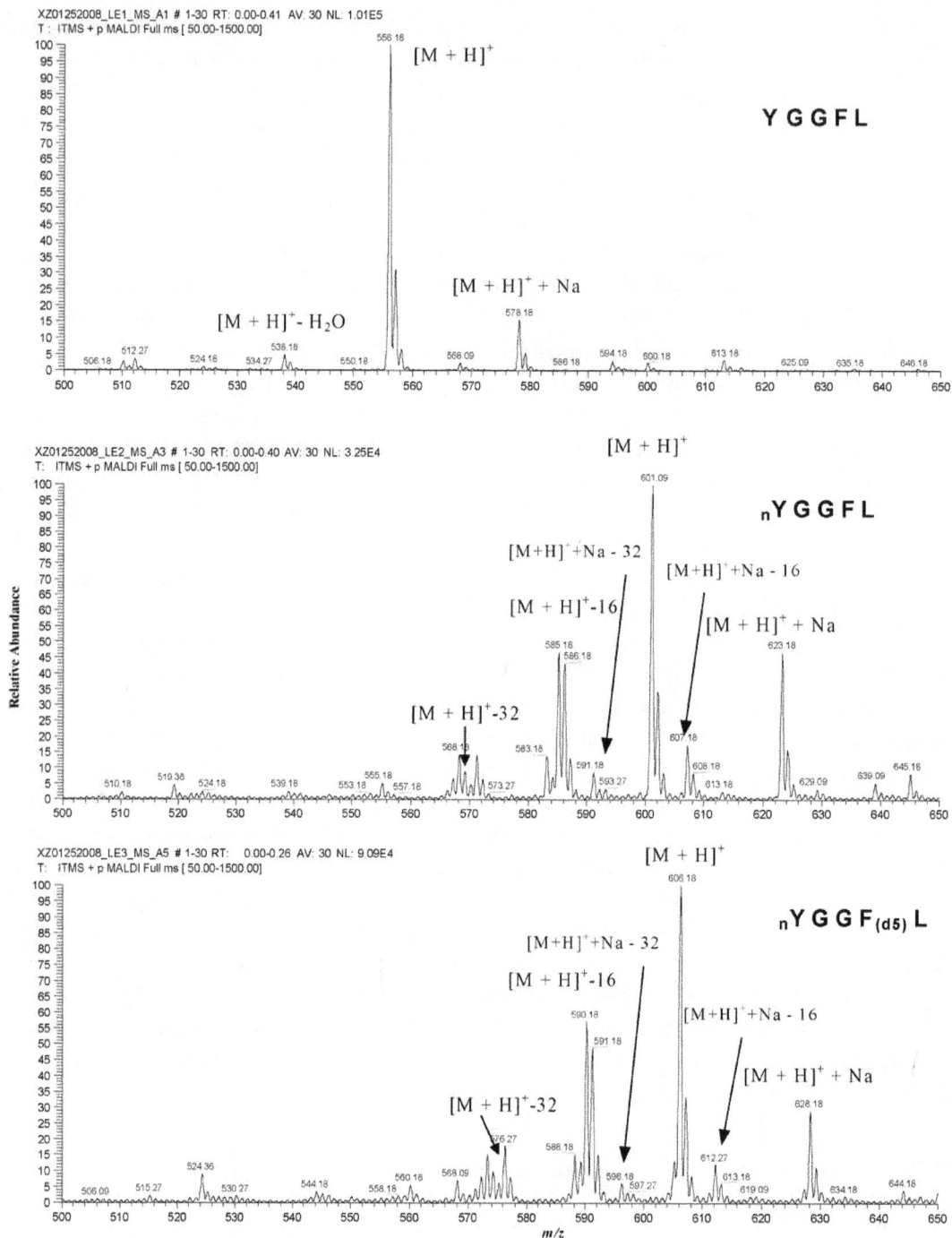

Figure 2: MS spectra of LE1 (top), LE2 (middle), and LE3 (bottom) with vMALDI-MS analysis. nY = nitro-Tyr. F(d5) = Phe residue with five 2H (d) atoms. Reproduced from Zhan and Desiderio (2009c) with permission from Elsevier Science, copyright 2009

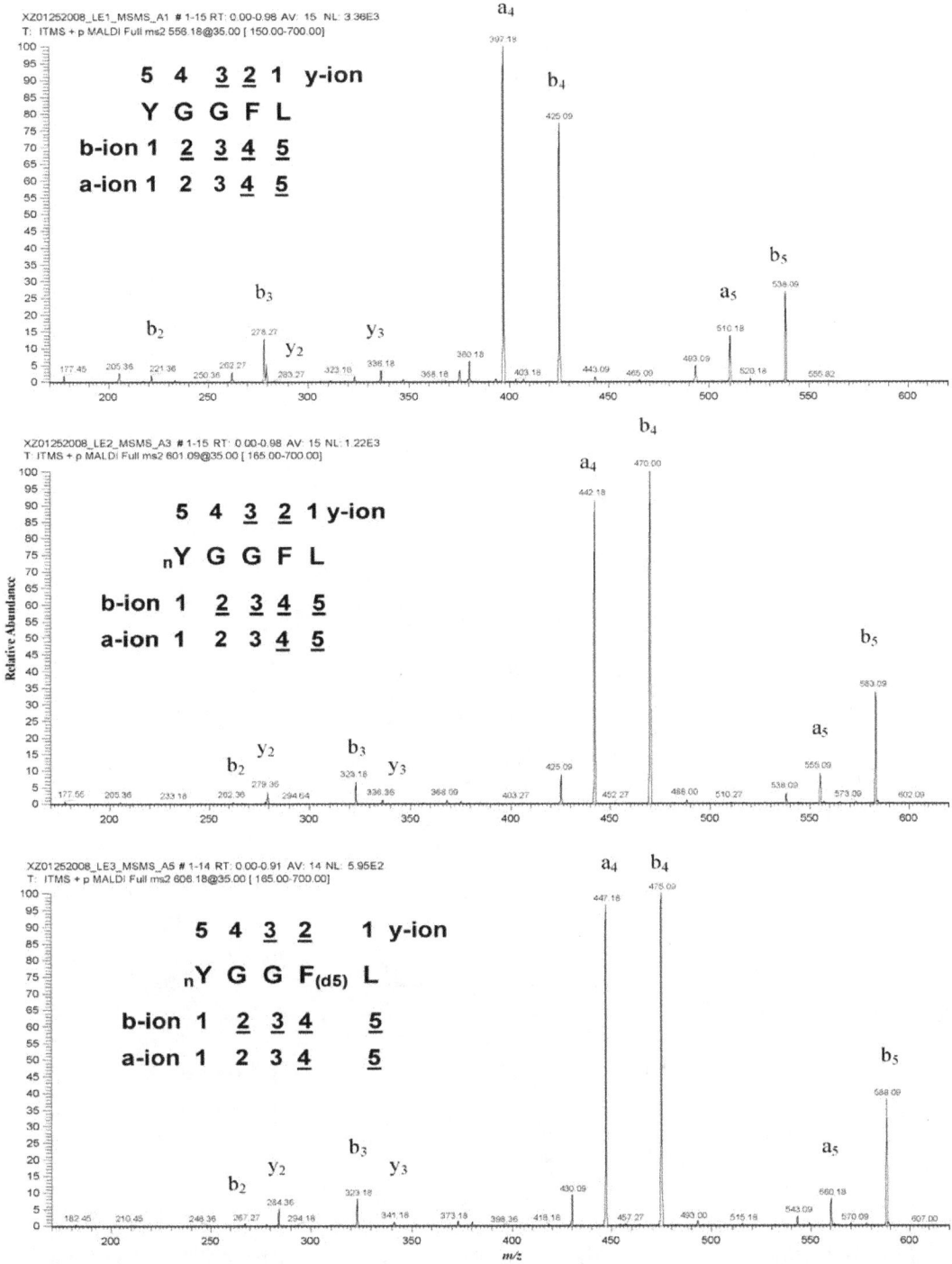

Figure 3: MS^2 spectra of LE1 (top), LE2 (middle), and LE3 (bottom) with vMAL-DI-MS/MS analysis. nY = nitro-Tyr. F(d5) = Phe residue with five 2H (d) atoms. Reproduced from Zhan and Desiderio (2009c) with permission from Elsevier Science, copyright 2009.

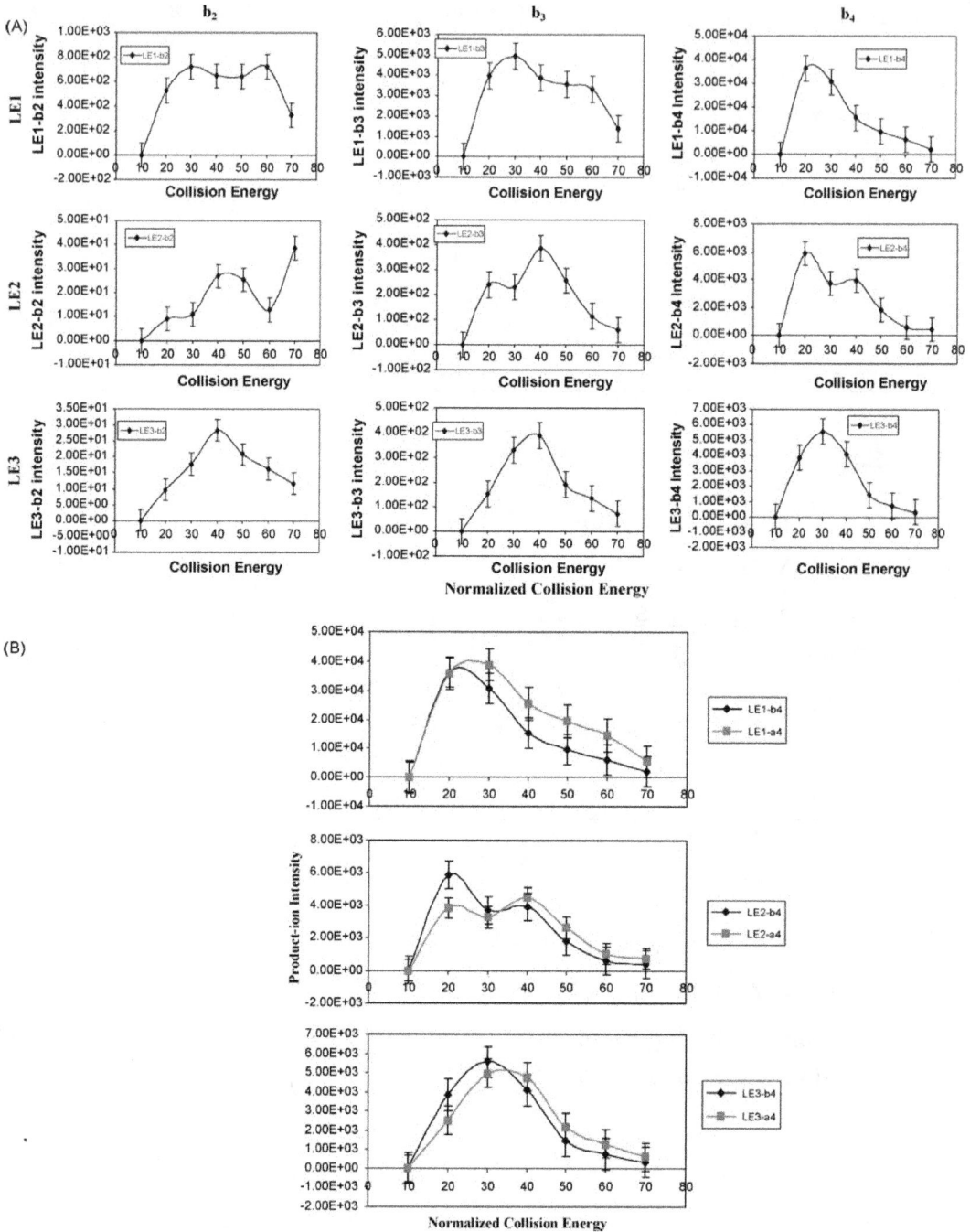

Figure 4: Effect of collision energy on fragmentation of nitropeptides. (A) Relationship between collision energy and product-ion intensity (n = 3). (B) Relationship between collision energy and product-ion b4 and a4 intensities (n = 3). Reproduced from Zhan and Desiderio (2009c) with permission from Elsevier Science, copyright 2009

Therefore, it is necessary to preferentially enrich nitroproteins/nitropeptides before MS analysis (Zhan & Desiderio, 2009a, Yeo *et al.*, 2008, Kim *et al.*, 2011, Lee *et al.*, 2009). Two preferential enrichment methods were used to study human pituitary and adenoma nitroproteomes, including 2DGE-based nitrotyrosine Western blot (Zhan & Desiderio, 2004 and 2007) and NTAC-based enrichment (Zhan & Dediderio, 2006).

2DGE-based nitrotyrosine Western blot (Zhan & Desiderio, 2004 and 2007) involved the following experiment procedure. Briefly, proteins were extracted from a post-mortem control pituitary and arrayed according to p*I* and M_r. The arrayed proteins were transferred to a PVDF membrane, incubated with anti-nitrotyrosine antibody, and visualized (Figure 5). *Ca.* 1000 protein spots were detected in the silver-stained 2D gel with a range of p*I* 3–10 and M_r 10–100 kDa) (Figure 5A). Thirty-two nitrotyrosine-positive Western blot spots were detected (Figure 5C) by comparison of digitized Western blot image (Figure 5C) to the negative-control (Figure 5D). Also, each nitrotyrosine positive Western blot spot (Figure 5C) was matched to the corresponding silver-stained 2D gel-spots (Figure 5A) so that the silver-stained gel-spots were excised for MS analysis. Therefore, even though abundance of a nitroprotein in a human tissue proteome is very low, 2DGE can separate and enrich each nitroprotein in a 2D gel spot to improve its immunodetection and MS-characterization.

The NTAC method (Zhan & Desiderio, 2006) (Figure 1) was used to preferentially enrich nitroproteins from a human pituitary adenoma proteome. Briefly, anti-nitrotyrosine antibodies were cross-linked to protein G beads, and incubated with a pituitary adenoma protein sample. Nitroproteins and nitroprotein–protein complexes were bound to the cross-linked anti-nitrotyrosine antibodies. Bound nitroproteins and nitroprotein–protein complexes were eluted to provide an enriched nitroprotein sample, and were subjected to trypsin digestion and MS/MS analysis. For our experiment, NTAC was an effective method to enrich nitroproteins from a human pituitary adenoma proteome and improve MS/MS identification of endogenous nitroproteins. A total of nine nitroproteins and three proteins that interact with nitroproteins were identified from a pituitary adenoma proteome (Zhan & Desiderio, 2006).

However, one must realize that 2DGE-based method has obvious limitations in the detailed protein analysis including deficiencies in the coverage of proteome, dynamic range, sensitivity and throughput, especially when a limited sample is processed (Zhan & Desiderio, 2005). Also, 2DGE-based Western blot is to relatively enrich and detect the nitrotyrosine-containing proteins, the non-nitrated tryptic peptides are much more than nitrated tryptic peptides, which will hinder the MS/MS characterization of nitrated tryptic peptides. Advantages of 2DGE-based Western blotting are that it can provide directly visualized image of nitroproteins and detect protein isoforms. NTAC-based MS/MS method has more advantages to overcome those limitations of 2DGE method, but it cannot provide the visualized image of nitroproteins and detect protein isoforms. The use of NTAC method to enrich the tryptic nitrated peptides, but not nitroproteins, would maximize the coverage of nitrotyrosine sites in a proteome.

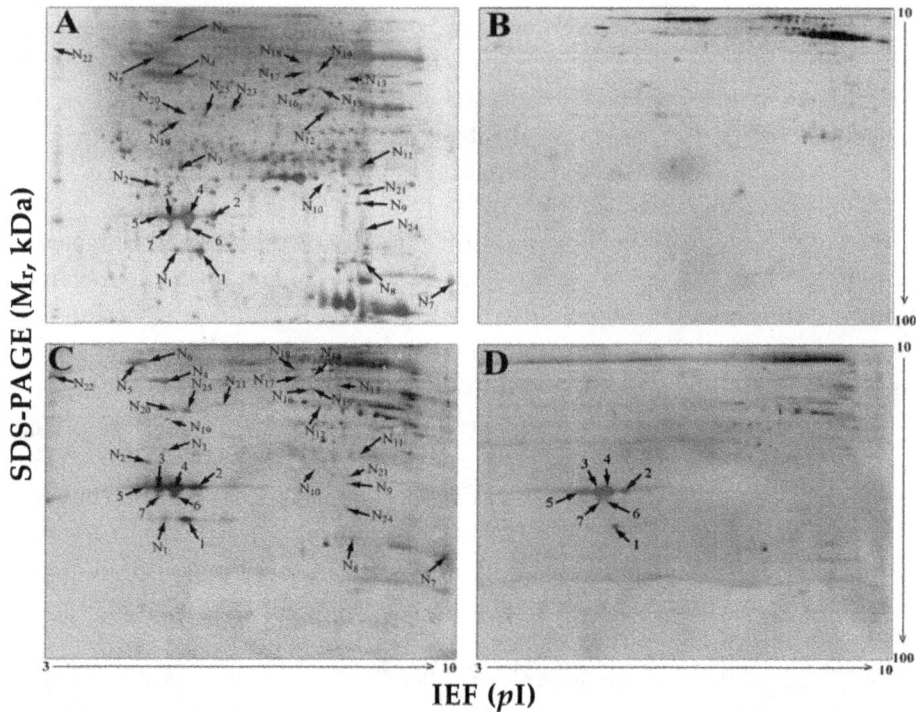

Figure 5: 2DGE-based Western blotting analysis of nitrotyrosine immunopositive proteins in a human pituitary (70 µg protein per 2D gel). (A) Silver-stained image on a 2D gel before transfer of proteins onto a PVDF membrane. (B) Silver-stained image on a 2D gel after transfer of proteins onto a PVDF membrane. (C) Western blot image of nitrotyrosine immunopositive proteins (anti-3-nitrotyrosine antibodies + secondary antibody). (D) Negative control of a Western blot to show cross-reaction of the secondary antibody (only the secondary antibody; no anti-3-nitrotyrosine antibody). Reproduced from Zhan and Desiderio (2007) with permission from Elsevier Science, copyright 2007

3.3   MS/MS Identification of Nitroproteins and Nitrated Sites in Human Pituitary and Adenoma

MS/MS is the essential method to obtain the amino acid sequence and nitration sites of a tryptic nitropeptide (Zhan & Desiderio, 2004, 2006 and 2007). A total of 32 2D gel spots were excised that corresponded to nitrotyrosine-positive Western blot spots from a post-mortem pituitary control tissue, and proteins were subjected to in-gel trypsin digestion and MS/MS analysis. Eight nitroproteins and eight nitrated sites were identified in pituitary control tissue (Table 1) (Zhan & Desiderio, 2004 and 2007), including actin, cGMP-dependent protein kinase 2, synaptosomal-associated protein, proteasome subunit alpha type 2, immunoglobulin alpha Fc receptor, stanniocalcin 1, mitochondrial co-chaperone protein HscB, and progestin and adipoQ receptor family member III. Those nitroproteins function in cellular immunity, neurotransmission, calcium and phosphate

Pituitary Adenoma		
	Protein name	nY site
Nitrated protein	Rho-GTPase-activating 5 [Q13017] (ARHGAP5)	Y^{550}
	Leukocyte immunoglobulin-like receptor A4 [P59901]	Y^{404}
	Zinc finger protein 432 [O94892]	Y^{41}
	PKA beta regulatory subunit [P31321] (PRKAR1B)	Y^{20}
	Sphingosine-1-phosphate lyase 1 [O95470]	Y^{356}, Y^{366}
	Centaurin beta 1 [Q15027]	Y^{485}
	Proteasome subunit alpha type 2 [P25787] (PSMA2)	Y^{228}
	Interleukin 1 family member 6 [Q9UHA7] (IL1F6)	Y^{96}
	Rhophilin 2 [Q8IUC4] (RHPN2)	Y^{258}
Nitroprotein-interacted protein	Interleukin-1 receptor-associated kinase-like 2 (IRAK-2) [O43187] (IRAK2)	
	Glutamate receptor interacting protein 2 [Q9C0E4] (GRIP2)	
	Ubiquitin [P62988] (UBB or UBC)	

Pituitary Control		
	Protein name	nY site
Nitrated protein	Synaptosomal-associated protein (SNAP91)	Y^{237}
	Ig alpha Fc receptor [P24071] (FCAR)	Y^{223}
	Actin [P03996] (ACTA2, ACTG2, ACTC1)	Y^{296}
	PKG 2 [Q13237] (PRKG2)	Y^{354}
	Mitochondrial co-chaperone protein HscB [Q8IWL3]	Y^{128}
	Stanniocalcin 1[P52823] (STC1)	Y^{159}
	Proteasome subunit alpha type 2 (PSMA2)	Y^{228}
	Progestin and adipoQ receptor family member III [Q6TCH7] (PAQR3)	Y^{33}

Table 1: Nitroproteins and non-nitrated proteins identified from a pituitary adenoma (Zhan & Desiderio, 2006), *and* control tissue (Zhan & Desiderio, 2004 and 2007). Note: nY = nitrotyrosine. Modified from Zhan and Desiderio (2004, 2006 and 2007) with permission from Elsevier Science, copyright 2004, 2006 and 2007. Reproduced from Zhan, Wang and Desiderio (2013) with permission from Hindawi Publishing Corporation open access journal and copyright remains with the authors.

metabolism, cellular structure and mobility, membrane receptor, co-chaperone in iron-sulfur cluster assembly in mitochondria, and the ATP/ubiquitin-dependent non-lysosomal proteolytic pathway.

The NTAC-enriched nitroprotein samples from a pituitary adenoma tissue were subjected to trypsin digestion and MS/MS analysis (Zhan & Desiderio, 2006). A total of nine nitroproteins and ten nitrated sites were identified (Table 1), including cAMP-dependent protein kinase type I-beta regulatory subunit, sphingosine-1-phosphate lyase 1, Rho-GTPase-activing protein 5, zinc finger protein 432, proteasome subunit alpha type 2, centaurin beta 1, leukocyte immunoglobulin-like receptor subfamily A member 4, interleukin 1 family member 6, and rhophilin 2. Three proteins including interleukin 1 receptor-associated kinase-like 2, ubiquitin, and glutamate receptor-interacting protein 2 were identified to interact with nitroproteins (Table 1), and form three nitroprotein–protein complexes, including nitrated interleukin 1 family member 6-interleukin 1 receptor-interleukin 1 receptor-associated kinase-like 2 (IL1F6-IL1R-IRAK2), nitrated proteasome-ubiquitin complex, and nitrated beta-subunit of cAMP-dependent protein kinase (PKA) complex (Zhan & Desiderio, 2006).

Those nine nitroproteins and three nitroproten-protein complexes were rationalized into a corresponding functional system (Figure 6) (Zhan & Desiderio, 2006). The nitrated S1P lyase 1 participates in sphingolipid metabolism to regulate cell proliferation, survival, and cell death as well as the immune system (Zhan & Desiderio, 2006, Maceykaa et al., 2002, Schwab et al., 2005, Hla, 2005). The nitrated proteasome-ubiquitin complex is an important enzymatic complex involved in the intracellular nonlysosomal proteolytic pathway (Zhan & Desiderio, 2006, Tamura et al., 1991, Kristensen et al., 1994). Nitrated CENT-beta 1 and nitrated PKAR1-beta are involved in the PKA signal pathway. IRAK-2 in the IL1-R complex and nitrated IL1-F6 are involved in the cytokine system. Nitrated LIRA4 might be involved in the immune system. Nitrated ZFP432 is involved in transcription regulatory systems. Nitrated RHOGAP5 and nitrated rhophilin 2 are involved in the GTPase signal pathway (Zhan & Desiderio, 2006).

3.4   Bioinformatics Recognition of the Functional Domains/Motifs of a Nitroprotein

Location of nitrotyrosine sites into a protein domain or motif would clarify biological activities of tyrosine nitration because functional and structural domains or motifs in a protein sustain a certain biological functions. Protein-domain analysis software such as ScanProsite (http://us.expasy.org/tools/scanprosite), Motifscan (http://myhits.isb-sib.ch/cgibin/motif_scan), Inter-ProScan (http://www.ebi.ac.uk/InterProScan), ProDom (http://prodom.prabi.fr/prodom/current/html/form.php), and Pfam (http://www.sanger.ac.uk/Software/Pfam) were effective tools that detect statistically significant domains in a nitroprotein and to locate each nitrated site within a protein domain (Zhan & Desiderio, 2006). It was used to analyze protein domains and motifs in each nitroprotein in a human pituitary adenoma proteome (Zhan & Desiderio, 2006). An interesting result demonstrated most nitrated sites occurred within important protein domains and motifs. Four examples were taken here in detail.

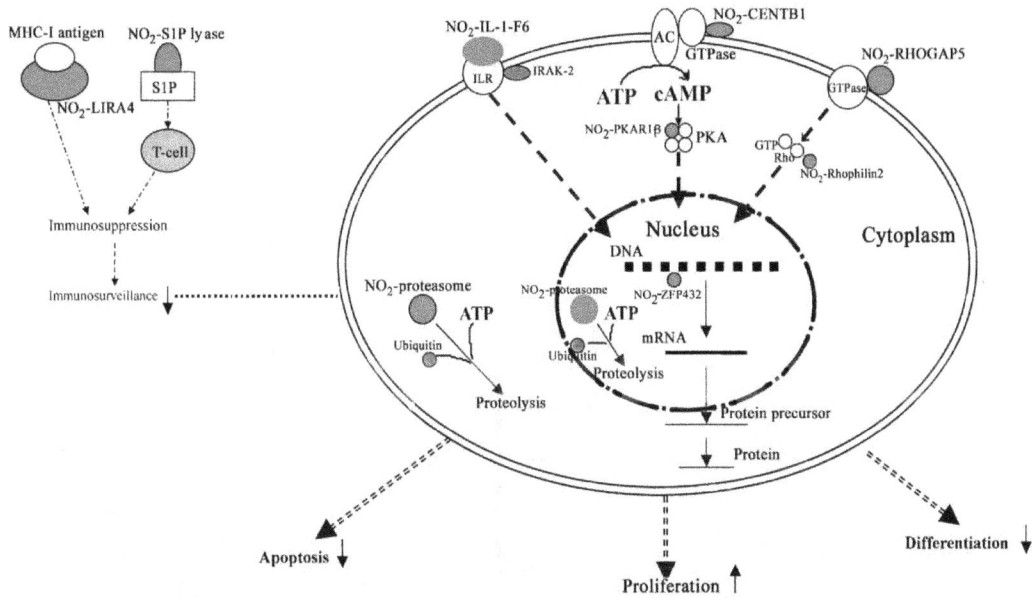

Figure 6: Experimental data-based model of nitroproteins and their functions in human nonfunctional pituitary adenomas. NO2-, nitroprotein. Reproduced from Zhan and Desiderio (2006) with permission from Elsevier Science, copyright 2006.

First, sphingosine-1-phosphate lyase 1 (S1P lyase 1) that was nitrated in human pituitary adenoma (Zhan & Desiderio, 2006) (Figure 7A) is a key enzyme to catalyze decomposition of S1P. Two nitrations (NO_2-^{356}Y and NO_2-^{366}Y) within the enzyme activity region would decrease the interaction intensity of enzyme:substrate (S1P lyase 1:S1P) and decrease the S1P decomposition because the nitro group ($-NO_2$) is an electron-withdrawing group that could decrease the level of enzyme-substrate binding. Study (Maceyka et al., 2002) demonstrates that sphingolipid metabolites including S1P, ceramide (Cer), and sphingosine (Sph) play an important role in the regulation of cell survival, proliferation, and cell death. Cer and Sph usually inhibit proliferation and promote apoptosis, whereas S1P stimulates growth and suppresses apoptosis. Because these metabolites are interconvertible, their relative levels determine cell fate. Nitration of S1P lyase 1 might increase the level of S1P relative to Cer and Sph, which would stimulate tumor cell proliferation and inhibit apoptosis.

Second, the Rho-GTPase-activating protein 5 (Figure 7B) contains four FF domains (Bedford & Leder, 1999) and one Rho-GAP domain. A nitration (NO_2-^{550}Y) within the region between two domains (FF4 and Rho-GAP) might impact on Rho-GTPase signal transduction (Zhan & Desiderio, 2006).

Third, zinc finger protein 432 (Figure 7C), a transcript factor, includes 16 C2H2-type zinc fingers binding DNA and one Kruppel-associated box (KRAB) domain that functions as a transcriptional suppressor (Payre &Vincent, 1998, Witzgall et al., 1994, Margolin et al., 1994). Nitration (NO_2-^{41}Y) within the KRAB domain might impair transcriptional suppression (Zhan & Desiderio, 2006).

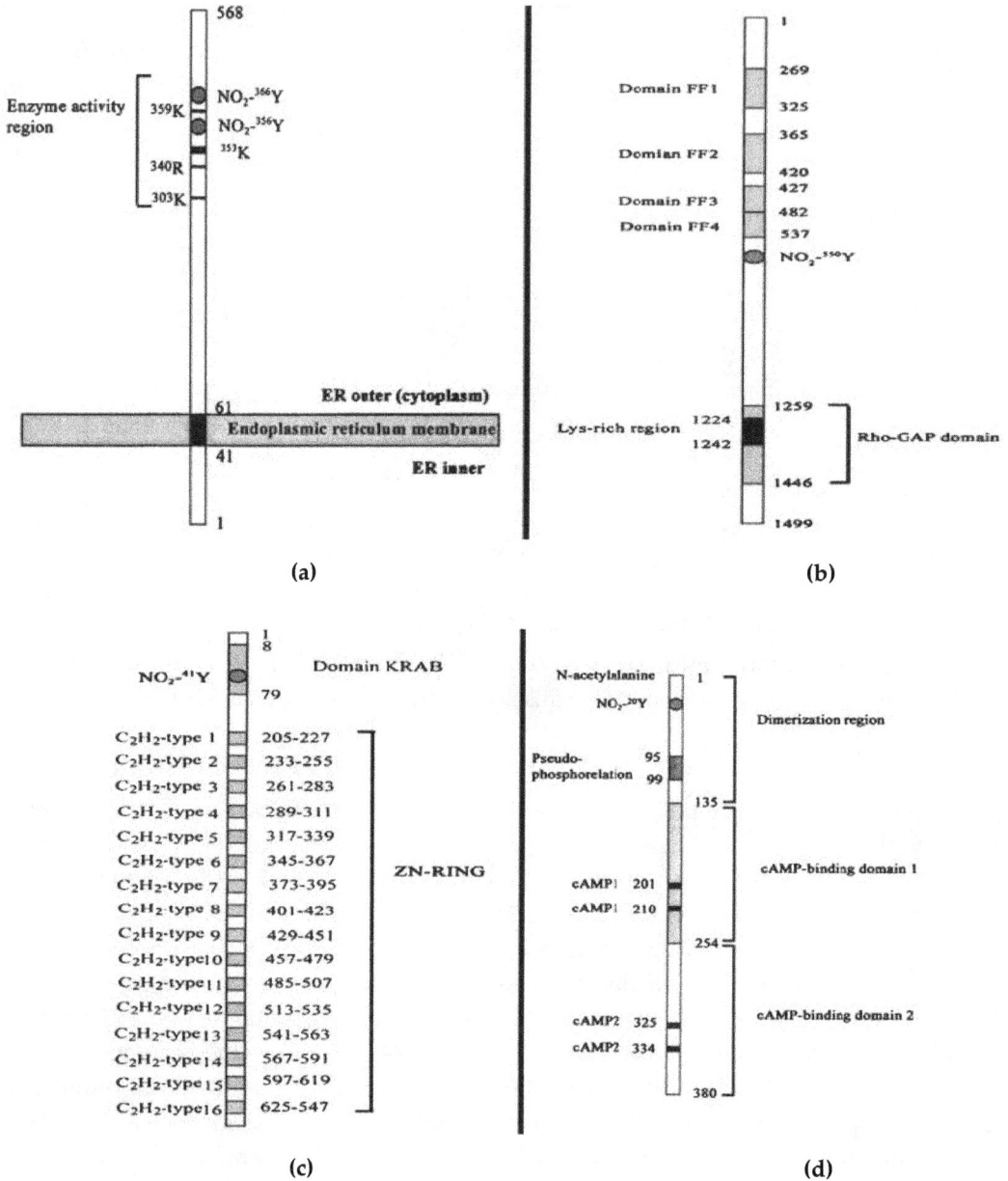

(a)

(b)

(c)

(d)

Figure 7: Nitration site and functional domains of four nitroproteins. (a) Sphingosine-1-phosphate lyase 1. The site ^{353}K is a pyridoxal phosphate-binding motif. (b) Rho-GTPase-activating protein 5. (c) Zinc finger protein 432. The KRAB domain is a transcriptional suppressor. The ZN-RING is a DNA-binding region. (d) cAMP-dependent protein kinase type I-beta regulatory subunit. Modified from Zhan and Desiderio (2006) with permission from Elsevier Science; reproduced from Zhan and Deiderio (2009a) with permission from Springer Science; and reproduced from Zhan, Wang and Desiderio (2013) with permission from Hindawi Publishing Corporation open access journal and copyright remains with the authors.

Fourth, The cAMP-dependent protein kinase type I-beta regulatory subunit (PKAR1-beta) (Figure 7D) contains one inhibitory region (pseudophosphorylation), one N-terminal dimerization domain, and two cAMP-binding domains. Each cAMP-binding domain contains two cAMP-binding sites. Nitration (NO_2-^{20}Y) within the dimerization region might affect dimerization of two regulatory chains to impair the functions of PKA (Zhan & Desiderio, 2006).

So the location of nitrated sites within the important protein domains/motifs provides an in-depth insight into the biological effects of tyrosine nitration on a protein.

3.5 Systems Biological Analysis of Signaling Pathway Networks that Involve Nitroproteins

Systems biology is a comprehensive analysis of all functionally interacting components of a biological system over time (Hood, 2003, Aderem, 2005, Hood & Tian, 2012). Compared to the traditional molecular biology methods that were used to study the role of a single gene, single protein, or single small-molecule model, the high-throughput "-omic" technologies including genomics, transcriptomics, proteomics, and metabolomics, drive the rapid development of systems biology to study a multiple-factor model of disease and to address the network of interaction and regulatory events that contribute to a disease (Zhan & Desiderio, 2010). Pathway biology is one important component of systems used to extensively analyze "-omic" data and to mine significantly signaling pathway networks and to address the biological significance of those "-omic" data.

IPA pathway analysis software was used to analyze signaling pathway networks that involve nitroproteins from human pituitary control (Zhan & Desideiro, 2004 and 2007) and adenoma tissues (Zhan & Desiderio, 2006). Those eight nitroproteins from a pituitary control and nine nitroproteins and three non-nitrated proteins that interact with nitroproteins from a pituitary adenoma tissue (Table 1) were used for IPA pathway analysis (Zhan & Desiderio, 2010). The results clearly showed that those pituitary adenoma nitroproteins and their complexes were involved in the tumor necrosis factor (TNF) and interleukin 1 (IL1) signaling networks (Figure 8A), which function in cancer, cell cycle, and reproductive system disease. Those nitroproteins in that network include IL1F6, PRKAR1B, ARHGAP5, PSMA2, and RHPN2, and the non-nitrated proteins that interact with nitroproteins include ubiquitin, GRIP2, and IRAK2. Three nitroprotein–protein complexes were identified: nitrated proteasome-ubiquitin complex, nitrated beta-subunit of PKA complex, and nitrated IL1F6-IL1 receptor-IL1 receptor-associated kinase-like 2 (IL1F6-IL1R-IRAK2) complexes. Those control pituitary nitroproteins were involved in the transforming growth factor beta 1 (TFGB1) and actin cellular skeleton signaling networks (Figure 8B), which function in gene expression, cellular development, and connective tissue development. Nitroproteins in that network include PRKG2, FCAR, actin, SNAP91, PAQR3, STC1, and PSMA2. Both networks (Figure 8A and B) include a beta-estradiol signal pathway, which indicates that hormone metabolism is involved in a normal pituitary and pituitary adenoma. It is consistent with the fact that NO is involved in pituitary hormone metabolism in normal physiology, and that a tumor interferes with hormone metabolism.

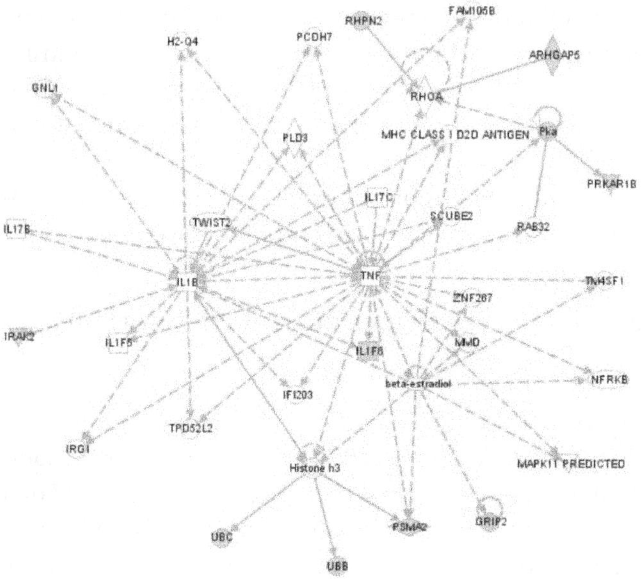

(A) Adenoma

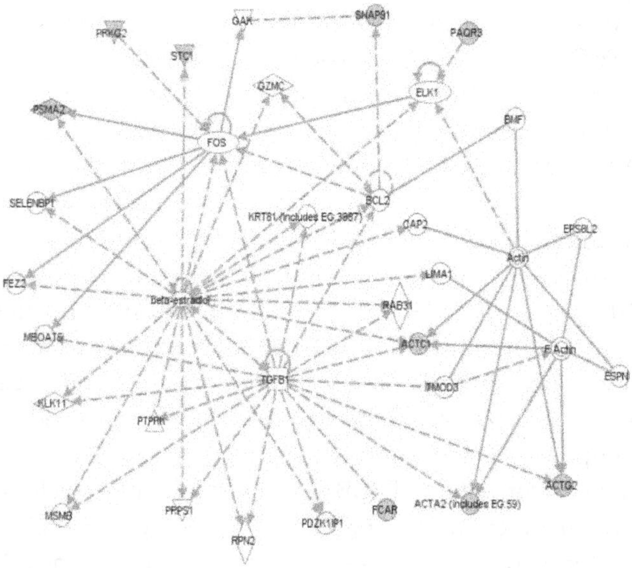

(B) Control

Figure 8: Significant signaling pathway networks mined from a nitroproteomic dataset. (A) Network is derived from adenoma nitroproteomic data and functions in cancer, cell cycle, reproductive-system disease. A gray node denotes an identified nitroprotein or protein that interacts with nitroproteins in our study. (B) Network is derived from control nitroproteomic data and functions in gene expression, cellular development, connective tissue development and function. A gray node denotes an identified nitroprotein in our studies. An orange solid edge denotes a direct relationship between two nodes (molecules: proteins; genes). An orange non-solid edge denotes an indirect relationship between two nodes (molecules: proteins; genes). The various shapes of nodes denote the different functions. A curved line means intracellular translocation; a curved arrow means extracellular translocation. Reproduced from Zhan and Desiderio (2010) with permission from BioMed Central open access journal and copyright remains with the authors, and reproduced from Zhan, Wang and Desiderio (2013) with permission from Hindawi Publishing Corporation open access journal and copyright remains with the authors.

Moreover, twelve statistically significant canonical pathways were mined from those pituitary adenoma nitroprotein data (Zhan & Desiderio, 2010), including the protein-ubiquitination pathway, p38 MAPK signaling, sonic-hedgehog signaling, cell-cycle G2/M DNA damage-checkpoint regulation, Toll-like receptor signaling, GABA-receptor signaling, the phototransduction pathway, amyloid processing, sphingolipid metabolism, LXR/RXR activation, IL-10 signaling, hypoxia signaling, and PXR/RXR activation (Zhan & Desiderio, 2010); and three statistically significant toxicity pathways were mined, including PXR/RXR activation, hepatic cholestasis, and LXR/RXR activation. Among those control pituitary nitroprotein data, twelve statistically significant canonical pathways were mined (Zhan & Desiderio, 2010), including VEGF signaling, regulation of actin-based motility by Rho, clatrin-mediated endocytosis, Fcγ receptor-mediated phagocytosis in NRF2-mediated oxidative-stress response, caveolar-mediated endocytosis, macrophages and monocytes, actin-cytoskeleton signaling, tight-junction signaling, leukocyte extravasation signaling, integrin signaling, and calcium signaling. No statistically significant toxicity pathways were mined.

Among four signaling pathway network systems (mitochondrial dysfunction, oxidative stress, cell-cycle dysregulation, and MAPK-signaling abnormality) that were tightly associated with pituitary adenomas (Zhan & Desiderio, 2010), three signaling pathway network systems (oxidative stress, cell-cycle dysregulation, and MAPK-signaling abnormality) are involved in protein nitration; for example, cell-cycle G2/M DNA damage checkpoint regulation, p38 MAPK signaling, and the NRF2-mediated oxidative stress response were discovered from pituitary adenoma nitroproteomic data (Zhan & Desiderio, 2010). Therefore, pathway systems analysis revealed that tyrosine nitration plays important roles in the pituitary tumorigenesis.

4   Conclusions

Protein tyrosine nitration is an important molecular event in pituitary adenoma, and is extensively associated with pituitary pathophysiological processes. Identification of nitroproeins and nitrated sites is an essential step to elucidate the functional roles of tyrosine nitration in a biological system. 2DGE-based nitrotyrosine Western blot coupled with MS/MS was used to detect 32 nitrotyrosine-positive gel-spots and eight nitroproteins and nitrated sites from a pituitary post-mortem tissue (Zhan & Desiderio, 2004 and 2007). NTAC-based enrichment coupled with MS/MS was used to identify nine nitroproteins and modified sites and three nitroprotein-interacting proteins from a pituitary adenoma tissue (Zhan & Desiderio, 2006), and most nitrotyrosine sites were located within important protein domains/motifs. Tyrosine nitration participated in three pathway network systems, including oxidative stress, cell-cycle dysregulation, and MAPK-signaling abnormality, that are significantly associated with pituitary adenomas (Zhan & Desiderio, 2010). Moreover, MALDI UV laser caused photodecomposition (loss of one or two oxygen atoms) of a nitro group of a nitropeptide. Recognition of the photodecomposition pattern could assist the interpretation of an MS spectrum of an endogenous nitropeptides. Those data clearly indicate that protein tyrosine nitration plays important roles in pituitary tumorigenesis.

However, the study of human pituitary adenoma nitroproteome is just at the beginning of our long-term program to elucidate the biological roles of tyrosine nitration in pituitary adenoma pathophysiology. Several aspects are worth studying: (1) Nitroproteomics of single-cell types of a pituitary adenoma will be necessary. A pituitary contains multiple cell types (Zhan & Desiderio, 2005). Those different cell types of pituitary adenomas could have not only a common mechanism in their formation but also some differences among different cell types of pituitary adenoma. Thus, it is important to study the same and different differentially expressed nitroproteins among the different cell types of pituitary adenomas, and to discover specific nitroprotein biomarkers for pituitary adenomas. (2) Quantitative nitroproteomics among different cell types of pituitary adenomas and controls are needed to determine nitroproteins that are unique to each cell type of pituitary adenoma. With precious LCM-enriched cell-types, isobaric tags for relative and absolute quantification (iTRAQ)-based quantitative proteomics and two-dimensional difference in-gel electrophoresis (2D-DIGE)-based quantitative proteomics would be the first method to analyze differentially expressed nitroproteins (DENPs) among different cell types of pituitary adenomas. (3) Structural biology is necessary to study three-dimensional spatial structure of a pituitary adenoma-related nitroprotein because it will be very easy to interpret the effect of tyrosine nitration on the 3D structure of a nitroprotein. Also, based on the 3-D structure and tyrosine nitration site and domain, it is possible for one to design a small drug towards the 3D structure and domain that contains tyrosine nitration. (4) A pituitary adenoma is a whole-body disease. In addition of pituitary adenoma tissue, cerebrospinal fluid (CSF) and blood plasma must be studied because some secreted proteins and peptides enter into the CSF and blood circulation in a pituitary adenoma patient (Zhan & Desiderio, 2010a). Also, CSF and blood specimens are much more accessible from patients and controls than pituitary tissues, and overcome the limitations of pituitary tissues (Zhan & Desiderio, 2010a). Any CSF and blood plasma nitroproteomic and nitropeptidomic variations would lead to the development of accurate biomarkers for predictive diagnosis, early-stage diagnosis, and measurement of prevention and therapy responses.

Acknowledgement

The authors acknowledge the financial supports from China "863" Plan Project (Grant No. 2014AA020610-1 to X.Z.), the Hunan Provincial Natural Science Foundation of China (Grant No. 14JJ7008 to X.Z.), the National Natural Science Foundation of China (Grant No. 81272798 and 81572278 to X.Z.), the Xiangya Hospital Funds for Talent Introduction (to X.Z.), and the National Institutes of Health, U.S.A. (RR16679 and NS 42843 to D.M.D.).

References

Aderem, A. (2005). Systems biology: its practice and challenges. Cell, 121, 511–513.

Aulak, K.S., Koeck, T., Crabb, J.W., & Stuehr, D. J. (2004). Dynamics of protein nitration in cells and mitochondria. American Journal of Physiology - Heart and Circulatory Physiology, 286, H30–H38.

Aulak, K. S., Miyagi, M., Yan, L., West, K. A., Massillon, D., Crabb, J. W., & Stuehr, D. J. (2001). Proteomic method identifies protein nitrated in vivo during inflammatory challenge. Proceedings of the National Academy of Science of the United States of America, 98, 12056–12061.

Beckman, J. S. (1996). Oxidative damage and tyrosine nitration from peroxynitrite. Chemical Research in Toxicology, 9, 836–844.

Bedford, M. T., & Leder, P. (1999). The FF domain: a novel motif that often accompanies WW domains. Trends in Biochemical Sciences, 24, 264–265.

Bocca, L., Valenti, S., Cuttica, C. M., Spaziante, R., Giordano, G., & Giusti, M. (2000). Nitric oxide biphasically modulates GH secretion in cultured cells of GH-secreting human pituitary adenomas. Minerva Endocrinologica, 25, 55–59.

Ceccatelli, S., Hulting, A. L., Zhang, X., Gustafsson, L., Villar, M., & Hokfelt, T. (1993). Nitric oxide synthase in the rat anterior pituitary gland and the role of nitric oxide in regulation of LH secretion. Proceedings of the National Academy of Science of the United States of America, 90, 11292–11296.

Cuttica, C. M., Giusti, M., Bocca, L., Sessarego, P., De Martini, D., Valenti, S., Spaziante, R., & Giordano, G. (1997). Nitric oxide modulates in vivo and in vitro growth hormone release in acromegaly. Neuroendocrinology, 66, 426–431.

Dalle-Donne, I., Scaloni, A., Giustarini, D., Cavarra, E., Tell, G., Lungarella, G., Colombo, R., Rossi, R., & Milzani, A. (2005). Proteins as biomarkers of oxidative/nitrosative stress in diseases: the contribution of redox proteomics. Mass Spectrometry Reviews, 24, 55–99.

Duvilanski, B. H., Zambruno, C., Seilicovich, A., Pisera, D., Lasaga, M., Diaz, M. C., Belova, N., Rettori, V., & McCann, S. M. (1995). Role of nitric oxide in control of prolactin release by the adenohypophysis. Proceedings of the National Academy of Science of the United States of America, 92, 170–174.

Haddad, I. Y., Pataki, G., Hu, P., Galliani, C., Beckman, J. S., & Matalon, S. (1994). Quantitation of nitrotyrosine levels in lung sections of patients and animals with acute lung injury. Journal of Clinical Investigation, 94, 2407–2413.

Halliwell, B., Zhao, K., & Whiteman, M. (1999). Nitric oxide and peroxynitrite. The ugly, the uglier and the not so good: a personal view of recent controversies. Free Radical Research, 31, 651–669.

Hla, T. (2005). Dietary factors and immunological consequences. Science, 309, 1682–1683.

Hood, L. (2003). Systems biology: integrating technology, biology, and computation.

Mechanisms of Ageing and Development, 124, 9–16.

Hood, L., & Tian, Q. (2012). *Systems approaches to biology and disease enable translational systems medicine. Genomics Proteomics Bioinformatics, 10, 181–185.*

Irie, Y., Saeki, M., Kamisaki, Y., Martin, E., & Murad, F. (2003). *Histone H1.2 is a substrate for denitrase, an activity that reduces nitrotyrosine immunoreactivity in proteins. Proceedings of the National Academy of Science of the United States of America, 100, 5634–5639.*

Khan, J., Brennan, D. M., Bradley, N., Gao, B., Bruckdorfeer, R., & Jacobs, M. (1998). *3-nitrotyrosine in the proteins of human plasma determined by an ELISA method. Biochemistry Journal, 330, 795–801.*

Kim, J. K., Lee, J. R., Kang, J. W., Lee, S. J., Shin, G. C., Yeo, W. S., Kim, K. H., Park, H. S., & Kim, K. P. (2011). *Selective enrichment and mass spectrometric identification of nitrated peptides using fluorinated carbon tags. Analytical Chemistry, 83, 157–163.*

Koeck, T., Fu, X., Hazen, S. L., Crabb, J. W., Stuehr, D. J., & Aulak, K. S. (2004). *Rapid and selective oxygen-regulated protein tyrosine denitration and nitration in mitochondria. The Journal of Biological Chemistry, 279, 27257–27262.*

Kristensen, P., Johnsen, A. H., Uerkvitz, W., Tanaka, K., & Hendil, K. B. (1994). *Human proteasome subunits from 2-dimensional gels identiWed by partial sequencing. Biochemical and Biophysical Research Communications, 205, 1785–1789.*

Lee, J. R., Lee, S. J., Kim, T. W., Kim, J. K., Park, H. S., Kim, D. E., Kim, K. P., & Yeo, W. S. (2009). *Chemical approach for specific enrichment and mass analysis of nitrated peptides. Analytical Chemistry, 81, 6620–6626.*

Lee, S. J., Lee, J. R., Kim, Y. H., Park, Y. S., Park, S. I., Park, H. S., & Kim, K. P. (2007). *Investigation of tyrosine nitration and nitrosylation of angiotensin II and bovine serum albumin with electrospray ionization mass spectrometry. Rapid Communications in Mass Spectrometry, 21, 2797–2804.*

Lloyd, R. V., Jin, L., Qian, X., Zhang, S., & Scheithauer, B. W. (1995). *Nitric oxide synthase in the human pituitary gland. American Journal of Pathology, 146, 86–94.*

Maceyka, M., Payne, S. G., Milstien, S., & Spiegel, S. (2002). *Sphingosine kinase, sphingosine-1-phosphate, and apoptosis. Biochimica et Biophysica Acta, 1585, 193–201.*

Mallozzi, C., D'Amore, C., Camerini, S., Macchia, G., Crescenzi, M., Petrucci, T. C., & Di Stasi, A. M. (2012). *Phosphorylation and nitration of tyrosine residues affect functional properties of synaptophysin and dynamin I, two proteins involved in exo-endocytosis of synaptic vesicles. Biochimica et Biophysica Acta, 1833, 110–121.*

Margolin, J. F., Friedman, J. R., Meyer, W. K. H., Vissing, H., Thiesen, H. J., & Rauscher III, F. J. (1994). *Kruppel-associated boxes are potent transcriptional repression domains. Proceedings of the National Academy of Science of the United States of America, 91, 4509–4513.*

McCann, S. M., Haens, G., Mastronardi, C., Walczewska, A., Karanth, S., Rettori, V., & Yu, W. H. (2003). *The role of nitric oxide (NO) in control of LHRH release that mediates gonadotropin release and sexual behaviour. Current Pharmaceutical Design, 9, 381–390.*

McCann, S. M., Karanth, S., Mastronardi, C. A., Dees, W. L., Childs, G., Miller, B., Sower, S., & Yu, W. H. (2001). Control of gonadotropin secretion by follicle-stimulating hormone-releasing factor, luteinizing hormonereleasing hormone, and leptin. Archives of Medical Research, 32, 476–485.

Miyagi, M., Sakaguch, H., Darrow, R. M., Yan, L., West, K. A., Aulak, K. S., Stuehr, D. J., Hollyfield, J. G., Organisciak, D. T., & Crabb, J. W. (2002). Evidence that light modulates protein nitration in rat retina. Molecular & Cellular Proteomics, 1, 293–303.

Payre, F., & Vincent, A. (1998). Finger proteins and DNA-specific recognition: distinct patterns of conserved amino acids suggest different evolutional modes. FEBS Letters, 234, 245–250.

Petersson, A. S., Steen, H., Kalume, D. E., Caidahl, K., & Roepstorff, P. (2001). Investigation of tyrosine nitration in proteins by mass spectrometry. Journal of Mass Spectrometry, 36, 616–625.

Pinilla, L., Gonzalez, L. C., Tena-Sempere, M., Bellido, C., & Aguilar, E. (2001). EVects of systemic blockade of nitric oxide synthases on pulsatile LH, prolactin, and GH secretion in adult male rats. Hormone Research, 55, 229–235.

Pinilla, L., Tena-Sempere, M., & Aguilar, E. (1999). Nitric oxide stimulates growth hormone secretion in vitro through a calcium- and cyclic guanosine monophosphate-independent mechanism. Hormone Research, 51, 242–247.

Riedel, W. (2000). Role of nitric oxide in the control of the hypothalamic– pituitary–adrenocortical axis. Zeitschrift Fur Rheumatologie, 59, II/36–42.

Sarver, A., Scheffler, N. K., Shetlar, M. D., & Gibson, B. W. (2001). Analysis of peptides and proteins containing nitrotyrosine by matrix-assisted laser desorption/ionization mass spectrometry. Journal of The American Society for Mass Spectrometry, 12, 439–448.

Scaloni, A. (2006). Mass spectrometry approaches for the molecular characterization of oxidatively/ nitrosatively modified proteins. In Redox Proteomics: From Protein Modification to Cellular Dysfunction and Diseases (Dalle-Donne, I., Scaloni, A., and Butterfield, D. A.,eds.), Wiley, Hoboken, NJ, 59–100.

Schwab, S. R., Pereira, J. P., Matloubian, M., Xu, Y., Huang, Y., & Cyster, J. G. (2005). Lymphocyte sequestration through S1P lyase inhibition and disruption of S1P gradients. Science, 309, 1735–1739.

Shigenaga, M. K., Lee, H. H., Blount, B. C., Christen, S., Shigeno, E. T., Yip, H., & Ames, B. N. (1997). Inflammation and NO(X)-induced nitration: assay for 3-nitrotyrosine by HPLC with electrochemical detection. Proceedings of the National Academy of Science of the United States of America, 94, 3211–3216.

Squadrito, G. L., & Pryor, W. A. (1998). Oxidative chemistry of nitric oxide: the roles of superoxide, peroxynitrite, and carbon dioxide. Free Radical Biology & Medicine, 25, 392–403.

Tamura, T., Lee, D. H., Osaka, F., Fujiwara, T., Shin, S., Chung, C. H., Tanaka, K., & Ichihara,

A. (1991). *Molecular cloning and sequence analysis of cDNAs for five major subunits of human proteasomes (multi-catalytic proteinase complexes). Biochimica et Biophysica Acta, 1089, 95–102.*

Torreilles, J., & Romestand, B. (2001). *In vitro production of peroxynitrite by haemocytes from marine bivalves: C-ELISA determination of 3-nitrotyrosine level in plasma proteins from mytilus galloprovincialis and crassostrea gigas. BMC Immunology, 2, 1.*

Ueta, Y., Levy, A., Powell, M. P., Lightaman, S. L., Kinoshita, Y., Yokota, A., Shibuya, I., & Yamashita, H. (1998). *Neuronal nitric oxide synthase gene expression in human pituitary tumours: a possible association with somatotroph adenomas and growth hormone-releasing hormone gene expression. Clinical Endocrinology (Ox.), 49, 29–38.*

Witzgall, R., O'Leary, E., Leaf, A., Oenaldi, D., & Bonventre, J. V. (1994). *The Kruppel-associated box-A (KRAB-A) domain of zinc Wnger proteins mediates transcriptional repression. Proceedings of the National Academy of Science of the United States of America, 91, 4514–4518.*

Yee, C. S., Seyedsayamdost, M. R., Chang, M. C., Nocerak D. G., & Stubbe, J. (2003). *Generation of the R2 subunit of ribonucleotide reductase by intein chemistry: Insertion of 3-nitrotyrosine at residue 356 as a probe of the radical initiation process. Biochemistry, 42, 14541–14552.*

Yeo, W. S., Lee, S. J., Lee, J. R., & Kim, K. P. (2008). *Nitrosative protein tyrosine modifications: biochemistry and functional significance. BMB Reports, 41, 194–203.*

Zhan, X., & Desiderio, D. M. (2003a). *A reference map of a human pituitary adenoma proteome. Proteomics, 3, 699–713.*

Zhan, X., & Desiderio, D. M. (2003b). *Spot volume vs. amount of protein loaded onto a gel: a detailed, statistical comparison of two gel electrophoresis systems. Electrophoresis, 24, 1818–1833.*

Zhan, X., & Desiderio, D. M. (2004). *The human pituitary nitroproteome: detection of nitrotyrosyl-proteins with two-dimensional Western blotting, and amino acid sequence determination with mass spectrometry. Biochemical and Biophysical Research Communications, 325, 1180–1186.*

Zhan, X., & Desiderio, D. M. (2005). *Comparative proteomics analysis of human pituitary adenomas: current status and future perspective. Mass Spectrometry Reviews, 24, 783–813.*

Zhan, X., & Desiderio, D. M. (2006). *Nitroproteins from a human pituitary adenoma tissue discovered with a nitrotyrosine aYnity column and tandem mass spectrometry. Analytical Biochemistry, 354, 279–289.*

Zhan, X., & Desiderio, D. M. (2007). *Linear ion-trap mass spectrometric characterization of human pituitary nitrotyrosine-containing proteins. International Journal of Mass Spectrometry, 259, 96–104.*

Zhan, X., & Desiderio, D. M. (2009a). *Mass spectrometric identification of in vivo nitrotyrosine sites in the human pituitary tumor proteome. Methods Molecular Biology, 566, 137–163.*

Zhan, X., & Desiderio, D. M. (2009b). Detection of nitrotyrosine-containing proteins. In The Protein Protocols Handbook Third Edition, J. M. Walkers (ed.), Humana Press, 1467–1490.

Zhan, X., & Desiderio, D. M. (2009c). MALDI-induced fragmentation of leucine enkephalin, nitro-Tyr-leucine enkaphalin, and d5-Phe-nitro-Tyr-leucine enkephalin. International Journal of Mass Spectrometry, 287, 77–86.

Zhan, X., & Desiderio, D. M. (2010). Signaling pathway networks mined from human pituitary adenoma proteomics data. BMC Medical Genomics, 3, 13.

Zhan, X., & Desiderio, D. M. (2010a). The use of variations in proteomes to predict, prevent, and personalize treatment for clinically nonfunctional pituitary adenomas. EPMA Journal, 1, 439–459.

Zhan, X., & Desiderio, D. M. (2011). Nitroproteins identified in human ex-smoker bronchoalveolar lavage fluid. Aging and Disease, 2, 100–115.

Zhan, X., Wang, X., & Desiderio, D. M. (2013). Pituitary adenoma nitroproteomics: current status and perspectives. Oxidative Medicine and Cellular Longevity, 2013: 580710.

Chapter 4

Purification and Biochemical Characterization of the DNA Strand-exchange Protein Dmc1 from Fission Yeast

Yasuto Murayama[1], Yumiko Kurokawa[2], Kentaro Ito[3],
Yasuhiro Tsutsui[3] and Hiroshi Iwasaki[3]

1 Introduction

Meiotic homologous recombination (HR) is initiated by DNA double-strand breaks (DSBs), which are created by a meiosis-specific topoisomerase-like protein, Spo11 (Figure 1A). The DSB ends are resected by a series of nucleases/helicase complexes, resulting in generation of single-stranded DNA (ssDNA) with 3′ overhangs (Mimitou & Symington 2009). The single-stranded ends are bound by a conserved RecA/Rad51-family recombinase to form nucleoprotein filaments that mediate strand invasion of homologous double-stranded DNA (dsDNA) regions, leading to D-loop formation (Sung & Klein 2006; Cox 2007). Strand invasion mediated by the RecA-/Rad51family recombinase follows DNA strand exchange between the complementary strand of the donor dsDNA and the recipient invading ssDNA, a reaction termed three-strand exchange. If strand exchange proceeds beyond the ss/ds junction of the recipient strand, an X-shape DNA structure (Holliday junction) is formed in a process that involves reciprocal strand exchange (also referred to as four-strand exchange). This event is followed by Holliday junction branch migration (Figure 1B).

[1] Chromosome Segregation Laboratory, Cancer Research UK, London Research Institute, UK

[2] Education Academy of Computational Life Science, Tokyo Institute of Technology, Japan

[3] Department of Biological Science, School of Bioscience and Biotechnology, Tokyo Institute of Technology, Japan

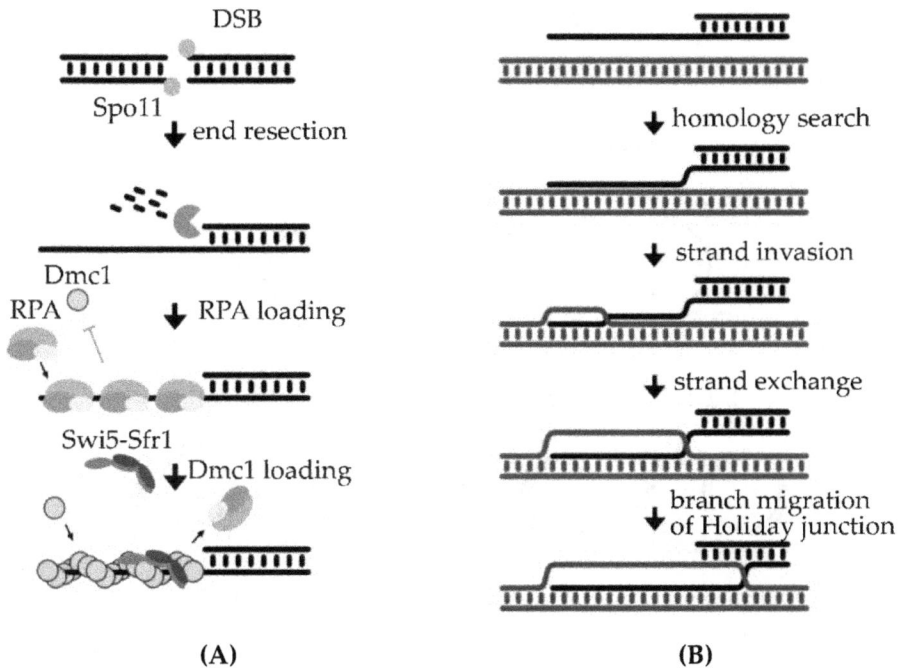

Figure 1 (A & B): Model of DNA strand exchange. **(A)** Dmc1 loading onto ssD-NA. DSB ends are processed in a specific order by helicases and nucleases, which generate ssDNA with 3′ overhangs. The ssDNA region is initially bound by RPA to prevent nucleolytic degradation. Dmc1 (or Rad51) is recruited to the ssDNA region with the aid of its accessory proteins, including the Swi5–Sfr1 complex. **(B)** The process of DNA strand exchange. First, the ssDNA region searches its intact complementary dsDNA. After pairing, the ssDNA invades and exchanges its complementary strand. Subsequent branch migration over the ss/dsDNA junction results in formation and branch migration of a Holliday junction.

DNA strand exchange driven by RecA/Rad51-family recombinases is a key step in homologous recombination. Two RecA/Rad51-family recombinases, Rad51 and Dmc1, mediate DNA strand exchange in eukaryotic cells. Rad51 functions in both vegetative and meiotic cells, whereas Dmc1 acts specifically in meiosis (Masson & West 2001; Sehorn & Sung 2004). Importantly, Dmc1 is critical for crossover between homologous chromosomes (Schwacha & Kleckner 1997; Hyppa & Smith 2010). Despite their distinct functional differences *in vivo*, both recombinases form very similar nucleoprotein filaments on ssDNA, and they have very similar biochemical properties (Sung 1994; Sehorn *et al.*, 2004).

Several accessory proteins are required for the DNA strand-exchange reaction mediated by RecA/Rad51-family recombinases (Sung & Klein 2006). In eukaryotic cells, ssDNA binding protein replication protein A (RPA) stimulates both Rad51- and Dmc1-mediated DNA strand exchange by resolving secondary structure in ssDNA and pre-

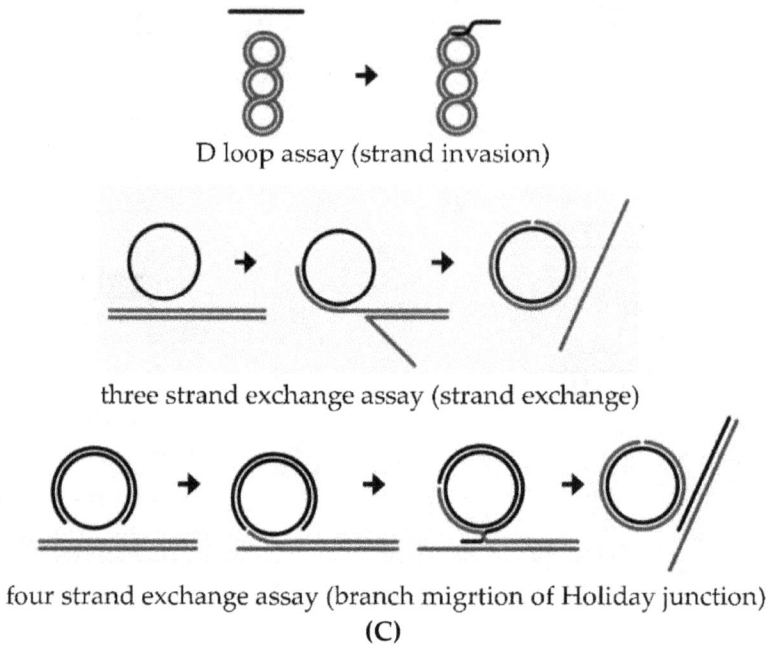

D loop assay (strand invasion)

three strand exchange assay (strand exchange)

four strand exchange assay (branch migrtion of Holiday junction)

(C)

Figure 1 (C): Model of DNA strand exchange. *In vitro* reconstitution assays for DNA strand exchange. The D-loop assay monitors strand invasion between a linear ssDNA and its complementary covalently closed circular DNA. The three-strand exchange assay reconstitutes the subsequent strand transfer or exchange between ssDNA and its recipient dsDNA. The four-strand exchange assay involves reciprocal dsDNA exchange via generation and branch migration of a Holliday junction.

venting the potential reverse reaction using displaced ssDNA on the donor DNA strand. However, RPA is an abundant protein in the cell, and its affinity for ssDNA is higher than those of Rad51. Consequently, RPA binds to ssDNA region before Rad51, and thereby prevents filament formation (Figure 1A). Likewise, bacterial ssDNA binding protein SSB shows the same positive and negative effects on RecA-mediated DNA strand exchange. A special class of accessory proteins called recombination mediators helps RecA/Rad51-family recombinases overcome inhibition by RPA/SSB. For example, Rad52, a representative recombination mediator of Rad51, physically interacts with both Rad51 and RPA, and promotes RPA displacement mediated by Rad51 filament formation (Sung 1997a; Benson *et al.*, 1998; New *et al.*, 1998; Shinohara & Ogawa 1998; Sugiyama & Kowalczykowski 2002; Kurokawa *et al.*, 2008). The fission yeast Swi5-Sfr1 complex is another type of accessory protein (Akamatsu *et al.*, 2003). The complex activates and stabilizes Rad51 filaments to promote the DNA strand-exchange reaction (Haruta *et al.*, 2006; Kurokawa *et al.* 2008). Likewise, Rad55-Rad57 complex and BRCA2 stabilize the Rad51 filament to overcome the inhibitory effects of RPA (Sung 1997b; Jensen *et al.*, 2010; Liu *et al.*, 2011). Despite these recent advances in our knowledge of

Rad51 filament dynamics, however, little is known about the accessory proteins of Dmc1.

Biochemical reconstitution of DNA strand exchange driven by Rad51 has elucidated several molecular mechanisms. D-loop formation, three-strand exchange, and four-strand exchange can be reconstituted in test tubes and monitored using appropriate biochemical assays (Cox 2007). As shown in Figure 1C, the D-loop assay monitors a strand-invasion step, whereas the three-strand exchange assay reconstitutes the subsequent strand transfer or exchange reaction. The four-strand exchange assay starts from three-strand exchange, and can monitor subsequent reciprocal DNA strand exchange. Using these assays, our group has revealed several important characteristics of the fission yeast Dmc1: 1) Dmc1 promotes formation and branch migration of Holliday junctions in a direction opposite to that of Rad51. 2) Swi5–Sfr1 stabilizes the Dmc1 filament and promotes RPA displacement by Dmc1. 3) Rad52 controls DNA strand exchange activity of Rad51 positively and that of Dmc1 negatively (Haruta *et al.* 2006; Murayama *et al.*, 2011; Murayama *et al.*, 2013). In this chapter, we describe the detailed procedures for purification of the fission yeast Dmc1 protein and the results we obtained with the purified protein in a conventional three-strand exchange assay.

2   Materials

2.1   Culture media

1. LB liquid medium: 1% tryptone, 0.5% yeast extract, and 1% NaCl, adjusted to pH 7.5 with NaOH.

2. LB agar (1.5%) plate

3. 50 mg/ml kanamycin and 34 mg/ml Chloramphenicol

4. 1 M isopropyl β-D-1-thiogalactopyranoside (IPTG)

2.2   *E. coli* Strain and Dmc1 Expression Plasmid

E. coli strain BL21-codonPlus (DE3)-RIPL (Agilent Technologies) and Dmc1-overproducing plasmid pYSTDmc1 (generated by cloning the *dmc1+* cDNA into pET28a).

2.3   Materials for Dmc1 Purification

1. R buffer: 20 mM Tris-HCl (pH 7.5), 1 mM dithiothreitol (DTT), 0.5 mM EDTA, 10% glycerol

2. 5% polyethyleneimine (pH 8.0)

3. Protease inhibitor cocktail (Roche)

4. SP Sepharose FF (packed manually in a XK 26/20 column)

5. Q Sepharose FF (packed manually in a XK 26/20 column)

6.   HiTrap Heparin HP (5 ml)

7.   HiLoad 16/600 Superdex 200 pg

8.   Resource Q (1 ml)

9.   Dialysis membrane (molecular weight cutoff of 10 kDa)

Note: all columns and resins were purchased from GE Healthcare.

2.4   Materials for *in vitro* Reconstitution Analyses

1.   ΦX174 virion DNA

2.   *Apa*LI-linearized ΦX174 dsDNA

3.   Strand-exchange buffer: 30 mM Tris-HCl (pH 7.5), 1 mM DTT, 3.5 mM MgCl$_2$, 2% glycerol, 125 mM NaCl (prepare 5× buffer for use)

4.   80 mM phosphocreatine

5.   80 U/ml creatine kinase

6.   100 mM ATP (dissolve in water and adjust to pH 7.5 with 1 M NaOH)

7.   6× DNA loading Dye: 30 mM Tris-HCl (pH 7.5), 0.25% bromophenol blue, 0.25% xylene cyanol, 15% Ficoll

8.   Stop solution: 30 mM Tris-HCl (pH 7.5), 30 mM EDTA, 5% SDS, 6.7 mg/ml proteinase K

9.   TAE buffer: 40 mM Tris-acetate (pH 8.0), 1 mM EDTA

10. 0.5 M EDTA (pH 8.0)

3   Methods

3.1   Protein Expression

1.   Transform the Dmc1 expression plasmid (see section 2.2) into *E. coli* strain BL21-codonPlus (DE3)-RIPL. Cultivate the resultant transformants at 37 °C overnight (12–15 h) on LB agar plates containing 50 μg/ml kanamycin and 34 μg/ml chloramphenicol.

2.   Inoculate ~20 transformant colonies into LB containing 50 μg/ml kanamycin and 34 μg/ml chloramphenicol and incubate with shaking at 37 °C (120 – 150 rpm, Innova 44, New Brunswick).

3.   When the optical density of the cultures at 600 nm reaches 0.4, induce protein expression by addition of IPTG to a final concentration of 1 mM. Place the cultures at 18 °C and continue to shake overnight (15 – 18 h).

4.   Harvest *E. coli* cells by centrifugation, wash once with 0.9% NaCl, and freeze the cell pellet in liquid nitrogen. The frozen cell pellet can be stored at –80 °C for at least 6 months.

3.2   Purification of Fission Yeast Dmc1

All procedures for protein purification should be performed at 4 °C.

1. Resuspend the *E. coli* cell pellets in 5 volumes of R buffer containing 0.2 M NaCl and protease inhibitor cocktail (Roche, without EDTA).

2. Disrupt cells by sonication (We use an XL2020 sonicator with a standard horn of the 12.7 mm-diameter tip (Misonix, Part # 200). We set the amplitude control knob to 7, which normally corresponds to 30% of the maximum output. One cycle contains 15 time pulses (1 second) with 1-second interval. We normally repeat the cycle for 5 times with 3-min interval. All procedures are applied on ice).

3. Clarify the cell lysate by centrifugation at 50,000×*g* for 1 h.

4. Gently add 5% polyethyleneimine (PEI) to the resultant cell lysate, with stirring, to a final concentration of 0.5%, and then incubate for 1 h.

5. Precipitate the PEI complex by centrifugation at 40,000×*g* for 30 min.

6. To elute Dmc1, resuspend the PEI pellet in R buffer containing 0.2 M ammonium sulfate. Disrupt the pellet using a spatula and incubate for an additional 1 h with stirring.

7. Precipitate the PEI complex by centrifugation at 40,000×*g* for 30 min.

8. Transfer the resulting supernatant, which contains Dmc1, to a new tube. Add ammonium sulfate with constant stirring to the supernatants at a final saturation concentration of 60% to precipitate proteins. Continue to stir for 1 h.

9. Pellet the salted-out proteins by centrifugation at 40,000×*g* for 30 min, and remove the supernatant.

10. Dissolve the salted-out proteins in 10 ml of R buffer containing 0.2 M KCl, and then dialyze against 2 L of the same buffer overnight (12 – 15 h).

11. Apply the dialyzed sample to a SP Sepharose FF column (20 ml) pre-equilibrated with R buffer containing 0.2 M KCl. Collect the flow-through fractions.

12. Dilute the SP Sepharose FF flow-through fractions with R buffer to a final concentration of 0.1 M KCl.

13. Load the sample onto a Q Sepharose FF column (20 ml) equilibrated with R buffer containing 0.1 M KCl.

14. Wash the column with three bed volumes (20 ml) of R buffer containing 0.1 M KCl.

15. Elute the bound proteins with a linear gradient of 0.1 – 0.6 M KCl in R buffer (10 bed volumes, 200 ml). Dmc1 should elute at ~0.4 M KCl.

16. Dilute the Q Sepharose eluate containing Dmc1 with R buffer to a final concentration of 0.1 M KCl (4-fold dilution).

17. Apply the sample to a heparin column equilibrated with R buffer containing 0.1 M KCl (GE Healthcare, HiTrap Heparin HP, 5 ml).

18. Wash the column with two bed volumes (10 ml) of R buffer containing 0.1 M KCl.

19. Elute the bound proteins with a linear gradient of 0.1 – 0.5 M KCl in R buffer (20

bed volumes, 100 ml). Dmc1 is eluted at ~0.3 M KCl.

20. Apply the heparin eluate to a HiLoad 16/600 Superdex 200 pg gel-filtration column (120 ml), and then separate the proteins by developing the column with R buffer containing 0.5 M KCl. Dmc1 is eluted at ~80 ml.

21. Dilute the Dmc1-containing fractions with R buffer to a final concentration of 0.1 M KCl.

22. Apply the resultant sample onto a Resource Q column (1 ml) equilibrated with R buffer containing 0.1 M KCl.

23. Wash the column with two bed volumes (2 ml) of R buffer containing 0.1 M KCl.

24. Elute the bound proteins with a linear gradient of 0.1 – 0.5 M KCl (40 bed volumes, 40 ml). Dmc1 is eluted at ~0.4 M KCl. Collect the peak fraction.

25. Dialyze the Resource Q peak fraction against R buffer containing 0.2 M KCl.

26. Determine the concentration of purified Dmc1; the extinction coefficient at 280 nm is 1.23×10^4 $M^{-1}cm^{-1}$. Purified Dmc1 can be stored in a deep freezer (–80 °C) after freezing the dialyzed aliquots in liquid nitrogen. We usually obtain 2 mg of Dmc1 from 10 L of the *E. coli* culture.

The summary of the purification is shown in Figure 2A.

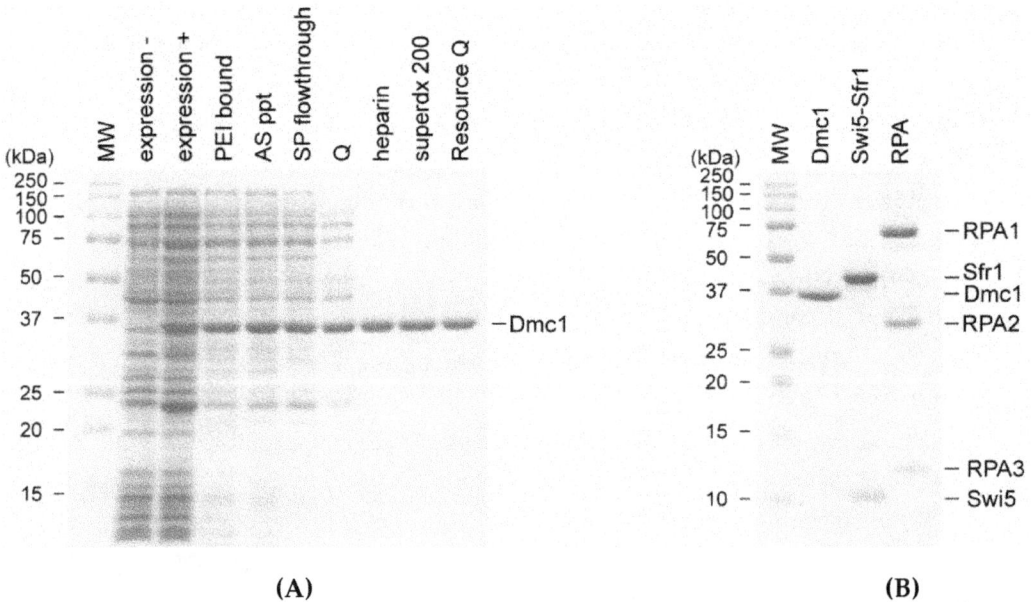

(A)   (B)

Figure 2: Protein purification. **(A)** Dmc1 purification. The gel image shows each step of Dmc1 purification. MW: molecular weight marker. Expression "–" or "+": supernatant after ultracentrifugation of *E. coli* cell lysate bearing pET28a (–) or pYSTDMC1 (+). Both cell lysates were prepared 18 h after addition of IPTG. PEI, polyethyleneimine; AS, ammonium sulfate. Aliquots of protein (5 μg) were analyzed by SDS-PAGE on a 12.5% gel. **(B)** Each purified protein (2 μg) was analyzed by SDS-PAGE on a 15% gel.

3.3   Other Proteins

Detailed procedures for purification of *S. pombe* Swi5–Sfr1 protein complex and RPA have been described previously (Murayama & Iwasaki 2011). The purified proteins are shown in Figure 2B. Concentrations of the purified Swi5–Sfr1 complex and RPA are determined based on extinction coefficients at 280 nm of 1.26×10^4 M^{-1} cm^{-1} and 9.89×10^4 M^{-1} cm^{-1}, respectively.

3.4   Preparation of DNA Substrates for *in vitro* Reactions

The *in vitro* DNA strand-exchange reaction described in this section monitors the strand exchange between a circular single-stranded DNA (cssDNA) and its complementary linear double-stranded DNA (ldsDNA). In our laboratory, we use commercially available ΦX174 virion for cssDNA, and Replicative form I DNA to prepare ldsDNA. As described in the protocols below, ΦX174 virion DNA solution is extracted with phenol to remove residual protein contamination, and ldsDNA is prepared by cutting RFI DNA with restriction enzymes.

3.4.1   Phenol Treatment of cssDNA

1.   Dissolve 150 μg of ΦX174 virion DNA in 500 μl TE.

2.   Extract the solution twice with phenol/chloroform/isoamyl alcohol (25:24:1) to remove proteins.

3.   Recover the virion DNA by ethanol precipitation.

4.   Dissolve the virion DNA in 200 μl of TE.

5.   Dialyze the DNA solution against 2 L of TE for 6 h at 4 °C with a float-type microdialyzer (Slide-A-Lyzer MINI Dialysis Units, 3500 MWCO [Thermo Scientific]).

6.   Calculate the virion DNA concentration by measuring absorbance at 260 nm, assuming 33 μg/ml per A_{260} unit.

3.4.2   Preparation of ldsDNA

1.   Digest 150 μg of ΦX174 RFI DNA with *Apa*LI in 500 μl reaction (We normally digest in 500 μl reaction mixture with 100 U of ApaLI at 37 ºC. After 3-hour incubation, the digestion was checked by agarose gel electrophoresis).

2.   Extract the solution twice with phenol/chloroform/isoamyl alcohol (25:24:1) to remove the restriction enzyme.

3.   Recover the DNA by ethanol precipitation.

4.   Dissolve the DNA in 200 μl of TE.

5.   Dialyze the DNA solution against 2 L of TE for 6 h at 4 °C.

6.   Calculate the ldsDNA concentration by measuring absorbance at 260 nm, assuming 50 μg/ml per A_{260} unit.

3.5   *In vitro* DNA Strand-exchange Reaction

The indicated concentrations of reagents, proteins, and DNA are the final concentrations. DNA concentrations are expressed in terms of total nucleotides. The final standard reaction volume is 10 μl.

1.   Mix Dmc1 (5 μM) and Swi5–Sfr1 (0.5 μM) in strand-exchange buffer containing 2 mM ATP, 8 mM phosphocreatine, and 8 U/ml creatine kinase in a 0.6 ml plastic tube on ice. (Add 1 μl of 10-fold concentrated protein solutions.)

2.   Add cssDNA (10 μM) and mix by pipetting. (Add 1 μl of 10-fold concentrated DNA dissolved in 10 mM Tris-HCl [pH 7.5].)

3.   Incubate at 30 °C for 10 min.

4.   Add RPA (1.5 μM) and mix by pipetting. (Add 1 μl of 10-fold concentrated protein solution.)

5.   Incubate at 30 °C for 10 min.

6.   Initiate DNA strand-exchange reaction by adding ldsDNA (10 μM; add 1 μl of 10-fold concentrated DNA dissolved in 10 mM Tris-HCl [pH 7.5]).

7.   Incubate at 30 °C for 90 min.

8.   Add 1.8 μl of the stop solution and mix by pipetting.

9.   Incubate at 30 °C for 15 min.

10.   Add 2.4 μl of 6× DNA loading Dye and mix by pipetting.

11.   Analyze the DNA samples by 1% agarose gel electrophoresis in TAE (3.5 V/cm for 120 min at room temperature). We routinely use a gel with a size of 6 cm x 11 cm.

12.   Soak the gel in SYBR Gold (1:30,000 dilution) dissolved in TAE for 2 h at room temperature.

13.   Wash the gel twice with TAE for 5 min with gentle shaking.

14.   Scan the gel image using a fluorescence imager (we use Fuji LAS-4000, Fuji Photo Film Co.)

15.   Quantitate the strand-exchange products using image analysis software (we use MultiGauge, Fuji Photo Film Co). Calculate the percentages of final products (NC, nicked circular) and intermediates (JM, joint molecules) as [NC]/([JM]/1.5+[NC]+[ldsDNA])×100 and ([JM]/1.5)/([JM]/1.5+[NC]+[ldsDNA])×100, respectively.

3.6   Measurement of Dmc1 ATPase Activity

The indicated concentrations of reagents, proteins and DNA are the final concentrations. DNA concentrations are expressed in terms of total nucleotides. The final standard reaction volume is 15 μl.

1.   Mix Dmc1 (5 μM) and Swi5–Sfr1 (0.5 μM) in strand-exchange buffer in a 0.6 ml plastic tube on ice. (Add 1 μl of 15-fold concentrated protein solutions.)

2. Add cssDNA (10 μM) to the mixture. (Add 1 μl of 15-fold concentrated DNA dissolved in 10 mM Tris-HCl [pH 7.5].)

3. Add a mixture of [g–^{32}P] ATP and cold ATP to a final concentration of 2 mM (10 kBq/reaction). (Add 1 μl of 15-fold concentrated ATP dissolved in water.)

4. Incubate at 30 °C and withdraw 2 μl aliquots at 0, 10, 20, 30, 45 and 60 min after ATP addition. Terminate the reaction by addition of 4 μl of 0.5 M EDTA.

5. Spot 1 μl of the samples onto a PEI-cellulose sheet (Merck).

6. Develop the sheet with 1 M formic acid/0.4 M LiCl in a thin-layer chromatography chamber.

7. Dry the developed sheet and scan the [^{32}P] signals using a phosphorimager (we use Fuji BAS2000, Fuji Photo Film Co).

8. Quantitate the hydrolyzed inorganic phosphate using image analysis software.

4   *In vitro* Dmc1-mediated DNA Strand Exchange

The *in vitro* DNA strand-exchange reaction monitors the transfer or exchange of the complementary strand of donor ldsDNA to the recipient cssDNA (Figure 1C). Pairing yields intermediates called joint molecules (JMs), and completion of strand-exchange produces nicked circular DNA as a final product. These products can be readily separated and analyzed by agarose gel electrophoresis. Using the *in vitro* DNA strand-exchange assay, we have shown that the fission yeast Swi5–Sfr1 complex stimulates Dmc1-mediated DNA strand exchange. Furthermore, we reported previously that Swi5–Sfr1 acts as Dmc1 loading factor on ssDNA by stabilizing the Dmc1 filament to promote displacement of pre-bound RPA (Murayama *et al.* 2013). During optimization of the *in vitro* conditions for Dmc1-mediated DNA strand exchange, we revealed several unique properties of Dmc1. In this section, we describe the optimization process.

4.1   Fission Yeast Dmc1 is a Heat-sensitive Protein

ssDNA-dependent ATPase activity is coupled to the efficiency of DNA strand exchange mediated by Dmc1 recombinase. To optimize the *in vitro* DNA strand-exchange reaction, we analyzed Dmc1 ATPase activity under various conditions. At 37 °C, at higher magnesium concentrations (> 2 mM), Dmc1 exhibited constant ATP hydrolysis for at least 1 h; however, at lower concentrations of magnesium (< 1 mM), Dmc1 lost its ATPase activity after a 1 h incubation (Figure 3). By contrast, Dmc1 exhibited similar ATPase activity at all magnesium concentrations analyzed when the reactions were carried out at 30 °C, which is much closer to the optimal temperature for fission yeast meiosis. These differences suggested that Dmc1 is a heat-sensitive protein. Consistent with this finding, we showed previously that Dmc1 ATPase is inactivated by 15-min preincubation at 37 °C (Murayama *et al.* 2013). These results indicate that Dmc1 is unstable at high temperature and low magnesium concentrations.

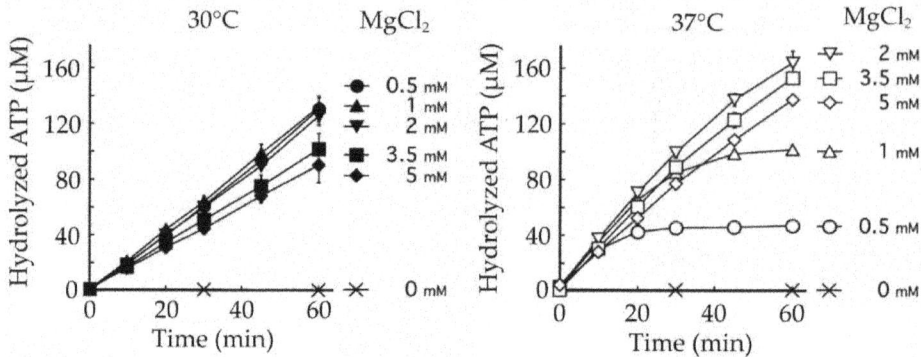

Figure 3: Dmc1 is a heat-sensitive protein. ssDNA-dependent ATPase activity of Dmc1 was analyzed in the presence of the indicated concentrations of MgCl$_2$ at 30 °C (**A**) or 37 °C (**B**). Aliquots were taken at the indicated time points, and samples were analyzed as described in the Methods.

4.2   Optimization of the Dmc1-mediated DNA Strand-exchange Reaction

Before 2010, many previously reported assays for budding yeast and human Dmc1 were conducted at 37 °C [representative ones are (Bugreev *et al.*, 2005; Sauvageau *et al.*, 2005)] and we had performed Dmc1-meidated strand exchange at 37 °C (Haruta *et al.* 2006). However, because we found that fission yeast Dmc1 is unstable at 37 °C but not 30 °C, we tried to carry out the DNA three-strand exchange reaction at 30 °C again (Murayama *et al.* 2013). In our "Dmc1 start" reaction, Dmc1 and cssDNA were initially mixed, followed by addition of RPA (Figure 4A). Consistent with the aforementioned analysis of the ATPase activity, high amount of DNA strand-exchange products were detected when the reaction was carried out at 30 °C in the presence of substoichiometric amounts of Swi5–Sfr1 (~10–20% concentration of Dmc1)(Murayama *et al.* 2013). At 30 °C, the optimal DNA:Dmc1 ratio was 2:1 (DNA concentration expressed as total nucleotides), whereas at 37 °C it was 1:1. Electron microscopy and crystal structure analyses revealed that the RecA homologues bound to DNA at a ratio of three nucleotides per protein monomer (Chen *et al.*, 2008; Sheridan *et al.*, 2008). The optimal DNA:Dmc1 ratio at 30 °C was closer to the DNA-binding ratio, implying that *in vitro* Dmc1 strand exchange more closely mirrors the physiological reaction at 30 °C than at 37 °C. When ΦX174 DNA substrates were used, about 35% of the input material was converted to strand-exchanged products. More than 80% product formation was observed when another set of DNA substrates based on "pSKsxAS", which is the pBluescript derivative containing 1.3 kb of the fission yeast *ade6+* fragment, were used under the same reaction conditions (Murayama *et al.* 2013). Although we have not yet identified the source of these differences in efficiency, it is clear that the overall characteristics of the reactions were the same in assays using the two different types of DNA substrates. As shown in Figure 1A, in living cells, RPA is considered to bind to ssDNA before Dmc1 (or Rad51). Therefore,

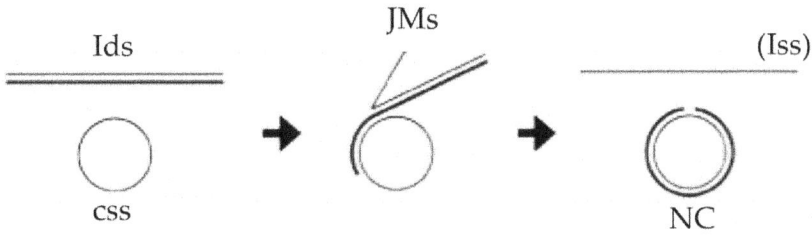

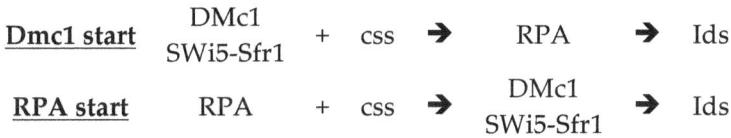

(A)

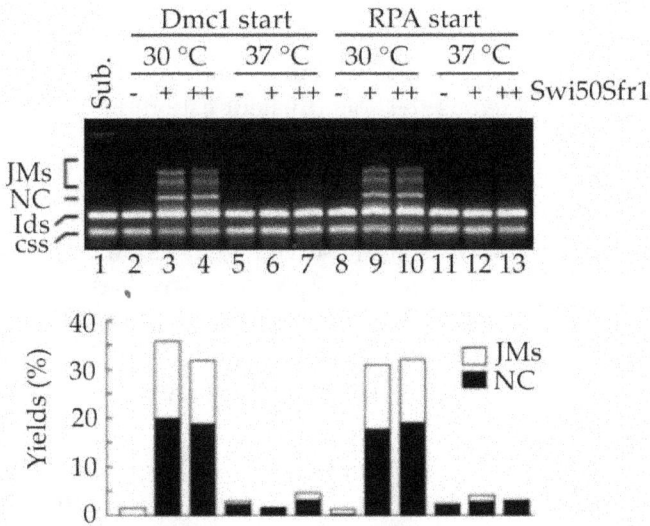

(B)

Figure 4: Dmc1-mediated DNA strand-exchange reaction. **(A)** Schematic of the three-strand exchange reaction. css, circular single-stranded DNA; lds, linear double-stranded DNA; NC, nicked circular DNA; JMs, joint molecules; lss, linear single-stranded DNA. **(B)** Gel images show the products of Dmc1-mediated three-strand exchange reaction in the absence and in the presence of Swi5-Sfr1 (0.5 μM or 3.5mM) performed at the indicated temperatures.. Sub, DNA substrates. **C.** Quantification of DNA strand-exchange products.

we carried out the DNA strand-exchange reaction using RPA-coated cssDNA (denoted as the "RPA start" reaction in Figure 4A). Although no products were detected in the absence of Swi5–Sfr1, Dmc1 efficiently promoted DNA strand exchange when the complex was present. These results suggested that Swi5–Sfr1 promotes Dmc1 loading onto RPA-coated ssDNA as a recombination mediator (Haruta *et al.* 2006; Murayama *et al.* 2013).

4.3   Calcium Ion Stimulates Dmc1-mediated DNA Strand Exchange in Fission Yeast

The calcium ion stimulates DNA strand exchange mediated by human or budding yeast Dmc1 (Bugreev *et al.* 2005; Lee *et al.*, 2005). In particular, the presence of the Ca^{2+} ion inhibits the ATPase activity of Dmc1, which requires the Mg^{2+} ion, and thereby promotes formation of the ATP-bound form of the Dmc1 filament, ultimately resulting in filament stabilization. Similarly, we reported previously that Swi5–Sfr1 stabilizes Dmc1 filaments on ssDNA, thereby promoting the DNA strand-exchange reaction (Murayama *et al.* 2013). To determine whether the Ca^{2+} ion also stimulates the activity of fission yeast Dmc1, we carried out the three-strand exchange reaction in the presence of the Ca^{2+} ion but in the absence of Swi5–Sfr1. In a time-course analysis, product formation was limited when the Mg^{2+} was added as the sole divalent cation. However, the reaction was stimulated by the further addition of small amounts of the Ca^{2+} ion (0.25 mM of $CaCl_2$) (Figure 5). On the other hand, strand exchange was not observed when Ca^{2+} (0.25 mM) was added as the sole divalent cation (data not shown). These results clearly indicated that the Ca^{2+} ion stimulates the DNA strand-exchange reaction mediated by fission yeast Dmc1. Consistent with our conclusions, Ploquin *et al.* reported that the Ca^{2+} ion stimulates the DNA strand-invasion activity of fission yeast Dmc1 (Ploquin *et al.*, 2007).

In this chapter we described a conventional method for biochemically reconstituting the Dmc1-mediated DNA-strand exchange reaction and provided an example of optimization of this reaction using fission yeast Dmc1. As mentioned above, we identified several biochemical properties of the fission yeast Dmc1. These findings were made possible by a fine optimization of the biochemical reaction conditions. As with any biochemical reaction, this fine-tuning of the *in vitro* reaction was critical for the success we achieved in characterizing the DNA strand-exchange reaction.

Acknowledgement

We are grateful to Y. Terada for preparation of the manuscript. The study performed in the laboratory of Dr. Iwasaki was supported in part by grants-in-aid for Scientific Research on Priority Areas from the Ministry of Education, Culture, Sports, Science, and Technology (MEXT) of Japan and for Scientific Research (A) from Japan Society for the Promotion of Science (JSPS), and by a research grant from the Takeda Science Foundation.

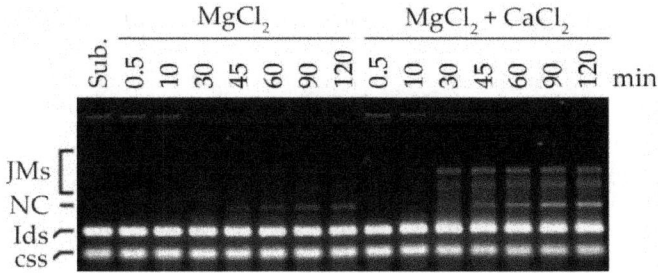

(A)

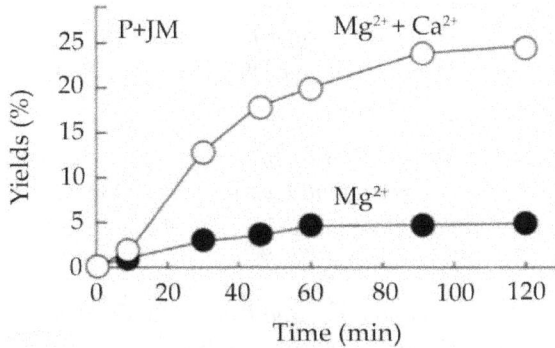

(B)

Figure 5: The calcium ion stimulates Dmc1-mediated DNA strand exchange. **(A)** Gel images show a time course of the DNA strand-exchange reaction in the presence of 3.5 mM MgCl₂ (left) or 3.5 mM MgCl₂ plus 0.25 mM CaCl₂ (left). Reactions (50 μl) were carried out at 30 °C, and aliquots (5 μl) were taken at the indicated time points. **BB)** Quantification of DNA strand-exchange products.

References

Akamatsu, Y., Dziadkowiec, D., Ikeguchi, M., Shinagawa, H., & Iwasaki, H. (2003). Two different Swi5-containing protein complexes are involved in mating-type switching and recombination repair in fission yeast. Proceedings of the National Academy of Sciences of the United States of America, 100, 15770–15775.

Benson, F. E., Baumann, P., & West, S. C. (1998). Synergistic actions of Rad51 and Rad52 in recombination and DNA repair. Nature, 391, 401–404.

Bugreev, D. V., Golub, E. I., Stasiak, A. Z., Stasiak, A., & Mazin, A. V. (2005). Activation of human meiosis-specific recombinase Dmc1 by Ca²⁺. The Journal of Biological Chemistry, 280, 26886–26895.

Chen, Z., Yang, H., & Pavletich, N. P. (2008). Mechanism of homologous recombination from the RecA-ssDNA/dsDNA structures. Nature, 453, 489–484.

Cox, M. M. (2007). Motoring along with the bacterial RecA protein. Nature Reviews Molecular Cell Biology, 8, 127–138.

Haruta, N., Kurokawa, Y., Murayama, Y., Akamatsu, Y., Unzai, S., Tsutsui, Y., & Iwasaki, H. (2006). The Swi5-Sfr1 complex stimulates Rhp51/Rad51 — and Dmc1-mediated DNA strand exchange in vitro. Nature Structural & Molecular Biology, 13, 823–830.

Hyppa, R. W., & Smith, G. R. (2010). Crossover invariance determined by partner choice for meiotic DNA break repair. Cell, 142, 243–255.

Jensen, R. B., Carreira, A., & Kowalczykowski, S. C. (2010). Purified human BRCA2 stimulates RAD51-mediated recombination. Nature, 467, 678–683.

Kurokawa, Y., Murayama, Y., Haruta-Takahashi, N., Urabe, I., & Iwasaki, H. (2008). Reconstitution of DNA strand exchange mediated by Rhp51 recombinase and two mediators. PLOS Biolology, 6(4), e88.

Lee, M. H., Chang, Y. C., Hong, E. L., Grubb, J., Chang, C. S., Bishop, D. K., & Wang, T. F. (2005). Calcium ion promotes yeast Dmc1 activity via formation of long and fine helical filaments with single-stranded DNA. The Journal of Biological Chemistry, 280, 40980–40984.

Liu, J., Renault, L., Veaute, X., Fabre, F., Stahlberg, H., & Heyer, W. D. (2011). Rad51 paralogues Rad55-Rad57 balance the antirecombinase Srs2 in Rad51 filament formation. Nature, 479, 245–248.

Masson, J. Y., & West, S. C. (2001). The Rad51 and Dmc1 recombinases: a non-identical twin relationship. Trends in Biochemical Sciences, 26, 131–136.

Mimitou, E. P., & Symington, L. S. (2009). DNA end resection: many nucleases make light work. DNA Repair (Amst), 8, 983–995.

Murayama, Y., & Iwasaki, H. (2011). An in vitro assay for monitoring the formation and branch migration of holliday junctions mediated by a eukaryotic recombinase. Methods in Molecular Biology, 745, 385–405.

Murayama, Y., Kurokawa, Y., Tsutsui, Y., & Iwasaki, H. (2013). Dual regulation of Dmc1-driven DNA strand exchange by Swi5-Sfr1 activation and Rad22 inhibition. Genes & Development, 27, 2299–2304.

Murayama, Y., Tsutsui, Y., & Iwasaki, H. (2011). The fission yeast meiosis-specific Dmc1 recombinase mediates formation and branch migration of Holliday junctions by preferentially promoting strand exchange in a direction opposite to that of Rad51. Genes & Development, 25, 516–527.

New, J. H., Sugiyama, T., Zaitseva, E., & Kowalczykowski, S. C. (1998). Rad52 protein stimulates DNA strand exchange by Rad51 and replication protein A. Nature, 391, 407–410.

Ploquin, M., Petukhova, G. V., Morneau, D., Dery, U., Bransi, A., Stasiak, A., Camerini-Otero, R. D., & Masson, J. Y. (2007). Stimulation of fission yeast and mouse Hop2-Mnd1 of the Dmc1 and Rad51 recombinases. Nucleic Acids Research, 35, 2719–2733.

Sauvageau, S., Stasiak, A. Z., Banville, I., Ploquin, M., Stasiak, A., & Masson, J. Y. (2005). *Fission yeast Rad51 and Dmc1, two efficient DNA recombinases forming helical nucleoprotein filaments. Molecular and Cellular Biology, 25, 4377–4387.*

Schwacha, A., & Kleckner, N. (1997). *Interhomolog bias during meiotic recombination: meiotic functions promote a highly differentiated interhomolog-only pathway. Cell, 90, 1123–1135.*

Sehorn, M. G., Sigurdsson, S., Bussen, W., Unger, V. M., & Sung, P. (2004). *Human meiotic recombinase Dmc1 promotes ATP-dependent homologous DNA strand exchange. Nature, 429, 433–437.*

Sehorn, M. G., & Sung, P. (2004). *Meiotic recombination: an affair of two recombinases. Cell Cycle, 3, 1375–1377.*

Sheridan, S. D., Yu, X., Roth, R., Heuser, J. E., Sehorn, M. G., Sung, P., Egelman, E. H., & Bishop, D. K. (2008). *A comparative analysis of Dmc1 and Rad51 nucleoprotein filaments. Nucleic Acids Research, 36, 4057–4066.*

Shinohara, A., & Ogawa, T. (1998). *Stimulation by Rad52 of yeast Rad51-mediated recombination. Nature, 391, 404–407.*

Sugiyama, T., & Kowalczykowski, S. C. (2002). *Rad52 protein associates with replication protein A (RPA)-single-stranded DNA to accelerate Rad51-mediated displacement of RPA and presynaptic complex formation. The Journal of Biological Chemistry, 277, 31663–31672.*

Sung, P. (1994). *Catalysis of ATP-dependent homologous DNA pairing and strand exchange by yeast RAD51 protein. Science, 265, 1241–1243.*

Sung, P. (1997a). *Function of yeast Rad52 protein as a mediator between replication protein A and the Rad51 recombinase. The Journal of Biological Chemistry, 272, 28194–28197.*

Sung, P. (1997b). *Yeast Rad55 and Rad57 proteins form a heterodimer that functions with replication protein A to promote DNA strand exchange by Rad51 recombinase. Genes & Development, 11, 1111–1121.*

Sung, P., & Klein, H. (2006). *Mechanism of homologous recombination: mediators and helicases take on regulatory functions. Nature Reviews Molecular Cell Biology, 7, 739–750.*

Chapter 5

Single DNA Molecule Sensing with Boron Nitride Nanopores

Zhi Zhou[1,2], Ying Hu[1,2], Xinyan Shan[1,2] and Xinghua Lu[1,2]

1 Introduction

Nanopore, as can be inferred from its name, is a nanometer-size pore positioned in a two-dimensional membrane. It functions as a tunnel for the transit of individual bio-molecules, including polymers, proteins, DNA and RNA. These molecules are charged and electrophoretic driven under a bias voltage. The passing of a single molecule through the nanopore, termed as translocation, can be detected by monitoring the transient change in ionic current. The transient current change is due to the blockade of molecule in the nanopore. It is believed that with sufficient measurement accuracy and precise molecule motion control, one can distinguish internal structure of a molecule that translocates through a nanopore, for example, base sequencing in a single DNA molecule. The central idea of nanopore is derived from coulter counter invented in 1950's (Graham, 2003) and it undergoes rapid development with the ongoing revolution in micro fabrication technology, such as focused ion beam microscope (FIB), electron beam lithography, and transmission electron microscope (TEM). The first nanopore experiment was reported in 1996 by Kasianowicz and co-workers with biological nanopore prepared in lipid bilayer membrane (Kasianowicz et al., 1996). Since then, nanopore has attracted great interest for its potential in low-cost fast label-free DNA sequencing application (Branton et al., 2008; Venkatesan & Bashir, 2011; Wanumu, 2012), and soon it emerges as a new tool to investigate single molecules.

[1] Beijing National Laboratory for Condensed-Matter Physics, Institute of Physics, Chinese Academy of Sciences, Beijing, China
[2] Collaborative Innovation Center of Quantum Matter, Beijing, China

There have been two categories of nanopores been reported, biological nanopores and solid state nanopores. Biological nanopores are generated with certain proteins exist in nature, such as alpha-Hemolysin (Bayley, 1999) and MspA (Butler *et al.*, 2008), while solid state nanopores are usually fabricated by drilling the pore on a thin solid film such as silicon nitride (SiN) membrane. Biological nanopores have shown great success in single molecules translocation experiments. Recent years, base discrimination (Manrao *et al.*, 2012) and DNA sequencing by decoding base quadromer (Laszlo *et al.*, 2014) have been demonstrated in biological nanopores made of specific proteins. Solid-state nanopores, however, are still more preferred for their higher stability, size control ability, modification of surface properties, and feasibility for devices integration. The first solid-state nanopore was fabricated in 2001 in silicon nitride membranes tens of nanometers thick (Li *et al.*, 2001), and significant progress has been made in detection of DNA translocation (Li *et al.*, 2003; Fologea *et al.*, 2005), and DNA motion control (Gershow & Golovchenko, 2007; Plesa *et al.*, 2013) in such nanopore devices.

Reducing the effective thickness of a solid-state nanopore is of significant meaning in increasing the lateral base sensitivity in a single DNA molecule and in reducing the complexity for base discrimination analysis. Therefore, atomic thick two-dimension materials have been considered as ideal candidates for the substrate of high-resolution nanopore devices. Very recently, inspired by the rapid development of novel atomic-thick 2D material (Geim & Novoselov, 2007; Golberg *et al.*, 2010; Radisavljevic *et al.*, 2011), nanopores have been successfully fabricated in a few single- or few-layer membranes, such as graphene (Garaj *et al.*, 2010; Merchant *et al.*, 2010; Schneider *et al.*, 2010), boron nitride (BN) layer (Liu *et al.*, 2013; Zhou *et al.*, 2013), and molybdenum sulfide (Liu *et al.*, 2014). High spatial resolution (Garaj *et al.*, 2010; Liu *et al.*, 2013; Liu *et al.*, 2014) of such ultimate thin nanopores show great promise for the DNA sequencing application. Atomic thick graphene layers, for example, have been employed in fabricating nanopore devices featured with high resolution and geometrical sensitivity (Garaj *et al.*, 2010; Garaj *et al.*, 2013). It has been noted through practical experiment that increasing the hydrophilicity of graphene nanopore is important to avoid clogging due to strong nonspecific hydrophobic interaction with DNA (Schneider *et al.*, 2013). Common hydrophilicity improvement methods such as UV ozone and oxygen plasmon treatment, however, are not applicable to graphene based nanopore devices because of carbon oxidization (Zhang *et al.*, 2012). By atomic-layer deposition of titanium dioxide (Merchant *et al.*, 2010) and self-assembled hydrophilic coating (Schneider *et al.*, 2013), the hydrophilicity of graphene nanopores can be improved but at the cost of increased effective thickness of the pores. New types of atomic thick nanopores with high hydrophilicity are thus strongly desired. As another atomic-thick 2D materials, hexagonal boron nitride (*h*-BN) has wide band gap energy of 5.97 *eV* (Watanabe *et al.*, 2004), low dielectric loss and low conductivity, good thermal conductivity (Pakdel *et al.*, 2012), and chemically stable with good oxidation resistance (Chen *et al.*, 2004). The single- and few-layer *h*-BN membranes can be obtained by cleavage (Lee *et al.*, 2010), epitaxial growth (Song *et al.*, 2010; Kim *et al.*, 2012), or chemical synthesis (Nag *et al.*, 2010), which provides a good candidate for nanopore devices fabrication.

In this chapter, we will present the fabrication, characterization, and application of nanopores fabricated on hexagonal boron nitride layers. By controlling the focal size of electron beam and drilling time, sub-2 nanometer BN nanopores can be fabricated with more than 50% yield. The BN nanopores possess strong oxidization-resistance which can bear UV-ozone treatment and results in significant improvement in hydrophilicity. The high hydrophilicity in treated BN nanopores reduces the non-specific hydrophobic interaction between the membrane and DNA molecules, results in less clogging in translocation experiments. Translocation signals through BN nanopores are observed and analyzed for both double strand DNA (dsDNA) and single strand DNA (ssDNA) molecules.

2   Fabrication of *h*-BN Nanopores

2.1   Nanopore Fabrication Process

The fabrication process of BN nanopores is schematically shown in Figure 1, which can be divided into three steps: growth of floating hexagonal boron nitride layers (Figure 1(a)), preparing of silicon nitride supporting windows (Figure 1(b)), and drilling nanopore in SiN supported *h*-BN layers (Figure 1(c)).

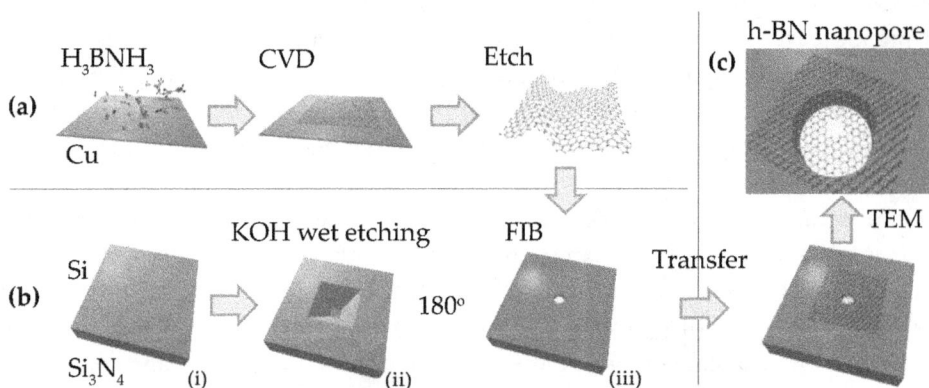

Figure 1: Fabrication process of *h*-BN nanopores. (a) The *h*-BN membrane is first grown on copper foils by chemical vapor deposition. Then, poly(methyl methacrylate) (PMMA) is coated on *h*-BN membrane, and the copper substrate is subsequently etched by FeCl₃, leaving *h*-BN/PMMA floating in solution. (b) Suspended SiN membrane (i.e. (iii)) on a pyramidal silicon pit (i.e. (i) & (ii)) is fabricated by anisotropic KOH etching. A 100–1000 nm sized hole is then drilled on center of SiN membrane. (c) The floating *h*-BN/PMMA flake is transferred on to the window, and PMMA is removed by acetone. A nanopore is then fabricated on the suspended *h*-BN membrane by focused electron beam in a transmission electron microscope. From reference (Zhou *et al.*, 2013)

As shown in Figure 1(a), the hexagonal boron nitride is grown by chemical vapor deposition (CVD) method (Kim *et al.*, 2012) on a 25 μm thick copper foil. The copper foil is firstly cleaned by acetone, ethanol, isopropanol, and deionized water, then placed into a quartz tube and heated to 1050 °C. Borane ammonia (BH_3-NH_3) carried by Ar/H_2 (200/200 *sccm*) mix gas es under atmospheric pressure, is decomposed on the copper surface and assembled to *h*-BN layers after 30 minutes growth. After cooling of the foil, a layer of poly(methyl methacrylate) (PMMA) is spin coated on the *h*-BN layers and cured at 145 °C for 5 minutes. By etching in 1 *M* (1 mol/L) iron(III) chloride for 12 hours, the underlying copper substrate is etched and floating *h*-BN/PMMA flacks are obtained.

As sketched in Figure 1(b), the SiN supporting window is prepared on a 500 μm thick silicon wafer with 50 nm thick low pressure chemical vapor deposited (LPCVD) SiN membrane on both sides (the top side is not shown to illustrate Si substrates). The wafer is first patterned by photolithography and reactive ion etching, exposing the underlying silicon substrate (window size 700 μm × 700 μm) on one side. Secondly, the exposed silicon is etched off in 22% *wt* KOH solution, leaving a 20–40 μm SiN window on the bottom side. A 100–1000 nm sized hole is drilled thereafter by focused ion beam (FIB).

The floating *h*-BN/PMMA flakes in Figure 1(a) are washed with deionized water several times, and then carefully transferred onto the SiN window in Figure 1(b), to cover the FIB drilled hole, washed by acetone to remove PMMA, rinsed in isopropyl alcohol, dried with nitrogen gas flow and finally it creates a suspended *h*-BN membrane. The nanopores are drilled in a TEM (JEM 2010F), operating under 200 *kV* voltage (Figure 1(c)) and a magnification of 800 *k*, by focusing electron beam on the *h*-BN membranes for less than 3 seconds.

2.2   Nanopore Size Control

For a nanopore device, the spatial resolution and sensitivity are critically determined not only by its thickness (Garaj *et al.*, 2010), but also by its size in diameter (Garaj *et al.*, 2013). As a demand for DNA sequencing application, the diameter of atomic thick *h*-BN nanopores shall be comparable to the dimension of DNA bases, typically sub-2 nm. With currently available nanofabrication facilities, it is possible but still as a challenge to drilling such small nanopores in ultra-thin membranes. In our practice, we find that by reducing the e-beam density to sub-200 pA/cm^2 and the drilling time to sub-1 second in a TEM, the pore size can be controlled down to less than 1 nm in *h*-BN membranes. Figures 2(a) and 2(b) show a 0.9 nm and a 1.3 nm *h*-BN nanopores, fabricated by focusing 200 pA/cm^2 electron beam onto a spot on the *h*-BN membranes. The diameter distribution of total twenty *h*-BN nanopores fabricated under 200 pA/cm^2 electron beams is shown in Figure 2(c), which presents a peak centered at 1.3 nm for nanopore diameter. About eleven nanopores have their diameters smaller than 2 nm, which gives a yield more than 50% in fabricating sub-2 nm *h*-BN nanopores. The variation in pore diameter may due to the non-precise hand control of the exposure time to the focused electron beam. With automatic electronic shutter, the precision in nanopore size can be improved further.

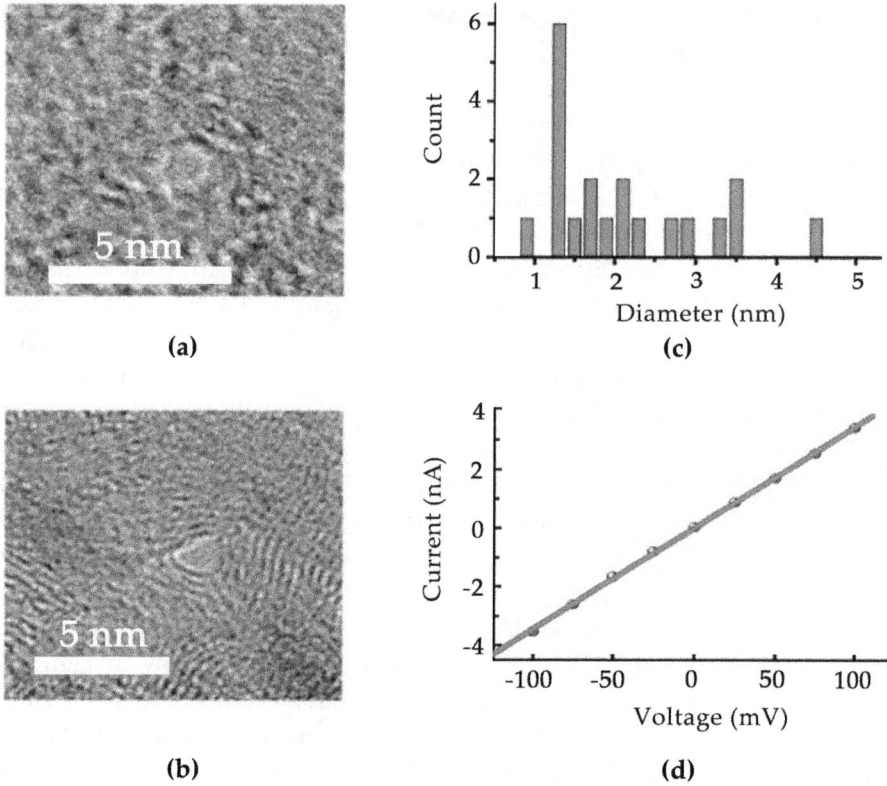

Figure 2: TEM images of a (a) 0.9 nm, and (b) 1.3 nm *h*-BN nanopores. (c): Diameter distribution of *h*-BN nanopores drilled with 200 pA/cm² electron beams (TEM model: JEM 2010F). (d): *I-V* curve of a typical 1.3 nm BN nanopore in 3 *M* KCl buffer. The fitted conductance is 34.4 nS (dark gray line).

The pore size can also be derived by its conductance in the electrolyte. In order to verify the size of these sub-2 nm *h*-BN nanopores, *I-V* curves are measured in 3 *M* KCl buffer solution. Typical *I-V* curve for a 1.3 nm nanopore is shown in Figure 2(d), with a linear fit (dark gray line). The fitted conductance value is 34.4 nS. The conductance of an ultra-small nanopore in buffer liquid can be calculated by following formula (Kowalczyk *et al.*, 2011),

$$G = \sigma \left(\frac{4l}{\pi d^2} + \frac{1}{d} \right)^{-1}, \tag{1}$$

where G is the nanopore conductance, σ is the conductivity of the bulk buffer (about 30 nS/nm for the 3 *M* KCl buffer), l is the effect thickness of the membrane (here we adopt the value of about 0.6 nm for a single layer *h*-BN, similar to that of single-layer graphene (Garaj *et al.*, 2010)), and d is the diameter of the nanopore (1.3 nm measured from TEM image). Therefore, the conductance is calculated to be 25 nS (corresponding to 1.6 nm effect hydrodynamic diameter), in the same order as the measured results.

3   Characterization of *h*-BN Nanopores

3.1   Structure of *h*-BN Layer and Nanopores

Typical TEM image of an *h*-BN nanopore is shown in Figure 3(a). The light gray area represents the suspended *h*-BN layer and the dark area is due to the SiN substrate underneath. An 8 nm nanopore is fabricated around the center of the suspended area, as indicated with a black arrow. Electron energy loss spectra (EELS) were taken on both the suspended *h*-BN layer (position indicated with gray circle) and the *h*-BN layer over the SiN membrane (black circle), as shown in Figure 3(b). Clear boron and nitrogen peaks appear in the spectrum of suspended *h*-BN layer (gray curve), while strong peaks of silicon and nitrogen are found in the spectrum taken over the SiN membrane (black curve). The carbon peak in the spectrum of suspended *h*-BN layer is due to the residual amorphous carbon contamination (possibly residual PMMA) during layer transfer. Figure 3(c) shows high-resolution TEM image of another nanopore (about 10 nm in diameter). The FFT of such TEM image shows clear six-fold symmetric spots (Figure 3(d)), indicating the hexagonal structure of the suspended *h*-BN layer. The circular pattern is due to the over-defocus of the electron beam.

Raman spectroscopy has been employed to further characterize the thickness of as-grown *h*-BN layers. Figure 3(e) shows a typical Raman spectrum of *h*-BN layer transferred onto a silicon wafer (to minimize the background luminescence from SiN), excited with a laser wavelength of 532 nm. It is known that the E_{2g} peak of a single-layer *h*-BN is centered at $1369 \pm 1\ cm^{-1}$, while that for the bi-layer and the bulk are centered at $1365 \pm 2\ cm^{-1}$ and $1366\ cm^{-1}$, respectively (Gorbachev *et al.*, 2011). The observed Raman peak in our samples is centered at $1369.3 \pm 0.1\ cm^{-1}$ (Figure 3(f)), indicating the presence of single-layer *h*-BN membrane. The small peaks at $1400\ cm^{-1}$ and $1600\ cm^{-1}$ are the third harmonic peaks of the silicon substrate (Lin *et al.*, 2007).

3.2   Hydrophilicity of *h*-BN layer

The hydrophilicity of a nanopore device is practically important to avoid clogging due to strong nonspecific hydrophobic interaction with biologic molecules (Schneider *et al.*, 2013).

For SiN nanopores, piranha solution (H_2SO_4: H_2O_2 = 3:1) and UV-ozone (UVO) treatment are commonly used methods to improve its hydrophilicity. Both methods oxidize the organic residuals on surface. For example, UVO induces ozone gas (O_3) in the environment by utilizing ultra-violet light, which is an effective oxidant to oxidize the organics and form hydrophilic hydroxyl group on most materials. Such methods, however, are not applicable for graphene nanopores since carbon atoms can be easily oxidized (Zhang *et al.*, 2012). Atomic-layer-deposition (ALD) of titanium dioxide (Merchant *et al.*, 2010) and self-assembled hydrophilic coating (Schneider *et al.*, 2013) has been employed to improve the hydrophilicity of graphene nanopores, which however increase the effective thickness of the nanopores. The apparent advantage of *h*-BN layer is its resistance to oxidation, which can be used to improve the hydrophilicity of *h*-BN nanopores.

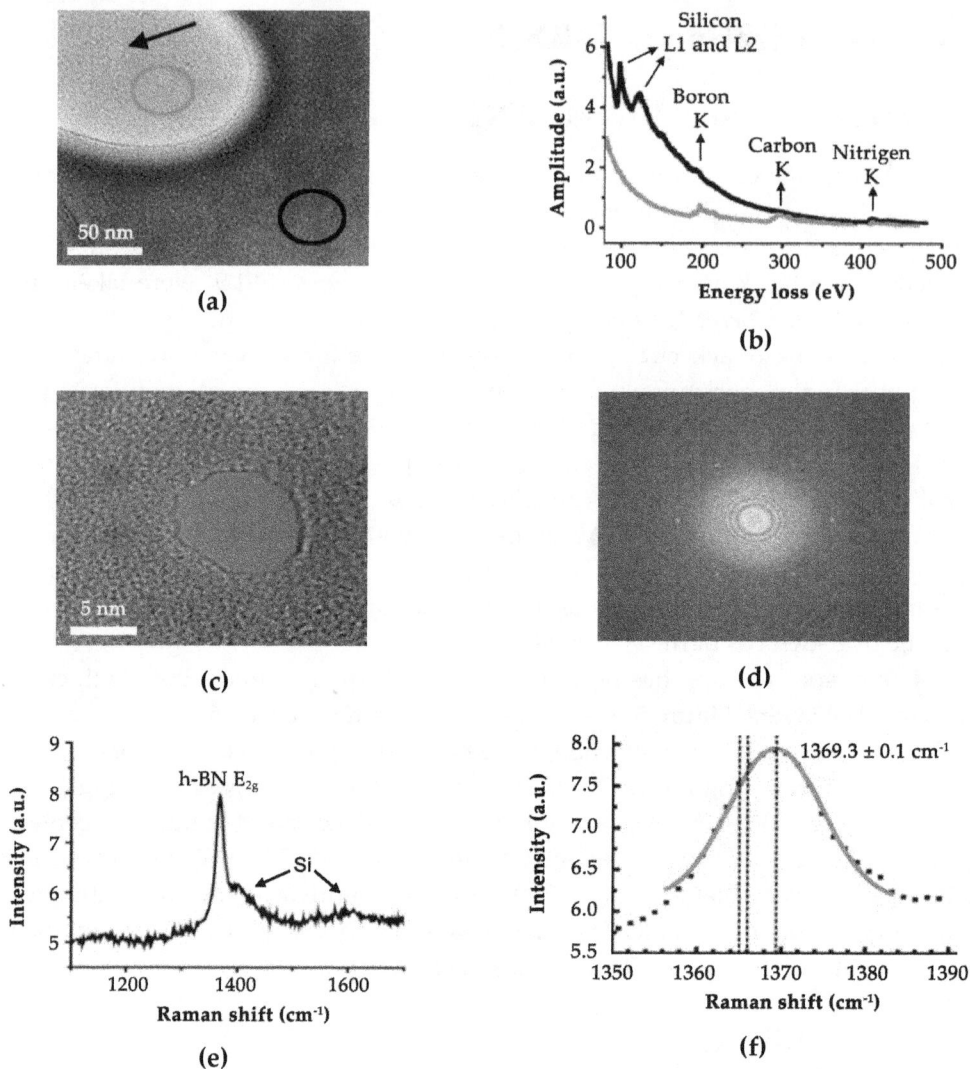

Figure 3: (a) TEM image of *h*-BN membrane (light gray area) supported by a SiN substrate (dark gray). The black arrow marks an 8 nm nanopore. (b) EELS taken in regions of suspended *h*-BN membrane and SiN substrate. Spectrums are taken at positions indicated by circles in (a). (c) High resolution TEM image of a 10 nm *h*-BN nanopore. (d) FFT of (c). The hexagonal structure of the suspended *h*-BN layer is represented by the clear six-fold symmetric spots. (e) Raman spectrum of *h*-BN layer transferred onto a Si substrate. (f) Zoom-in Raman spectrum of E_{2g} peak of an *h*-BN layer. The peak center locates at 1369.3 ± 0.1 *cm⁻¹* as derived from fitting with a Gaussian line profile. The dashed lines at 1365, 1366, and 1369 *cm⁻¹* indicate the peak positions for bulk, double layer, and single layer *h*-BN, respectively. From reference (Zhou *et al.*, 2013).

The hydrophilicity of *h*-BN layer is characterized by the contact angle of an electrolyte droplet (1 *μL* 1 *M* KCl-TE) on surface. For comparison, we measured the contact angles of SiN surface and graphene membrane as well. Figure 4 shows the measured contact angles on SiN surface (50 nm thick), UVO treated SiN surface, *h*-BN layer, UVO treated *h*-BN layer, and graphene. The *h*-BN layer (both treated and untreated) and graphene are transfer onto a SiN substrate for the characterization. Each measurement is carried out with more than 10 samples. The measurements on treated samples are taken immediately after 15-minute UVO treatment (Jelight Company Inc., model No. 42–220). The untreated *h*-BN layer gives a contact angle of 57°, close to that on SiN surface (54°). The contact angle on UVO treated *h*-BN layer decreases to 26°. Such good wetting property can last for at least 30 minutes in ambient lab environment, long enough for device assembling in a typical nanopore experiment. We note that the UVO treated SiN membrane shows the lowest contact angle of 6° and the graphene surface produce a contact angle of 67°, highest among all materials characterized in our experiment.

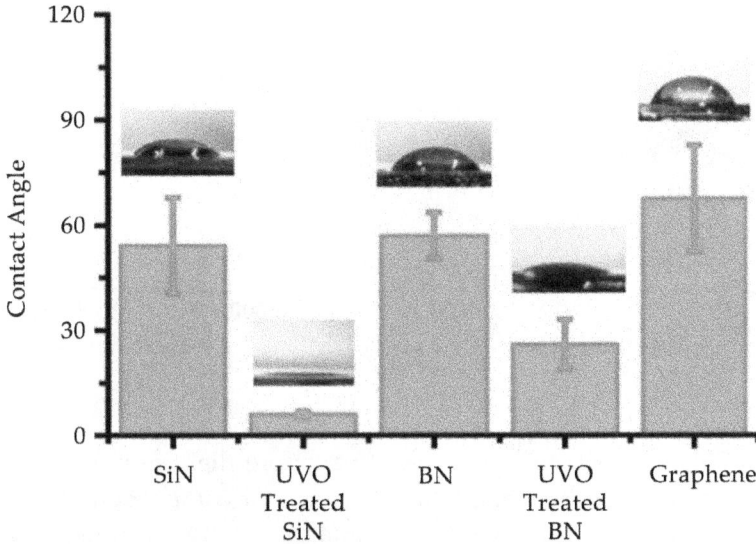

Figure 4: Contact angles of 1 *M* KCl-TE droplet on SiN (54°), UVO treated SiN (6°), BN membrane (57°), UVO treated BN membrane (26°) and graphene membrane (67°). The inset images are typical microscopic images of electrolyte droplets on these surfaces. From reference (Zhou *et al.*, 2013).

3.3   Noise Spectrum in *h*-BN Nanopore Device

The noise level of the nanopore system can be described by the following equation (Rosenstein & Shepard, 2013):

$$S_n(f) = \frac{A_1 I^2}{f} + A_2 + A_3 Cf + A_4 (Cf v_n)^2,$$ (2)

where f is frequency, $S_n(f)$ is the total power spectral density for bandwidth f, I is base current, and A_1 is a dimensionless parameter, C is the system capacitance, v_n is the voltage noise of the amplifier and A_2, A_3, and A_4 are constants. The first term is $1/f$ noise, the second term is white noise (composed of Johnson noise and shot noise), and the last two terms are capacitive noise. The $1/f$ noise dominates the noise level in the low-frequency region. The noise spectrum can be derived by fast Fourier transform (FFT) of real-time current traces in single molecule translocation experiment. Figure 5(a) presents the power spectrum of an h-BN nanopore on a 200 nm SiN window (light gray line) and a graphene nanopore on similar window (dark gray line). Both spectra are fitted with equation (2). The fitted parameter A_1 for the h-BN nanopore is 6.7×10^{-7}, about 8 times smaller than that of the graphene nanopore (5.0×10^{-6}). The spectra are taken with nanopores with similar pore diameter and device structure (for example: membrane area and supporting window size). The base current is 15 nA for both spectra. The reduction in $1/f$ noise possibly arises from the cleaner and more hydrophilic surface (Merchant *et al.*, 2010) of the h-BN layer treated by UVO.

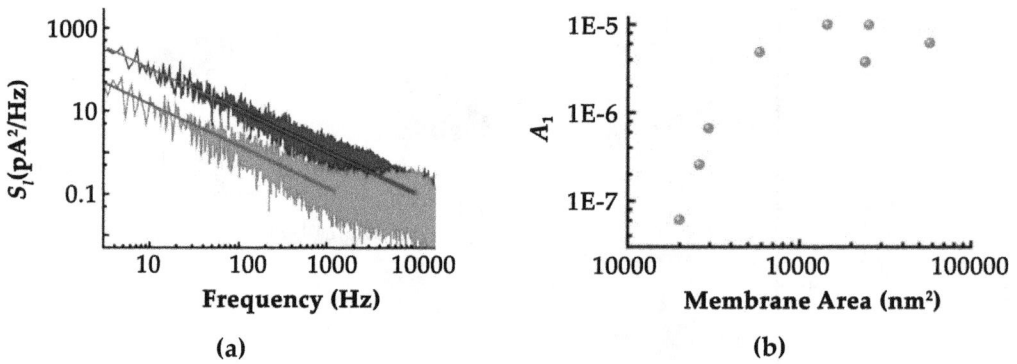

(a)   (b)

Figure 5: (a) Noise spectrums of an h-BN nanopore (light gray) and a graphene nanopore (dark gray) with similar chip structure for comparison. Base current is 15 nA and both spectrums are fitted with equation (2). (b) The fitted parameter A_1 as a function of membrane area. Adopted from reference (Zhou *et al.*, 2013).

It is found that the $1/f$ noise in h-BN nanopore is closely related to the area of the suspended membrane. Figure 5(b) plots the value of A_1 as a function of membrane area, which is obtained by subtracting nanopore area from the SiN window area. For a smaller 180 nm window, the value reduces to 2.6×10^{-7}; and for a bigger 550 nm window, it increases to 3.75×10^{-6}. This observation is consistent with previous report where the $1/f$ noise of a graphene nanopore is related to the size of the supporting SiN window (Garaj *et al.*, 2013). In addition, the h-BN nanopores are more stable for smaller supporting SiN window. Reducing window size is not only good for minimizing the $1/f$ noise but also help increase the fabrication yield of h-BN nanopores.

4   DNA Translocation through *h*-BN Nanopores

4.1   Experiment Setup

The basic experiment setup for DNA translocation through a nanopore is illustrated in Figure 6(a). The *h*-BN nanopore device is assembled in saline solution reservoir (1 *M* KCl, room temperature, pH = 7.8) with a pair of silver chloride (Ag/AgCl) electrodes on both sides. A bias voltage *V* is supplied to drive ions and charged molecules through the nanopore and the ionic current is monitored in real time. The ionic current is detected by an Axopatch preamplifier (200B) at acquisition rate of 250 *kHz*, followed by a 30 *kHz* 4-pole Bessel filter. When negatively charged DNA molecules are added to the reservoir, they will be electrophoretic driven towards the nanopore. The translocation of the DNA molecule through the nanopore induces a transient conductance change, as shown in Figure 6(b). Typically, a transient current drop in the ionic current is observed. The nanopore presents a relatively high conductance at the "open pore" state, and low conductance at the "blocked pore" state. The recorded translocation events are analyzed in a Matlab GUI program. The program allows us to view the events one by one and only those events with signal-to-noise ratio (SNR) higher than 8 are selected for analysis.

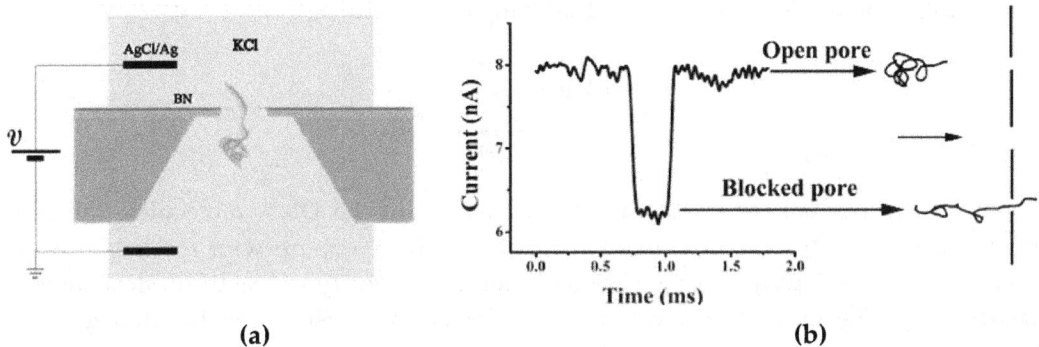

Figure 6: (a) Schematic of nanopore device and experiment setup. (b) Typical current trace of a DNA translocation event through an *h*-BN nanopore. The current is reduced when the molecule blocks the nanopore during translocation. The "open pore" and "blocked pore" are associated with the states that a DNA molecule is out of or in the nanopore.

4.2   dsDNA Translocation through *h*-BN Nanopore

Figure 7(a) shows the *I-V* curve of a 4 nm *h*-BN nanopore in 1 *M* KCl buffer (containing 10 *mM Tris*-HCl and 1 *mM* EDTA, *pH* around 8.0). The linear fit derives the nanopore conductance of 23 nS, corresponding to effect hydrodynamic diameter of 2.9 nm. The double strand λ-DNA (48.5 kbp) molecules were pre-warmed to 70 °C for 1 minute to reduce possible secondary structures. After the DNA molecules are injected into the reservoir, translocation events are observed in current traces as downward transient spikes, shown in Figure 7(b). Normally hundreds of translocation events can be observed before the nanopore becomes clogged. The duration of translocation events varies widely from 0.1 ms to 2 s. Three typical translocation events of different translocation durations are plotted in Figure 7(c) with zoomed-in details. To investigate the statistical behavior of dsDNA translocation through the h-BN nanopore, we plot the conductance blockade (ΔG) versus duration (Δt) of each translocation event in Figure 7(d). The drive voltage for this data set is 150 mV. The right panel of Figure 7(d) is the histogram of conductance blockade, fitted with a single Gaussian peak (red line). The center of fitted curve represents an averaged conductance blockade of 2.8 nS for unfolded dsDNA molecules. No translocation event of folded DNA is observed in this device since the pore size is too small for the folded dsDNA molecules to pass through. The averaged conductance blockade is invariant as the driving voltage changes from 150 mV to 250 mV, as shown in the inset of Figure 7(d). This is consisted with the translocation model, where the conductance drop is determined by the blockade area and the conductance of DNA molecules.

To investigate the DNA translocation dynamics in the h-BN nanopore, we plot the histogram of translocation duration Δt on the upper side of the scatter plot in Figure 7(d). The histogram of translocation duration is then fitted with density functions of 1D biased diffusion model (Li & Talaga, 2010; Ling & Ling, 2013):

$$P(t) = N \frac{L \times \exp\left(-\dfrac{(L-vt)^2}{4Dt} \right)}{t\sqrt{4\pi Dt}}, \tag{3}$$

where N is a normalized constant, L is the length of the DNA molecules (the effect thickness of the h-BN membrane 0.6 nm is negligible compare with the length of unfolded λ-DNA 16.5 μm), D and v are diffusion and velocity of electrophoresis motion, respectively. The mean translocation speed for DNA translocation is fitted to be 5.5 μm/ms, as the gray curve in the upper panel of Figure 7(d), similar to that in previous report on λ-DNA translocation through graphene nanopores (Schneider $et\ al.$, 2010). The fitted diffusion constant is 8 μm^2/ms, which is significantly larger than the bulk value of λ-DNA. The histogram data do not match the fitting curve perfectly. Translocation events with duration time less than 1 ms (as contained in the black circle in the scatter plot) may be contributed by DNA fragments, while those events with much longer duration time (contained in the orange circle in the scatter plot) are due to dsDNA-nanopore interaction. For quantitative analysis, we discriminate elongated DNA translocation events as those events longer than the peak duration time by 1.5 σ, where σ is the full width at the half maximum (FWHM) of the fitted curve. The translocation time of elongated events in Figure 7(d) is more than 6 ms. The percentage of elongated events adds up to 65% of all data points in the figure. The averaged translocation time of the elongated events is 108 ms, about 40 times longer than that of normal events. The anomalously long translocation time, as well as the high percentage, of elongated events indicates a pretty strong interaction between dsDNA molecules and the h-BN nanopore.

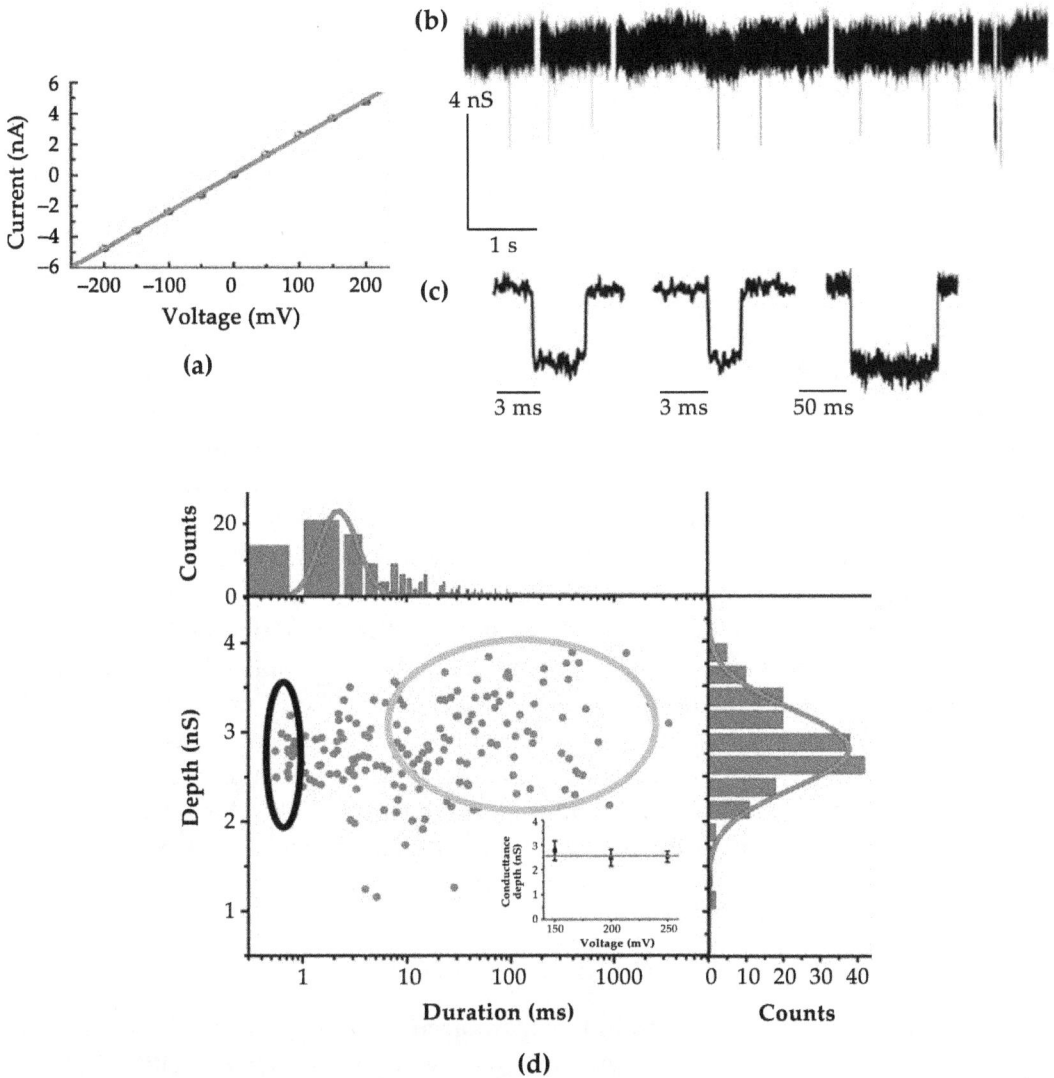

Figure 7: (a) *I-V* curve of a 4 nm *h*-BN nanopore with a linear fit (gray line). The fitted conductance is about 23 nS. (b) Current trance with λ-DNA translocation events. (c) Zoomed-in details of three typical translocation events with different translocation duration. (d) Scatter plot of the conductance blockade (ΔG) versus the event duration (Δt). The right panel is the histogram of conductance blockade fitted with Gaussian function; while the upper panel is the histogram of event duration fitted with 1D biased diffusion model. The events in black circle originate from DNA segments and those in orange circle are delayed events due to strong dsDNA-nanopore interaction. The inset shows the conductance blockade as a function of bias voltage from 150 to 250 *mV*. From reference (Zhou *et al.*, 2013).

Slowing down DNA translocation speed allows electronics to detect DNA molecules with sufficient time or low bandwidth. This is essential since the bandwidth of a state-of-the-art current preamplifier is usually below MHz. Thus it is of special interest to explore the effect of interaction between DNA molecules and the h-BN nanopore. For this purpose, we further tested the dsDNA translocation through h-BN nanopores of different sizes. Figures 8(a) and 8(b) show the scatter plot of the selected unfolded dsDNA translocation events through a moderate 10 nm h-BN nanopore (Figure 8(a)) and a big 30 nm h-BN nanopore (Figure 8(b)). The multi-level events are not plotted for better comparison with the results in the 4 nm BN nanopore. Bias voltage of 150 mV and λ-DNA are used for the experiment with the 10 nm nanopore; bias voltage of 200 mV and 10 kbp DNA are used for the 30 nm nanopore. The right side panels are conductance blockade histogram fitted with Gaussian curves, while the top side panels are histogram of translocation duration fitted with 1D biased diffusion model. The average conductance blockade is 2.1 nS for the 10 nm h-BN nanopore (a) and 2.4 nS for the 30 nm h-BN nanopore (b). Significant portion of translocation events through the 10 nm h-BN nanopores are slowed down due to interaction with the nanopore. For the 30 nm h-BN nanopore, only very small percentage of the translocation events displays elongated translocation time.

Multi-level translocation events are observed in these two nanopores, indicating folded or partial folded translocation states due to the large nanopore diameter. Typical translocation events are shown in Figures 8(c) and 8(d) for the 10 nm and 30 nm h-BN nanopores, respectively. By analyzing duration time of all unfolded events, the percentage of translocation events undergoes dsDNA-nanopore interaction is about 71% in the 10 nm h-BN nanopore and about 20% in the 30 nm nanopore. The elongated translocation time is 16 ms (5 times of normal events) for the 10 nm nanopore and 0.85 ms (3 times of normal events) for the 30 nm nanopore.

4.3   ssDNA Translocation through h-BN Nanopore

Detecting translocation of single strand DNA molecules through a nanopore is a basic step towards DNA base sequencing. At current stage, most experiments with solid state nanopores are carried out with double strand DNA. There are very few studies on the translocation of single strand DNA through atomic thick solid state nanopores. We herein investigate the translocation of single strand DNA through atomic thick h-BN nanopores. The ssDNA sample used in our experiment is prepared by random amplification from a virus template, which has several hundred base pairs. After purification, the ssDNA sample is diluted with KCl buffer (1 M KCl, 10 mM Tris-HCl, 5 mM MgCl$_2$, and pH = 9.0). Figure 9(a) shows a typical current trace of 20 μm ssDNA translocation though a 20 nm h-BN nanopore. Figure 9(b) shows zoomed-in details of a few typical translocation events of ssDNA through h-BN nanopore. To demonstrated, the events were further filtered with a 10 kHz Bessel filter.

The scatter plot of the conductance blockade versus translocation duration is presented in Figure 9(c). One would expect that the conductance blockade of ssDNA be half of that for the dsDNA, similar to that demonstrated in graphene nanopores (Garaj

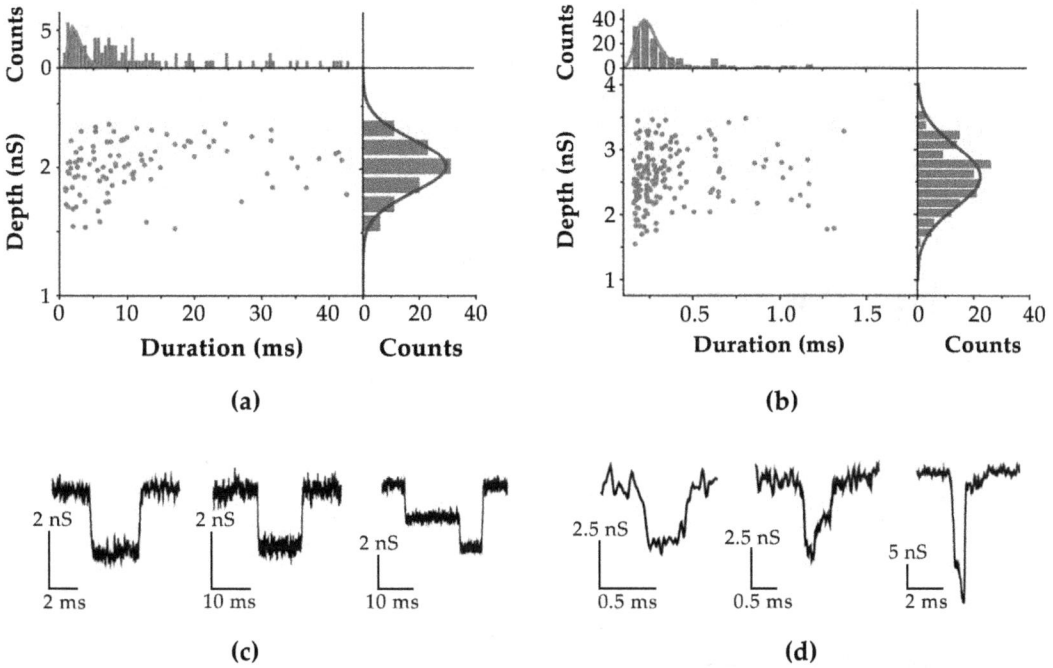

Figure 8: Scatter plot of dsDNA translocation events through (a) a 10 nm and (b) a 30 nm *h*-BN nanopore. Bias voltage of 150 *mV* and λ-DNA are used for the experiment with 10 *nm* nanopore; bias voltage of 200 *mV* and 10 *kbp* DNA are used for the 30 nm nanopore. The right side panels are conductance blockade histogram with Gaussian curve fitting (black line) and top side panels are translocation duration histograms fitted with 1D biased diffusion model. The average conductance blockade is 2.1 nS for (a) and 2.4 nS for (b). (c–d) Typical unfolded and partial folded translocation events through the 10 nm and 30 nm *h*-BN nanopores. From reference (Zhou *et al.*, 2013).

et al., 2013). However, from the right panel of Figure 9(c), we derive the averaged conductance blockade of 6.9 nS (gray curve) for translocation of ssDNA molecules through this 20 nm *h*-BN nanopore. This is apparently larger than the conductance blockade for the dsDNA translocation through *h*-BN nanopores of similar sizes. This discrepancy is attributed to the as formed entangled blob structure, as reported in silicon nitride nanopores previously (Kowalczyk *et al.*, 2010). The top panel is histogram of events duration, fitted with 1D biased diffusion model (equation (3)). The fitted diffusion constant is 0.15 μm²/*ms* with velocity around 3 μm/*ms*.

5   Discussion

Base discrimination between poly(A), poly(C), and poly(T) (homogeneous chain of adenine, cytosine and thymine, respectively) was realized recently with sub-2 nm nanopores in silicon nitride membrane (Venta *et al.*, 2013). However, due to its thickness of 5–8 nm, such nanopore embraces more than 10 bases simultaneously and the signal analysis is challenging due to the average effect. Fabricating sub-2 nm nanopores in atomic thick membranes such as the *h*-BN layer in our study, shows great potential for base discrimination in a single ssDNA molecule.

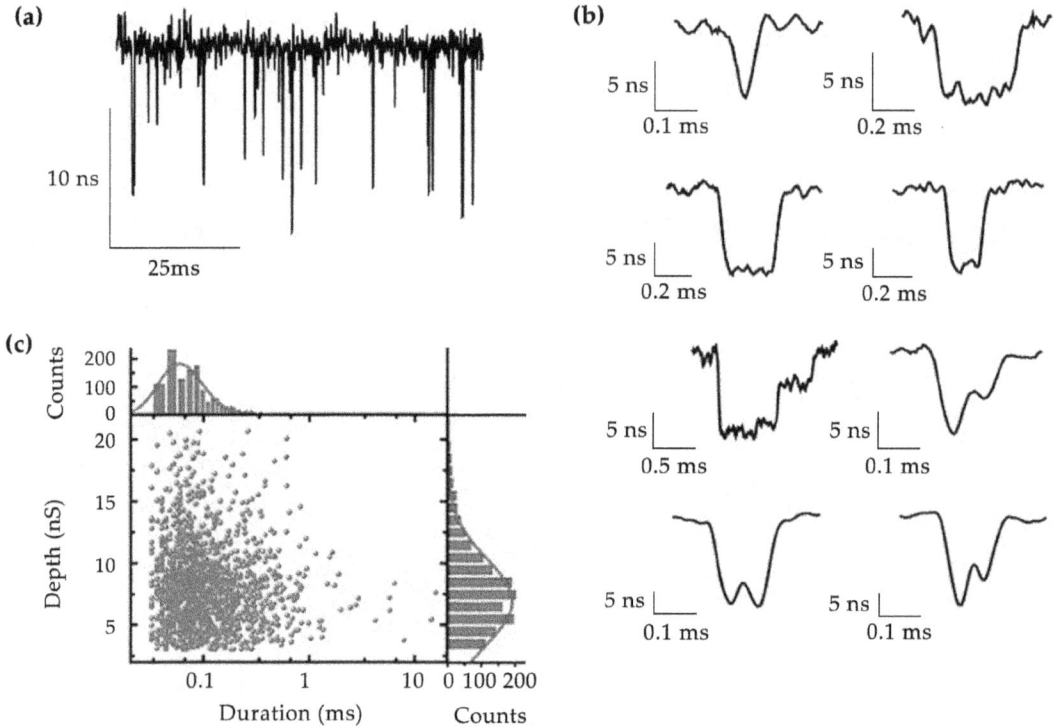

Figure 9: (a) Current trace of ssDNA translocation though a 20 nm *h*-BN nanopore. (b) Typical translocation events with zoomed-in details. (c) Scatter plot of conductance blockade versus translocation duration of ssDNA translocation events. The applied bias voltage is 100 *mV*, the concentration of ssDNA is 20 μm, and the *pH* of the electrolyte is 9.0. The right panel is the conductance blockade with Gaussian fit (black line); while the top panel is the histogram of event duration, fitted with 1D biased diffusion model.

One of the obstacles for DNA sequencing with solid-state nanopores is the fact that the velocity of DNA translocation is too fast for measurement with electronics available nowadays. The typical duration for one base pair is about tens of nanosecond to several micro-second, demanding a current detecting bandwidth of several *MHz* to one hundred *MHz*, which are several orders of magnitude higher than the bandwidth of electronics generally used in nanopore experiments (for example, Axopatch 200B). Hence, developing high-speed electronics and reducing the velocity of DNA translocation is crucial for reading out the single base information. Repeat-measurement can also improve the accuracy but sacrifices the sequencing efficiency. Phi29 DNA polymerase was recently employed to control the DNA's motion and the DNA translocation velocity was slowed down dramatically (Cherf *et al.*, 2012). By virtue of such technology, DNA sequencing with MspA nanopore has achieved great progress (Manrao *et al.*, 2012). Such studies illustrate a new path towards DNA sequencing by incorporating functional biomaterials with solid state membranes.

Design optimized device structure is an additional direction that needs attention. In high bandwidth measurements, the noise level will be dominated by the capacitive noise. The disadvantage of ultrathin membrane is their relatively high capacitance. Smart design and integration of ultimate thin *h*-BN nanopore device with the electronic system are of great demand, through which the electronic noise can be greatly reduced.

Acknowledgement

This work is supported by National Basic Research Program of China under Grant No. 2012CB933002 and Strategic Priority Research Program (B) of the Chinese Academy of Sciences, Grant No. XDB07030100. X. Shan acknowledges the financial aid from Open Research Fund Program of the State Key Laboratory of Low-Dimensional Quantum Physics under Grant No. KF201201. X. Lu thanks the support from Hundred Talent Program of Chinese Academy of Sciences.

References

Bayley, H. (1999). *Designed membrane channels and pores. Current Opinion in Biotechnology, 10, 94–103.*

Branton, D., Deamer, D. W., Marziali, A., Bayley, H., Benner, S. A, Butler, T., Ventra, M. D., Garaj, S., Hibbs, A., Huang, X., Jovanovich, S. B, Krstic, P. S, Lindsay, S., Ling, X. S., Mastrangelo, C. H, Meller, A., Oliver, J. S, Pershin, Y. V, Ramsey, J M., Riehn, R., Soni, G. V, Tabard-Cossa, V., Wanunu, M., Wiggin, M., & Schloss, J. A (2008). *The potential and challenges of nanopore sequencing. Nature Biotechnology, 26, 1146–1153.*

Butler, T. Z., Pavlenok, M., Derrington, I. M., Niederweis, M., & Gundlach, J. H. (2008). *Single-molecule DNA detection with an engineered MspA protein nanopore. Proceedings of the National Academy of Sciences of the United States of America, 105, 20647–20652.*

Chen, Y., Zou, J., Campbell, S. J., & Caer G. L. (2004). *Boron nitride nanotubes: Pronounced resistance to oxidation. Applied Physics Letters, 84, 2430–2432.*

Cherf, G. M., Lieberman, K. R, Rashid, H., Lam, C. E, Karplus, K., & Akeson, M. (2012). *Automated forward and reverse ratcheting of DNA in a nanopore at 5-Å precision. Nature Biotechnology, 30, 344–348.*

Dekker, C. (2007). *Solid-state nanopores. Nature Nanotechnology, 2, 209–215.*

Fologea, D., Gershow, M., Ledden, B., McNabb, D. S., Golovchenko, J. A., & Li, J. (2005). *Detecting Single Stranded DNA with a Solid State Nanopore. Nano Letters, 5, 1905–1909.*

Garaj, S., Hubbard, W., Reina, A., Kong, J., Branton D., & Golovchenko, J. A. (2010). *Graphene as a subnanometre trans-electrode membrane. Nature, 467, 190–193.*

Garaj, S., Liu, S., Golovchenko, J. A., & Branton, D. (2013). *Molecule-hugging graphene nanopores. Proceedings of the National Academy of Sciences of the United States of America, 110, 12192–12196.*

Geim, A. K., & Novoselov, K. S. (2007). *The rise of graphene. Nature Materials, 6, 183–191.*

Gershow, M., & Golovchenko, J. A. (2007). *Recapturing and trapping single molecules with a solid-state nanopore. Nature Nanotechnology, 2, 775–779.*

Golberg, D., Bando, Y., Huang, Y., Terao, T., Mitome, M., Tang, C., & Zhi, C. (2010). *Boron Nitride Nanotubes and Nanosheets. ACS Nano, 4, 2979–2993.*

Gorbachev, R. V., Riaz, I., Nair, R. R., Jalil, R., Britnell, L., Belle, B. D., Hill, E. W., Novoselov, K. S., Watanabe, K., Taniguchi, T., Geim, A. K., & Peter Blake. (2011). *Hunting for Monolayer Boron Nitride: Optical and Raman Signatures. Small, 7, 465–468.*

Graham, M. D. (2003). *The Coulter principle: Foundation of an industry. Journal of the Association for Laboratory Automation, 8, 72–81.*

Kasianowicz, J. J., Brandin, E., Branton, D., & Deamer, D. W. (1996). *Characterization of individual polynucleotide molecules using a membrane channel. Proceedings of the National Academy of Sciences of the United States of America, 93, 13770–13773.*

Kim, K. K., Hsu, A., Jia, X., Kim, S. M., Shi, Y., Hofmann, M., Nezich, D., Rodriguez-Nieva, J. F., Dresselhaus, M., Palacios, T., & Kong, J. (2012). *Synthesis of Monolayer Hexagonal Boron Nitride on Cu Foil Using Chemical Vapor Deposition. Nano Letters, 12, 161–166.*

Kowalczyk, S. W., Grosberg, A. Y., Rabin, Y., & Dekker, C. (2011). *Modeling the conductance and DNA blockade of solid-state nanopores. Nanotechnology, 22, 315101.*

Laszlo, A. H., Derrington, I. M., Ross, B. C., Brinkerhoff, H., Adey, A., Nova, I. C., Craig, J. M., Langford, K. W., Samson, J. M., Daza, R., Doering, K., Shendure, J. & Gundlach, J. H. (2014). *Decoding long nanopore sequencing reads of natural DNA. Nature Biotechnology, 32, 829–833.*

Lee, C., Li, Q., Kalb, W., Liu, X., Berger, H., Carpick, R. W., & Hone, J. (2010). *Frictional Characteristics of Atomically Thin Sheets. Science, 328, 76–80.*

Li, J., & Talaga, D. S (2010). *The distribution of DNA translocation times in solid-state nanopores. Journal of Physics: Condensed Matter, 22, 454129.*

Li, J., Stein, D., McMullan, C., Branton, D., Aziz, M. J. & Golovchenko, J. A. (2001). *Ion-beam sculpting at nanometre length scales. Nature, 412, 166–169.*

Li, J., Gershow, M., Stein, D., Brandin, E., & Golovchenko, J. A. (2003). *DNA molecules and configurations in a solidstate nanopore microscope. Nature Materials, 2, 611–615.*

Lin, Q., Painter, O. J., & Agrawa, G. P. (2007). *Nonlinear optical phenomena in silicon waveguides: Modeling and applications.* Optics Express, 15, 16604–16644.

Ling, D. Y, & Ling, X. S. (2013). *On the distribution of DNA translocation times in solid-state nanopores: an analysis using Schrödinger's first-passage-time theory.* Journal of Physics: Condensed Matter, 25, 375102.

Liu, S., Lu, B., Zhao, Q., Li, J., Gao, T., Chen, Y., Zhang, Y., Liu, Z., Fan, Z., Yang, F., You, L., & Yu, D. (2013). *Boron Nitride Nanopores: Highly Sensitive DNA Single-Molecule Detectors.* Advanced Materials, 25, 4549–4554.

Liu, K., Feng, J., Kis, A., & Radenovic, A. (2014). *Atomically Thin Molybdenum Disulfide Nanopores with High Sensitivity for DNA Translocation.* ACS Nano, 8, 2504–2511.

Manrao, E. A, Derrington, I. M, Laszlo, A. H, Langford, K. W, Hopper, M. K, Gillgren, N., Pavlenok, M., Niederweis, M., & Gundlach, J. H (2012). *Reading DNA at single-nucleotide resolution with a mutant MspA nanopore and phi29 DNA polymerase.* Nature Biotechnology, 30, 349–353.

Merchant, C. A., Healy, K., Wanunu, M., Ray, V., Peterman, N., Bartel, J., Fischbein, M. D., Venta, K., Luo, Z., Johnson, A. T. C., & Drndić, M. (2010). *DNA Translocation through Graphene Nanopores.* Nano Letters, 10, 2915–2921.

Nag, A., Raidongia, K., Hembram, K. P. S. S., Datta, R., Waghmare, U. V., & Rao, C. N. R. (2010). *Graphene Analogues of BN: Novel Synthesis and Properties.* ACS Nano, 4, 1539–1544.

Pakdel, A., Zhi, C., Bando, Y., & Golberg, D. (2012) *Low-dimensional boron nitride nanomaterials.* Materials Today, 15, 256–265.

Plesa, C., Cornelissen, L., Tuijtel, M. W, & Dekker, C. (2013). *Non-equilibrium folding of individual DNA molecules recaptured up to 1000 times in a solid state nanopore.* Nanotechnology, 24, 475101.

Radisavljevic, B., Radenovic, A., Brivio, J., Giacometti, V., & Kis, A. (2011). *Single-layer MoS₂ transistors.* Nature Nanotechnology, 6, 147–150.

Rosenstein, J. K., & Shepard, K. L. (2013). *Temporal Resolution of Nanopore Sensor Recordings.* 35th Annual International Conference of the IEEE EMBS. 4110–4113.

Schneider, G. F., Kowalczyk, S. W., Calado, V. E., Pandraud, G., Zandbergen, H. W., Vandersypen, L. M. K., & Dekker, C. (2010). *DNA Translocation through Graphene Nanopores.* Nano Letters, 10, 3163–3167.

Schneider, G. F., Xu, Q., Hage, S., Luik, S., Spoor, J. N.H., Malladi, S., Zandbergen, H., & Dekker, C. (2013). *Tailoring the hydrophobicity of graphene for its use as nanopores for DNA translocation.* Nature Communications, 4, 2619.

Song, L., Ci, L., Lu, H., Sorokin, P. B., Jin, C., Ni, J., Kvashnin, A. G., Kvashnin, D. G., Lou, J., Yakobson, B. I., & Ajayan, P. M. (2010). *Large Scale Growth and Characterization of Atomic Hexagonal Boron Nitride Layers.* Nano Letters, 10, 3209–3215.

Venkatesan, B. M., & Bashir, R. (2011). Nanopore sensors for nucleic acid analysis. Nature Nanotechnology, 615–624.

Venta, K., Shemer, G., Puster, M., Rodríguez-Manzo, J. A., Balan, A., Rosenstein, J. K., Shepard, K., & Drndić, M.(2013). Differentiation of Short, Single-Stranded DNA Homopolymers in Solid-State Nanopores. ACS Nano, 7, 4629–4636.

Wanunu, M. Nanopores: A journey towards DNA sequencing. Physics of Life Reviews, 9, 125– 158.

Watanabe, K., Taniguchi, T., & Kanda, H. (2004). Direct-bandgap properties and evidence for ultraviolet lasing of hexagonal boron nitride single crystal. Nature Materials, 3, 404–409.

Zhang, E. X., Newaz, A. K. M., Wang, B., Zhang, C. X., Fleetwood, D. M., Bolotin, K. I., Schrimpf, R. D., Pantelides, S. T., & Alles, M. L. (2012). Applied Physics Letters, 101, 121601.

Zhou, Z., Hu, Y., Wang, H., Xu, Z., Wang, W., Bai, X., Shan, X., & Lu, X. (2013). DNA Translocation through Hydrophilic Nanopore in Hexagonal Boron Nitride. Scientific Reports, 3, 3287

Chapter 6

Protein Purification and Analysis Led to New Roles to the α_1–β_1 (and α_2–β_2) Interface of Human Hemoglobin Molecule

Yoshiaki Sugawara[1], Yoko Abe[2], Ikumi Ohgushi[2], Eriko Ueno[2],
Mai Okazakid[2], Mai Yamada[2], Aya Okamoto[2], Mariko Miyake[2],
Fusako Fukami[2], Asako Suzuki[3], Yayoi Yukuta[3],
Etsuko Kadono[3] and Ai Yano[3]

1 Introduction

Cellular life is reliant upon rapid and efficient responses to internal and external conditions, wherein basic molecular events associated with these processes are the structural transitions of the proteins (structural protein allostery) involved (Vitagliano *et al.*, 2008). Therefore, deeper understanding of the structural basis of protein allostery is of paramount importance to characterize these processes. The human hemoglobin (Hb) molecule ($\alpha_2\beta_2$) holds a special position in these structural transitions. Hb ($\alpha_2\beta_2$; alternatively, a dimer of $\alpha\beta$ protomers) has two types of $\alpha\beta$ interface, *i.e.*, $\alpha_1\beta_1$ (and $\alpha_2\beta_2$) and $\alpha_1\beta_2$ (and $\alpha_2\beta_1$). The latter α_1–β_2 (and α_2–β_1) interface is known to be associated with cooperative O_2 binding, and exhibits principal roles if the molecule goes from its deoxygenated to oxygenated quaternary structure. However, the role of the former α_1–β_1 (and α_2–β_2) interface has been unclear for a long time.

In this regard, important and intriguing observations have been accumulating while paying attention to the α_1–β_1 (and α_2–β_2) interface. Hence, a new graze could be

[1] Department of Health Science, Prefectural University of Hiroshima, Japan
[2] Department of Health Science, Hiroshima Prefectural Women's University, Japan
[3] Department of Human Life Science, Hiroshima Women's University, Japan

focused on the $\alpha_1-\beta_1$ (and $\alpha_2-\beta_2$) interface. With respect to the $\alpha_1-\beta_1$ (and $\alpha_2-\beta_2$) interface, a new role was attributed first as stabilizing the HbO_2 tetramer against acidic autoxidation (oxidation of ferrous heme iron by bound O_2) (Tsuruga *et al.*, 1998; Yasuda, *et al.*, 2002). That is, the $\alpha_1-\beta_1$ (and $\alpha_2-\beta_2$) interface produces a conformational constraint in the β chain whereby the distal (E7) histidine (His) residue is tilted slightly away from the bound O_2 so as to prevent proton-catalyzed displacement of O_2^- (superoxide anion or more properly superoxide anion radical, O_2^{-}) by a solvent water molecule. The β chains thus acquire pH-dependent delayed autoxidation in the HbO_2 tetramer. The next role was suggested by our studies searching for similar phenomena in normal human erythrocytes under mild heating (Sugawara *et al.*, 2009; 2010; 2011; 2013). It seemed that tilting of the distal (E7) His in turn triggered degradation of the Hb molecule to hemichrome, and subsequent clustering of Heinz bodies within the erythrocyte. Thus, it was suggested that the Hb molecule controls removal of erythrocytes from the blood circulation via triggering degradation of the Hb molecule to hemichrome, and subsequent clustering of Heinz bodies within the erythrocytes depending on the internal and extraneous conditions of the erythrocyte, including pH and temperature. In our recent publication (Sugawara *et al.*, 2011), we reviewed and summarized current interpretations of the oxidative behavior of human Hb and the related results. We emphasized the correlation between the oxidative behavior of human Hb and its inseparably related instability (degradation) of the Hb molecule to hemichrome (hemichrome formation) as well as the involvement of the $\alpha_1-\beta_1$ (and $\alpha_2-\beta_2$) interface of the Hb molecule.

On the basis of the findings and arguments appeared in *Appl. Sci.* 2011:1:13–55 (Sugawara *et al.*), in this chapter, we deliberately aim to deal with necessary basic methods in protein purification and analysis that led us to grasp new roles assigned to the $\alpha_1-\beta_2$ (and $\alpha_2-\beta_1$) interface of the human hemoglobin molecule: one is for stabilizing the HbO_2 tetramer against acidic autoxidation; and the other is for controlling the fate (removal) of its own erythrocyte from the blood circulation. The Hb molecule seems to adequately differentiate between the two types of function (dual roles) responsible for the $\alpha_1-\beta_1$ (and $\alpha_2-\beta_2$) interface from physiological to cellular. In both the $\alpha_1-\beta_1$ (and $\alpha_2-\beta_2$) interface produces a conformational constraint in the constructed chains of the Hb molecule via tilting of the distal (E7) His residues.

2   Human HbO_2 Purification and its Biphasic Autoxidation Curves Observed in Acidic Solutions

The dynamics of the reaction of Hb with O_2 provide them particularly suitable O_2 carriers (Figure 1). In this O_2 binding process of Hb, the iron remains in the ferrous state so that the reaction is an oxygenation, not an oxidation. However, once the molecule is oxygenated, the resultant species (HbO_2) must undergo oxidation by the bound O_2 to the ferric met-form. If HbO_2 is oxidized, the product (ferric metHb) cannot be oxygenated in its present form. *In situ*, the resultant metHb is reduced back to the ferrous state by an intra-erythrocytic nicotinamide adenine dinucleotide (NADH)-dependent reducing system (Scott, *et al.*, 1965; Hultquist & Passon, 1971; Sugita, *et al.*, 1971).

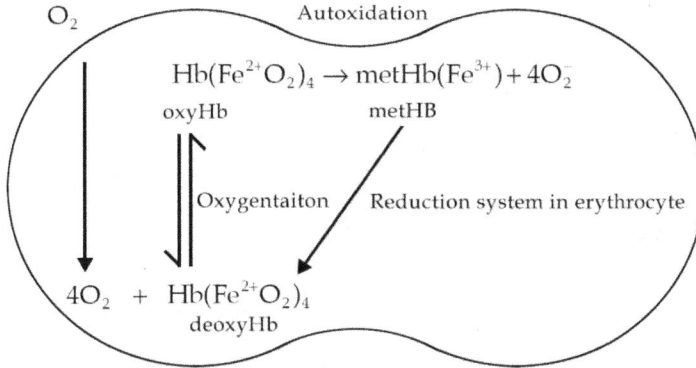

Figure 1: Dynamics of the reaction between Hb and O₂ make the Hb molecule a particularly suitable O₂ carrier.

Since the early works of Brooks (1931; 1935), the oxidative process of ferrous heme iron by bound O_2 (*i.e.*, autoxidation) of human Hb (HbO_2) has been investigated by several workers. Among others, Monsouri and Winterhalter (1973) and Tomoda *et al.* (1981) observed that the rate of autoxidation is strongly dependent upon the pH values of solutions. The study of Monsouri and Winterhalter (1973) also showed that autoxidation of human HbO_2 exhibited a biphasic nature with a initial fast (k_A^f) reaction, followed by a second slower (k_A^s) reaction, when observed in acidic solutions. Following the method of Monsouri and Winterhalter (1973) our previous ultraviolet-visible (UV/Vis) spectroscopic study (Sugawara *et al.*, 1993) indicated that this biphasic behavior seen in acidic solutions disappeared if the pH of solutions was more than 8, and became $k_A^f = k_A^s$.

We deal first with the biphasic nature of the autoxidation of human HbO_2 seen in acidic solutions as well as its purification on the basis of our previous report (Sugawara *et al.*, 1993). This is because the pH-dependent biphasic nature of autoxidation was the starting point that led us to uncover a new function of the α₁–β₁ (and α₂–β₂) interface of the Hb molecule.

HbO_2 was prepared from freshly drawn samples of human blood (total, 50–80 mL) obtained from healthy donors (Sugawara *et al.*, 1993). Samples were centrifuged at 2,400 × g for 10 min to remove supernatant plasma and buffy coats. The erythrocytes obtained were washed five times with ice-cooled 0.9% NaCl solution (saline) by centrifugation and hemolyzed by adding the same volume of ice-cooled distilled water. The hemolysate was then fractionated with ammonium sulfate between 20% saturation and 70% saturation at pH 6.8. After dialysis, this solution was passed through two Sephadex G-50 columns (5 × 90 cm) equilibrated with 10 mM Tris-HCl (pH 8.6). The effluent Hb fraction was further separated using a diethylaminoethyl (DEAE)-cellulose column (3 × 15 cm) equilibrated with 10 mM Tris-HCl (pH 8.6) and washed sequentially with step-wise changing of buffer solutions as follows: (i) 60 mM Tris-HCl (pH 8.0); (ii) 100 mM Tris-HCl (pH 7.5); finally (iii) 100 mM NaCl with 100 mM Tris-HCl (pH 8.0). HbO_2 (human adult) was eluted out as the major fraction with 60 mM Tris-HCl (pH 8.0) and used in the experiments after dialyzing against 5 mM Tris-HCl buffer (pH 8.5). Note here that Sephadex G-50 (fine) was a product of Pharmacia (Uppsala, Sweden), and DEAE-cellulose was purchased from Whatman (Maidstone, UK).

The autoxidation reaction was measured by UV/Vis spectroscopic means in 0.1 M buffer over a wide pH range (5.3–10.5) at 37 °C. Two milliliters of solution containing 0.2 M buffer was placed in a test tube and incubated in a waterbath maintained at 37 ± 0.1 °C using a NESLAB temperature control system (Model RTE-100 or 111 or 210; NESLAB Instruments, Inc., Portsmouth, NH, USA). The reaction was started by adding the same volume of fresh HbO_2 solution (50–125 μM in heme contents). The reaction mixture was then quickly transferred to a spectrophotometric cell (Spectrocell, Type Inject-A-Cell; Funakoshi Co., Tokyo, Japan) with a screwcap stopper. Changes in absorption at 450–650 nm were recorded on the same chart at measured time intervals. Spectra were recorded using an UV/Vis spectrophotometer (JASCO, Model Ubest-50 or V-560 or V-570; Japan Spectroscopic Co., Tokyo, Japan), equipped with a thermostatically controlled (within ± 0.1 °C) cell holder. At the final state of each run, Hb molecules were all completely converted to the ferric met form by addition of potassium ferricyanide. The buffers used were: acetate for pH 4.5–5.5, 2-(N-morpholino) ethanesulfonic acid monohydrate (MES) for pH 5.0–6.75, N-2-hydroxyethylpiperazine-N'-2-ethanesulfonic acid (HEPES) for pH 6.55–8.3, 2-(cyclohexylamino) ethanesulfonic acid for pH 8.2–10.2, and 3-cyclohexylaminopropanesulfonic acid for pH 10.0–10.5.

Figure 2 shows an example of the UV/Vis spectrophotometric changes over time from 450 nm to 650 nm for autoxidation of human HbO_2 when observed in 0.1 M MES buffer (pH 5.3) at 37 °C. In this reaction process, HbO_2 was autoxidized to its ferric met form through thetendency of the bound O_2 to oxidize ferrous heme iron (II) with generation of superoxide ani- on radical ($O_2^{\cdot-}$ or simply designated as O_2^-):

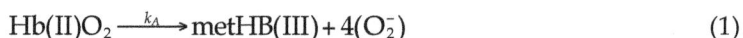

$$Hb(II)O_2 \xrightarrow{\;k_A\;} metHB(III) + 4(O_2^-) \tag{1}$$

Here k_A represents the observed rate constant of the reaction at a given pH and temperature. The reaction process was followed in each experimental run by the ratio ($[HbO_2]_t/[HbO_2]_0$) of HbO_2 concentration after time t to that at time $t = 0$ that was monitored by the absorbance ratio of $(A_t - A_\infty)/(A_0 - A_\infty)$ at 576 nm (α-peak of HbO_2). The ratio was then plotted against time. Each curve shown in Figure 3 represents the $-\ln([HbO_2]_t/[HbO_2]_0)$ *versus* time plot (first-order plot) for this phenomenon. In acidic solutions (Figure 3(a)), the reaction was biphasic and can be described by first-order kinetics containing two rate constants as follows:

$$d[HbO_2]/dt = P \cdot \exp(-k_A^f \cdot t) + (1 - P) \cdot \exp(-k_A^s \cdot t). \tag{2}$$

This equation was originally proposed by Monsouri & Winterhalter (1973), where k_A^f and k_A^s represent first-order rate constants for the initial fast oxidation and the second slower oxidation, respectively, and P is the molar fraction of the initial fast component. In Figure 3(a), solid lines represent the best fitting derived by the least-squares method using the equation to each run. However, as shown in Figure 3(b), when the pH of solutions is more than 8, a plot of $-\ln([HbO_2]_t/[HbO_2]_0)$ *versus* time showed a single-phase reaction with a single first-order rate constant, although curve fittings could be

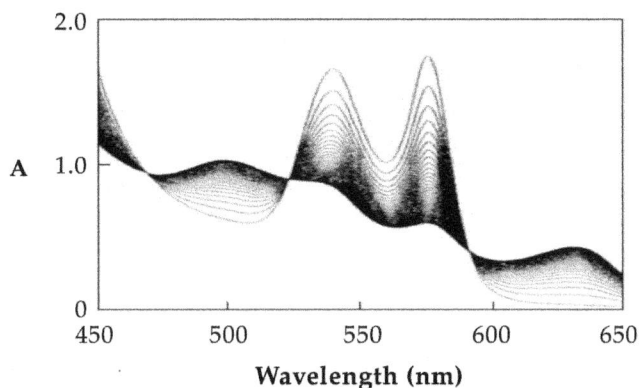

Figure 2: UV/Vis spectral changes over time from 450 nm to 650 nm following human HbO$_2$ autoxidation, redrawn from Sugawara *et al.* (2011). The changes were monitored in 0.1 M 2-(N-morpholino) ethanesulfonic acid monohydrate (MES) buffer (pH 5.3) at 37 °C. Conditions: HbO$_2$ concentration was 125 µM (in heme contents); and the scanning interval was 30 min.

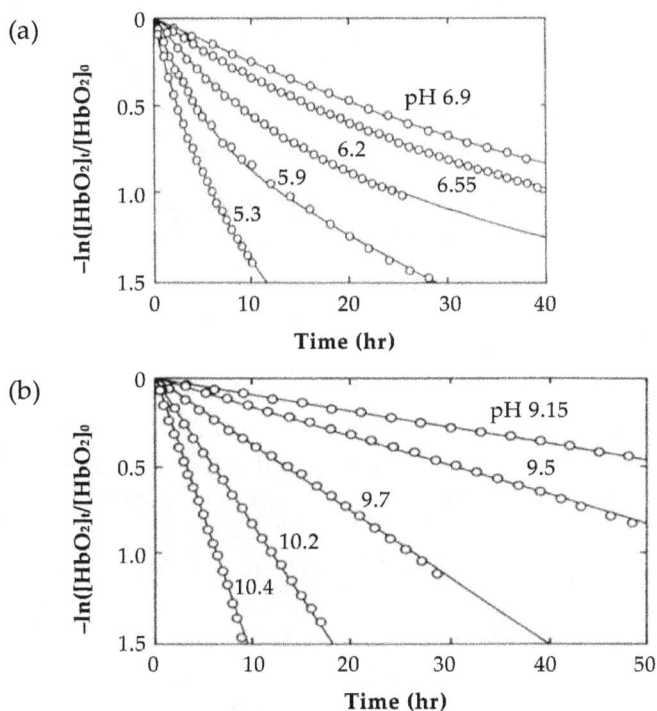

Figure 3: A −ln([HbO$_2$]$_t$/[HbO$_2$]$_0$) *versus* time plot (first-order plot) for human HbO$_2$ autoxidation, redrawn from Sugawara *et al.* (2011). (a) Acidic autoxidation seen in acidic-to-neutral pH ranges and (b) alkaline autoxidation in alkali solutions. Solid lines represent the least-squares fitting to experimental data in each run. Conditions: HbO$_2$ concentration was 50–125 µM (in heme contents); and the reaction proceeded in 0.1 M buffer at 37 °C.

made using the same equation under conditions of $P = 0.5$ and $k_A^f = k_A^s$. Thus, it was shown that the biphasic behavior seen in acidic solutions gradually disappeared with increasing pH of solutions and completely disappeared if the pH of solutions was more than 8.

In this way, the kinetic parameters and molar fraction of the initial fast component (P) for the biphasic nature of human HbO_2 autoxidation were established in each run in 0.1 M buffer at 37 °C (Table 1).

pH	P	$k_A^f (h^{-1})$	$k_A^s (h^{-1})$	k_A^s / k_A^f
5.3	0.47	0.438	0.078	0.178
5.9	0.48	0.270	0.030	0.111
6.2	0.48	0.134	0.0154	0.115
6.55	0.49	0.070	0.010	0.142
6.9	0.53	0.0465	0.0073	0.157
9.15	0.50	0.0095	0.0095	1.0
9.5	0.50	0.0184	0.0184	1.0
9.7	0.50	0.0381	0.0381	1.0
10.2	0.50	0.080	0.080	1.0
10.4	0.50	0.157	0.157	1.0

Table 1: Summary of kinetic parameters for the autoxidation of human HbO_2 in 0.1 M buffer obtained by least-squares fitting to the experimental data in each run, redrawn from Sugawara *et al.* (2011).

It was evident that the values of P varied from 0.47 to 0.53. This means that HbO_2 was autoxidized with half of the component via the reaction process with the initial fast reaction with k_A^f and the other half via the procedure with the second slower rate (k_A^s). Thus, autoxidation of human HbO_2 may be written as follows:

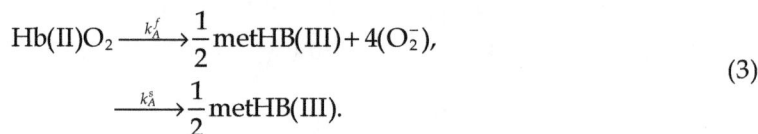

$$Hb(II)O_2 \xrightarrow{k_A^f} \frac{1}{2}metHB(III) + 4(O_2^-),$$

$$\xrightarrow{k_A^s} \frac{1}{2}metHB(III).$$

(3)

To clarify the processes behind this phenomenon, the obtained values of k_A^s / k_A^f were plotted against the pH of solutions (Figure 4). In Figure 4, the solid line shows that the computed curve obtained by the least-squares method fitted the experimental data over the whole range of pH 5–10.5, where a single dissociable group, AH with K_a, was as sumed to be involved in the reaction:

$$HbO_2 \xleftrightarrow{K_a} HbO_2(A^-).$$

(4)

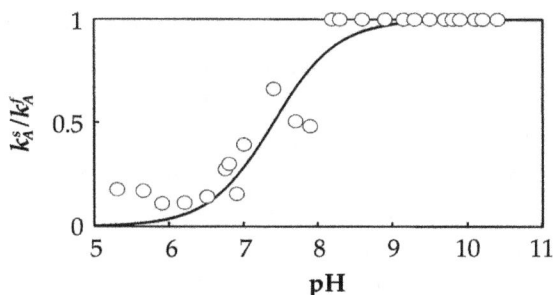

Figure 4: A k_A^s / k_A^f *versus* pH plot for human HbO_2 autoxidation, redrawn from Sugawara *et al.* (2011). The solid line stands for the best-suited fitting under the assumption that a single, dissociable group, AH with K_a, can be involved in the reaction. This was achieved with the setting $pK_a = 7.4$.

For neutral amino acids, acid-base equilibrium is usually given by the dissociation constant: $AH \leftrightarrow A^- + H^+$ and thus $K_a = [A^-] \cdot [H^+]/[AH]$. The best fitting was achieved when $pK_a = 7.4$ (at 37 °C). In this regard, Hermans & Rialdi (1965) and Fasman (1976) reported microcalorimetric ionization data on amino-acid residues for sperm whale myoglobin (Mb) in which they assigned the His residue with values of $pK_a = 6.62$, the standard Gibbs energy $(\Delta G°) = 37.7$ kJ· mol^{-1}, the enthalpy $(\Delta H°) = 29.7$ kJ· mol^{-1}, and the entropy $(\Delta S°) = -26.8$ J· mol^{-1}· K^{-1}. It is unwise to identify a dissociation group only by its pK_a value because of the anomalies often found in proteins. Hence, we confirmed that AH must be a His residue assuming that the primary and tertiary structures of α and β subunits are remarkably similar to each other and to Mb. This fact provides information for the existence of a pH-sensed molecular device that can manifest the biphasic autoxidation of the HbO_2 tetramer via participation of a single amino-acid residue with $pK_a = 7.4$ (at 37 °C).

3   Chain Separation of the Constituted Chains from Human HbO₂ and Rate Measurements of the Chains

To not only elucidate the pH-dependent biphasic characteristics of human HbO_2 autoxidation but also to clarify how the Hb molecule can prompt the range of fast (k_A^f) and slow (k_A^s) components against pH values of the solutions, chain separation of the constituted chains from the parent molecules is essential. This section looks into the results of our study investigating chain separation of α and β chains from the HbO_2 tetramer and their rate measurements (Sugawara *et al.*, 2011).

Isolation of α and β chains from the parent molecules was made using sodium *p*-hydroxymercuribenzoate (*p*-MB) by a one-column method using carboxymethyl (CM)-cellulose and alternatively by a two-column method. The following procedure was for two-column method; details for the one-column method can be found in Sugawara *et al.* (2003). One-hundred milligrams of *p*-MB were dissolved in 2 mL of 0.1 M NaCl and neutralized with 1 M CH₃COOH. This was reacted with 10 mL of HbO₂ solution in 30 mM phosphate buffer, pH 6.0, in the presence of 0.1 M NaCl. To obtain the $\alpha_{p\text{-MB}}$ chains, the mercurated HbO₂ solution was adjusted to pH 8.2 by filtration through a Sephadex G-25 column (25 × 40 cm) equilibrated with 15 mM HEPES buffer (pH 8.2). The resultant solution was then passed through a DEAE-cellulose column (3 × 12 cm) equilibrated with the same buffer. Under these chromatographic conditions, the $\alpha_{p\text{-MB}}$ chains were readily eluted out because the unreacted HbO₂ and mercurated β chains were retained on top of the column at this pH. With respect to separation of the $\beta_{p\text{-MB}}$ chains, the pH of the mercurated HbO₂ solution was adjusted to 6.7 using a Sephadex G-25 column (25 × 40 cm) equilibrated with 10 mM phosphate buffer (pH 6.7) and the solution applied on a CM-cellulose column (3 × 12 cm) equilibrated with the same buffer. Under these conditions, only the $\beta_{p\text{-MB}}$ chains were eluted completely. Measurement of the autoxidation rate for the isolated chains was identical to the procedure of rate measurements for HbO₂. Remind about that Sephadex G-25 (fine) was a product of Pharmacia (Uppsala, Sweden), and CM-cellulose (CM-32) was purchased from Whatmann (Maidstone, UK).

According to the method of Boyer (1954), free sulfhydryl groups of the regenerated α or β chains were titrated UV/Vis spectrophotometrically at 250 nm with p-MB in 0.1 M buffer, pH 7.0. The details of regeneration of SH groups from mercuribenzoated α and β chains can be seen in Yasuda et al. (2002). The resulting contents were 1.0 (1.05 ± 0.08) for the α chain and 2.0 (2.01 ± 0.08) for the β chain, respectively, as might be expected from the number of cysteines located at positions $\alpha 104(\text{G11})$, $\beta 93(\text{F9})$ and $\beta 112(\text{G14})$ for HbA (Yasuda et al., 2002).

Figure 5 shows the pH profiles for the autoxidation rate of the isolated $\alpha_{p\text{-MB}}$ and $\beta_{p\text{-MB}}$ chains. With reference to the rates (k_A^s and k_A^f) of the parent molecules calculated from biphasic autoxidation curves, the isolated chains were shown to be oxidized much more rapidly to the ferric met-form over the entire pH range (5–10.5) because the reaction followed simple, first-order kinetics as follows:

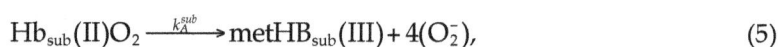

$$\text{Hb}_{\text{sub}}(\text{II})\text{O}_2 \xrightarrow{k_A^{sub}} \text{metHB}_{\text{sub}}(\text{III}) + 4(\text{O}_2^-),\tag{5}$$

where Hb$_{\text{sub}}$ represents each subunit of the Hb molecule. It was also shown that the rate of the initial first component (k_A^f) of the parent molecules was found to lie closer to the values of k_A for the isolated $\alpha_{p\text{-MB}}$ and $\beta_{p\text{-MB}}$ chains if the pH of solutions was less than 6.

Similar pH profiles were obtained for p-MB-removed chains, i.e., the α_{SH} and β_{SH} chains. p-MB can be removed from the $\alpha_{p\text{-MB}}$ and $\beta_{p\text{-MB}}$ chains by incubation with 2-mercaptoethanol, as described elsewhere (Tsuruga, et al., 1998). In separated-chain solutions, the protein is known to exist in equilibrium of $\alpha \leftrightarrow \alpha_2$ or $\beta \leftrightarrow \beta_4$, respectively. Under our experimental conditions, the monomeric form (87%) was present in the separated α chain, whereas the tetrameric form (99%) was predominant in the β chain. This estimation was made on the basis of the results by McDonald et al. (1987).

Thus, it became evident that the isolated α and β chains could be oxidized much more readily over the measured pH range (5–10.5) when compared with the respective rates of the parent molecules as a reference. With respect to the difference in the rate between the isolated individual chains, this seemed to be within reasonable experimental errors in the values of $\alpha_{p\text{-MB}}$ and $\beta_{p\text{-MB}}$ chains, and the α_{SH} and β_{SH} chains.

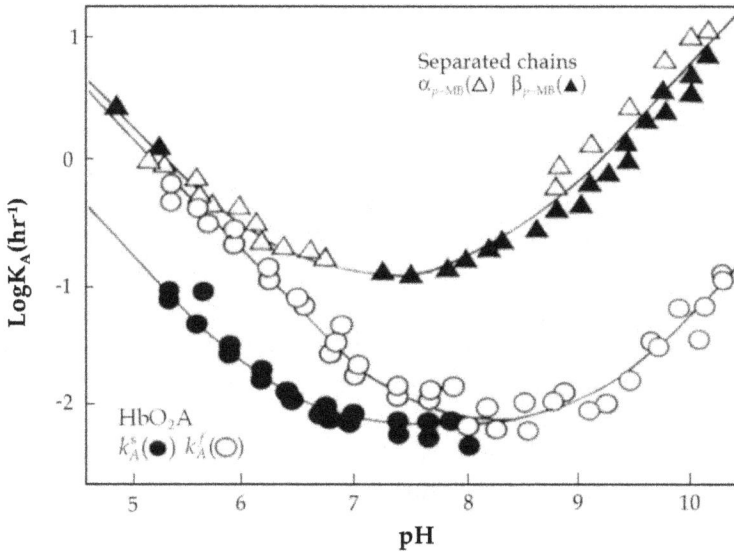

Figure 5: Logarithmic values of first-order rate *versus* pH plot for autoxidation of the isolated α ($\alpha_{p\text{-MB}}$) and β ($\beta_{p\text{-MB}}$) chains with a reference to the relevant values (k_A^f and k_A^s) of the parent molecules, redrawn from Sugawara *et al.* (2011). Conditions: the concentration of isolated α and β chains was 50 µM (in heme contents); the reaction rate was measured in 0.1 M buffer at 37 °C.

4   UV/Vis Spectroscopic Procedure for Detecting Innate Instability of the Hb Molecule and its Degradation to Hemichrome

Autoxidation seems to be inseparably related to the instability of the Hb molecule and its degradation to hemichrome. It has been suggested that the oxidation (autoxidation) process of Hb may be associated with transformation of the oxidized molecule (high-spin Fe^{3+}) into hemichrome, the formation of which can result in the accumulation of soluble and insoluble hemichromes and precipitation (Rchmilewitz, *et al.*, 1969; Rchmilewitz, *et al.*, 1971; Rchmilewitz, 1974; Winterbourn & Carrell, 1974; Macdonald, 1994; Rifkind, *et al.*, 1994). Formation of hemichrome is enhanced in separated α and β chains (Rchmilewitz, *et al.*, 1971; Rifkind, *et al.*, 1994; Brounori, *et al.*, 1975; Tomoda, *et al.*, 1978a; McDonald, *et al.*, 1987; Sugawara *et al.*, 2003). In our UV/Vis spectroscopic study (Sugawara *et al.*, 2003), it was shown that human HbO_2 from healthy donors tended to degrade to produce hemichrome even at close to physiological temperatures and pH. This section looks about the innate molecular instability of Hb, which triggers degradation of the molecule to hemichrome. This process is readily detected through UV/Vis spectroscopic observation during the entire process of autoxidation of human HbO_2 (Sugawara *et al.*, 2003).

Figure 6 indicates how autoxidation is inseparably related to the instability of the Hb molecule and its degradation to hemichrome. Figure 6(a) shows the spectrophotometric changes over time from 450 nm to 650 nm when fresh HbO_2 was placed in o.1 M MES buffer (pH 5.0) at 37 °C. It proceeded without showing any hemichrome formation during the entire process. Contrary to this, the situations demonstrated in Figure 6 (b–d) are very different. Figure 6(b) illustrates the observed UV/Vis spectra with time for hemichrome formation during autoxidation of HbO_2 when HbO_2 was incubated in 0.1 M MES buffer (pH 6.5) at 40 °C. HbO_2 was autoxidized to its ferric met form. However, sudden disruption of the spectra was observed during the late stage of the reaction whereby hemichrome formation could be detected by elevation of the baseline and a shift in isosbestic points caused by precipitation. Similarly it took place at the intermediate stage in 0.1 M HEPES buffer (pH 8.0) at 40 °C in the case of Figure 6(c), while at the initial stage in the case of Figure 6(d) in which immediately after fresh HbO_2 was transfer to the cuvette in 0.1 M HEPES buffer (pH 7.0) at 45 °C.

In brief, hemichrome formation could be readily detected even in HbO_2 at every stage during the course of autoxidation (*i.e.*, during the initial, intermediate, and final stages) while varying the temperature of the solution from 35 °C to 55 °C and the pH from 4.5 to 10.5. As its occurrence was a function of not only the pH and temperature of the solution, but also of the progress of the autoxidation of HbO_2, in Figure 7, we attempted to categorize the phenomenon into the following four cases in terms of $[HbO_2]_{t=E.P.}/[HbO_2]_0$:

1. $t = 0$ or $[HbO_2]_{t=E.P.}/[HbO_2]_0 = 1 \leq t_{E.P.} < [HbO_2]_{t=E.P.}/[HbO_2]_0 = 0.75$;

2. $[HbO_2]_{t=E.P.}/[HbO_2]_0 = 0.75 \leq t_{E.P} < [HbO_2]_{t=E.P.}/[HbO_2]_0 = 0.25$;

3. $t_{E.P.} \leq [HbO_2]_{t=E.P.}/[HbO_2]_0 = 0.25$;

4.   no hemichrome formation during the entire process.

Here E.P. is the observed emergence point of hemichrome formation in each run. $[HbO_2]_{t=E.P.}/[HbO_2]_0$ is the ratio of HbO_2 concentration after time $t = E.P.$ to that at time $t = 0$ and can be monitored by the absorbance ratio of $(A_t - A_\infty)/(A_0 - A_\infty)$ at 576 nm (α-peak of HbO_2). $[HbO_2]_{t=E.P.}/[HbO_2]_0 = 0.5$ represents equal mixtures of HbO_2 and metHb, *i.e.*, the midpoint of the autoxidation reaction. Hence, case (1) means that hemichrome formation was noticeable at the initial stage of autoxidation. Accordingly, case (2) indicates its occurrence at the intermediate stage, and case (3) at the final stage. In Figure 7, the symbols used correspond to: ● for case (1), ▲ for case (2), △ for case (3) and ○ for case (4). To determine if the phenomenon was represented by case (3) or case (4), the reaction mixture was converted to metHb by the addition of small amounts of ferricyanide and maintained at the given temperature for 2 days to see if hemichrome precipitation occurred.

Thus, the findings suggested that human HbO_2 was highly susceptible to hemichrome formation, even under physiological pH and temperature. Certainly, the broken lines in Figure 7(a) show that the threshold for this HbO_2 susceptibility to hemichrome in relation to pH and temperature. When compared with the tetrameric parent molecule, the isolated α ($\alpha_{p\text{-MB}}$) and β ($\beta_{p\text{-MB}}$) chains were found to have much higher suscep-

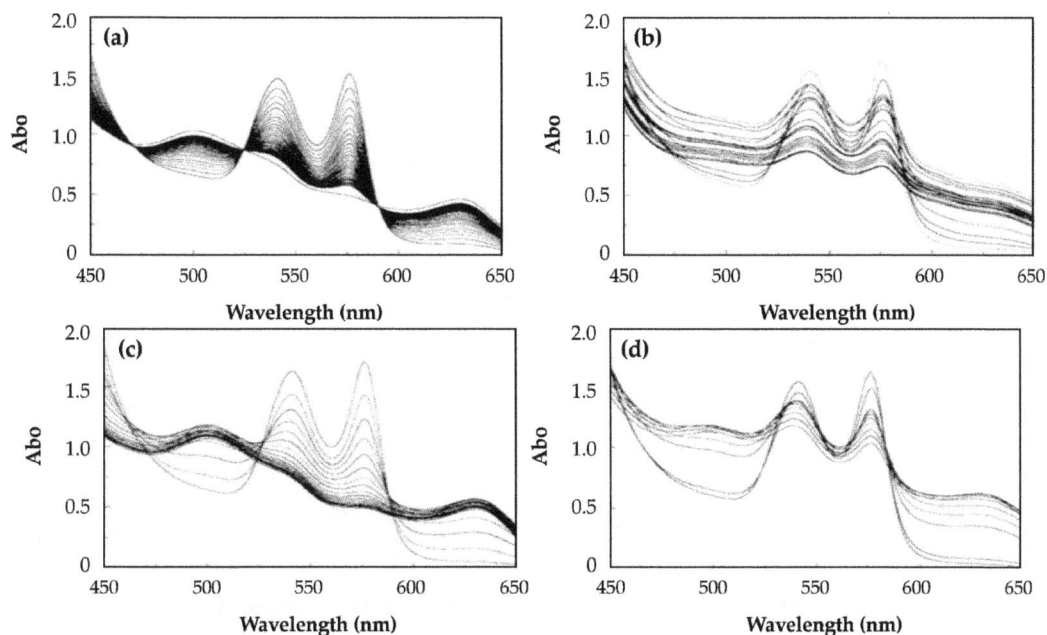

Figure 6: Hemichrome formation associated with human HbO₂ autoxidation, redrawn from Sugawara *et al.* (2011). UV/Vis spectral changes over time for hemichrome formation associated with human HbO₂ autoxidation in which the reaction was monitored (a) in 0.1 M MES buffer (pH 5.0) at 37 °C and scanning interval = 15 min; (b) in 0.1 M MES buffer (pH 6.5) at 40 °C and scanning interval = 150 min; (c) in 0.1 M HEPES buffer (pH 8.0) at 40 °C and scanning interval = 150 min; (d) in 0.1 M HEPES buffer (pH 7.0) at 45 °C and scanning interval = 60 min. Conditions: HbO₂ concentration was 235 µM (in heme contents).

tibilities to hemichrome formation, and showed individual pH–temperature diagrams (Figure 7(b)). The occurrence of hemichrome can be described as follows:

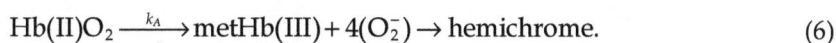

$$Hb(II)O_2 \xrightarrow{k_A} metHb(III) + 4(O_2^-) \rightarrow hemichrome. \tag{6}$$

We must be careful when evaluating the data of the isolated chains shown in Figure 5. Because of the instability of Hb molecules and their relationship to hemichrome, the first-order rate constant for the isolated chains was established in each experimental run using only the initial slope of the $-\ln([Hb_{sub}O_2]_t/[Hb_{sub}O_2]_0)$ *versus* time plot. Once hemichrome precipitation arose, one could not get the endpoint spectrum (the ferric met form) of the reaction, whereby Hb molecules in the reaction mixture should be all completely converted to the ferric met form by addition of potassium ferricyanide. Hence, measurement must be confined within the initial range, in which existence of isosbestic points of the spectra that means non-occurrence of hemichrome formation during the entire reaction process was surely guaranteed.

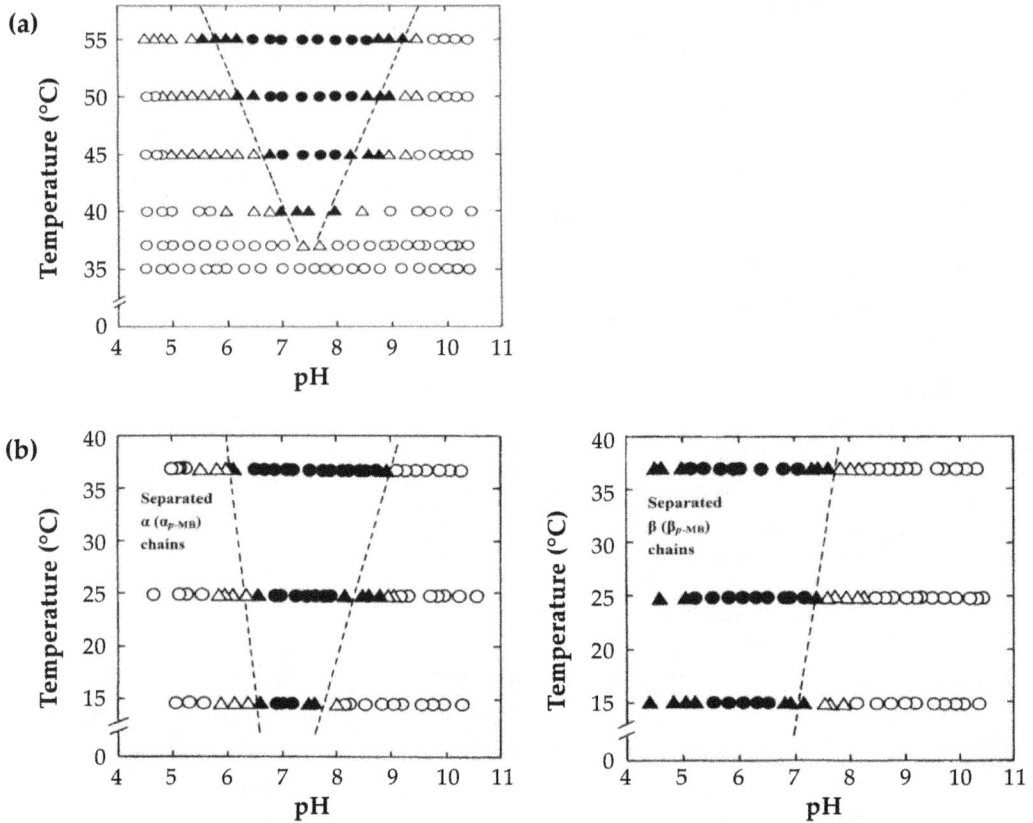

Figure 7: Hemichrome formation associated with human HbO$_2$ autoxidation, re-drawn from Sugawara *et al.* (2013). (a) pH–temperature diagram for HbO$_2$ autoxidation. (b) pH–temperature diagrams for the autoxidation of isolated α and β chains. The symbols used are as follows: ●– hemichrome formation noticeable at the initial stage during the course of autoxidation; ▲– at the intermediate stage; △– at the final stage; ○– autoxidation reaction proceeded with no hemichrome formation during the entire process.

5   Hemichrome Formation Test for Monomeric Bovine Heart Myoglobin (MbO$_2$)

As mentioned above, human HbO$_2$ was supposed to be highly susceptible to hemichrome formation (even under physiological pH and temperature) in terms of pH- and temperature-dependent hemichrome emergence detected by UV/Vis spectroscopy. Moreover, the isolated α ($\alpha_{p\text{-}MB}$) and β ($\beta_{p\text{-}MB}$) chains were shown to degrade much more readily to produce hemichrome over the measured pH and temperature ranges, when compared with the tetrameric parent molecule. Along with this line, the question may be arisen as to whether the monomeric myoglobin (MbO$_2$) have similar propensity of human HbO$_2$ to hemichrome.

Regarding to this issue, a series of experiments using UV/Vis spectroscopic observation for hemichrome emergence (hemichrome emergence tests) were undertaken for monomeric bovine heart MbO_2 (Sugawara *et al.*, 2003). At first, these tests were conducted in 0.1 M buffer over the same range of pH (pH 4.5 to 10.5) and temperature (35 to 55 °C). However, our attempts failed to recognize any hemichrome emergence in this pH and temperature range. In order to further check this point, we made an attempt to expand our tests to temperature region exceeding 55 °C. In this respect, we employed thermal denaturation measurement for MbO_2 using differential scanning calorimetry (DSC). Ultimately we engaged in these tests over a wide temperature range for bovine heart MbO_2 from physiological to temperatures just before thermal unfolding (Sugawara *et al.*, 2003).

Mb was isolated from bovine heart muscle, in which the essential step was chromatographic separation of MbO_2 from metMb on a DEAE-cellulose column. According to our previous method (Shikama & Sugawara, 1978; Sugawara & Shikama, 1979), Mb was extracted over night at pH 8.0 from the minced muscle of fresh bovine heart with 1.5 volumes of ice-coold distilled water. All procedures were carried out at low temperature (0–4 °C) as far as possible. The extract was fractionated with ammonium sulfate between 70 and 100% saturation at pH 6.9 in the presence of 5×10^{-4} M ethylenediaminetetraacetic acid (EDTA). The precipitate was centrifuged down at 30,000 g for 15 min and dissolved in a minimum volume of 5 mM Tris-Hcl buffer, pH 8.4, and the solution was then dialyzed against the same buffer containing 5×10^{-4} M EDTA. The crude Mb solution which contained a large amount of hemoglobin (bovine) was applied to a couple of Sephadex G-50 columns (5 × 90 cm) equilibrated with 5 mM Tris-HCl [tris(hydroxymethyl)aminomethane hydrochloride] buffer, pH 8.4. The column was then eluted with the same buffer to separate myoglobin completely from hemoglobin, and the effluent Mb solution was dialyzed against 5 mM Tris-HCl buffer (pH 8.4) containing 5×10^{-4} M EDTA. At this stage about 60% of the Mb solution was in the oxy-form (MbO_2). The dialyzed Mb solution was applied to a DEAE-cellulose column (4 × 15 cm) which had been equilibrated with 5 mM Tris-HCl buffer, pH 8.4. The column was washed with a large volume of 15 mM Tris-HCl buffer, pH 8.4 until the brown-colored band of metMb was eluted out completely. The oxy-form (MbO_2) was then eluted out with 30 mM mM Tris-HCl buffer, pH 8.4. In this oxy-form (MbO_2) isolation procedure, Sephadex G-50 (Pharmacia, Uppsala, Sweden; fine) and DEAE-cellulose (Whatman, Maidstone, UK; De-32) were used.

Thermal denaturation of bovine heart Mb was assessed by differential scanning calorimetry in terms of T_d, the temperature at which the transition is half complete. A non-adiabatic calorimeter (DSC, Seiko I & E DSC-10/SSC-570 Thermal Controller Model, Tokyo, Japan) was used at a heating rate of 1 °C/min and at protein concentrations of 1.5–5.5 mg/mL. After treatment of the raw DSC data, in which correction of the sample curve for changes of slope observed in a run with buffer in each cell was made by subtracting the buffer curve from the protein curve point by point, the linear portions of the corrected curve corresponding to pre- and post-transition base lines were extrapolated to T_d. T_d was also determined by successive area measurements until the vertical line drawn at T_d divided the peak area into two halves. The area under heat capacity curve was determined by means of a planimeter.

Figure 8(a) is an example of DSC scanning for MbO_2 in 0.1 M HEPES buffer at pH 7.4. In terms of T_d, that is, the temperature at which the thermal unfolding is half complete, Figure 8(b) gives an upper limit temperature to examine whether hemichrome formation associated with autoxidation can be observed in monomeric MbO_2 or not, although the concentration (0.91 mM) used for DSC measurement was 100 times higher than that of our hemichrome emergence test.

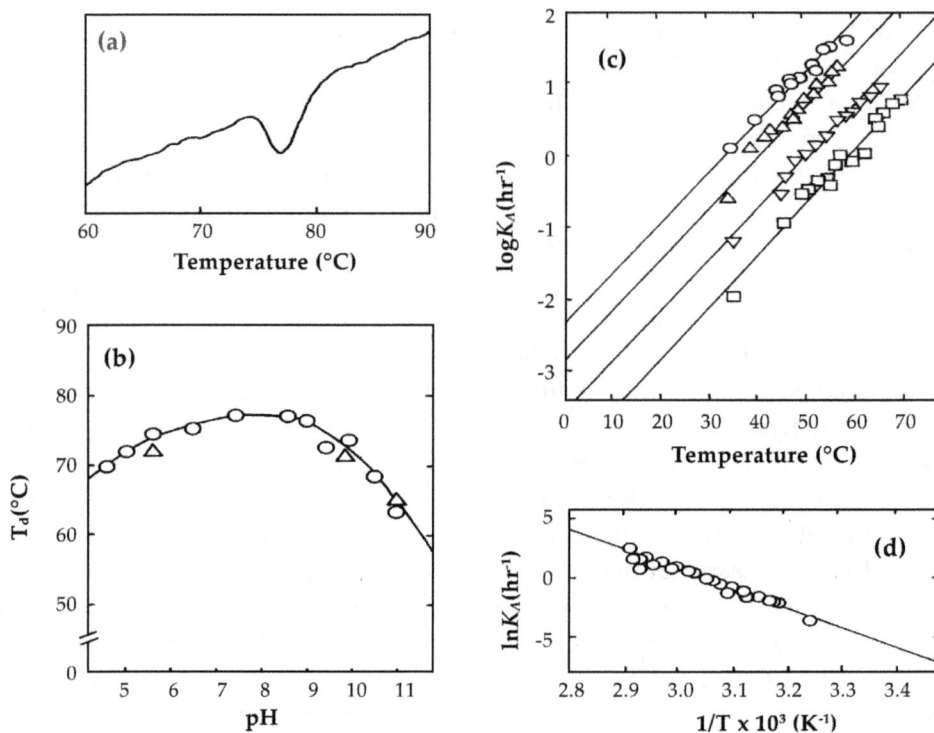

Figure 8: Hemichrome formation test for monomeric bovine heart Mb, redrawn from Sugawara *et al.* (2013). (a) Tracing of DSC curve for unfolding of bovine heart MbO_2 in 0.1 M HEPES buffer at pH 7.4. Protein concentration was 2.35 mg·ml^{-1} (0.91 mM). (b) By means of DSC, the properties of thermal unfolding of bovine heart MbO_2 and metMb were depicted as a function of pH and temperature in terms of T_d (*i.e.*, the temperature at which the transition is half complete). Protein concentration was 1.5 - 5.5 mg·ml^{-1} (0.91 to 5.81 mM). O: MbO_2, △: metMb. (c) Temperature dependence of first-order rate constants, k_A of autoxidation of bovine heart MbO_2. The autoxidation was measured in 0.1 M buffer at a given pH and temperature under air saturated condition. The resulting data of pH 5.0 in 0.1 M MES buffer (O), 6.0 in 0.1 M MES buffer (△), 7.0 in 0.1 M HEPES buffer (∇) and 9.0 in 0.1 M CHES buffer (□) were plotted against a given temperature. MbO_2 concentration was 97μM. (d) Arrhenius plot of k_A, measured in 0.1 M HEPES buffer at pH 7.4.

Considering an upper limit temperature in each run, our search for detecting possible hemichrome emergence was carried out by varying pH of the solution from 4.5 to 10.5 and varying the temperature from the physiological level to the level just before thermal unfolding. Typical examples are shown in Figure 8(c, d), where k_A represents the observed first-order rate constant of autoxidation of MbO_2 at a given pH and temperature. In air-saturated buffers, MbO_2 is oxidized by the bound O_2 to its ferric met form (metMb) with generation of O_2^- as essentially in the same manner as HbO_2:

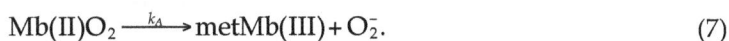

$$Mb(II)O_2 \xrightarrow{k_A} metMb(III) + O_2^-. \tag{7}$$

Here k_A is given by:

$$d[MbO_2] / dt = k_A \cdot [MbO_2]. \tag{8}$$

In the hemichrome emergence tests, the ratio of MbO_2 concentration after time t to that at time $t = 0$ was monitored by absorbance change, for instance, at α-peak (581 nm) of MbO_2. In each run, k_A in hr^{-1} was determined from the slope of linear plots of $-\ln([MbO_2]_t/[MbO_2]_0)$ *versus* time and plotted against temperature of the solution in Figure 8(c) and against the inverse of the absolute temperature, that is Arrhenius plots in Figure 8(d). In these figures, our experimental data gave a single straight line against the temperature examined at constant pH of the solution. This implies that there was no hemichrome emergence (formation) under these circumstances. This point was also confirmed by the resulting activation energy, E_A. From the slope of each straight line on Arrhenius plots shown in Figure 8(d), E_A was calculated and appeared to be almost constant, i.e., 121.55 ± 14.38 KJ·mol^{-1} (29.08 ± 3.44 Kcal·mol^{-1}) over the pH range of 4.5 to 10.5 and at the temperature range greater than or equal to 35 °C. These were in good agreement with those observed by Gotoh and Shikama (1974), where E_A is almost constant with the value of 26.5 Kcal·mol^{-1} (110.77 KJ·mol^{-1}) over pH range of 5 to 10 using bovine heart MbO_2 based on the measurements of the rate at 0, 15, 25, and 30 °C.

We, therefore, concluded that the monomeric bovine heart Mb (MbO_2) did not show any propensity for hemichrome formation over a wide pH range of 4.5 to 10.5 and over a wide temperature range from physiological to temperatures just before thermal unfolding. Contradictorily, in the tetrameric human HbO_2, higher susceptibilities to hemichrome formation were pronounced as well as occurrence of hemichrome emergence even under physiological pH and temperature. It seemed that this can be the most significant feature of human HbO_2 as O_2^- carrying protein in the blood.

6   UV/Vis Spectrophotometric, Isoelectric-Focusing Electrophoretic and Polyacrylamide Gel Electrophoretic Studies for the Autoxidation of Human HbO₂

In this section, we focus on our findings resulting from UV/Vis spectrophotometric, isoelectric-focusing electrophoretic and polyacrylamide gel electrophoretic measurements for autoxidation of human HbO_2 (Sugawara *et al.*, 2011). This is because it has been demonstrated that the reaction process of the HbO_2 autoxidation should be reflected by the presence of intermediate Hb with valency hybrids such as $(\alpha^{2+}\beta^{3+})_2$ and $(\alpha^{3+}\beta^{2+})_2$ (Tomoda *et al.*, 1981) and a different oxidation rate due to different Hb chains (Mansouri & Winterhalter, 1973). In our experiment (Sugawara *et al.*, 2011), we employed isoelectric-focusing electrophoresis on an ampholine plate gel as for detecting the valency hybrid intermediates. Simultaneously, as soon as chain separation was achieved using p-MB, 7.5% polyacrylamide gel electrophoresis was undertaken for a series of samples to analyze the oxidized ratio of the constituted chains after time t to that at time $t = 0$. A schematic diagram of this simultaneous multi-measurements technique is represented by Figure 9.

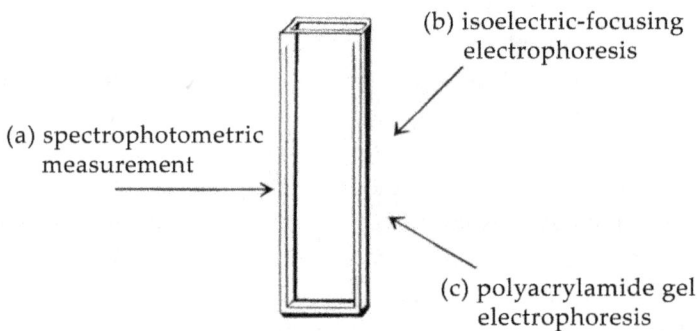

(b) isoelectric-focusing electrophoresis

(a) spectrophotometric measurement

(c) polyacrylamide gel electrophoresis

Figure 9: Schematic diagram of our simultaneous multi-measurements technique for observing the autoxidation of human HbO_2.

The experiment was carried out in 0.05 M phosphate buffer (pH 5.0) in the presence of 20% (v/v) glycerol at 37 °C after setting the HbO_2 concentration to 1.25 mM (heme content). We employed a nearly tenfold higher HbO_2 concentration than the usual HbO_2 concentration so that the reaction was monitored using a 1-mm photometric cell instead of a conventional 1-cm cell. Glycerol was used as a protein stabilizer to prevent hemichrome formation during the entire time course of the experiment. For these UV/Vis spectrophotometric, isoelectric-focusing electrophoretic and polyacrylamide gel electrophoretic measurements, an appropriate volume of 0.1 M buffer solution was placed in a test tube and incubated in a waterbath maintained at 37 ± 0.1 °C using a NESLAB temperature control system (Model RTE-1111). The reaction was started by adding the same volume of HbO_2 solution preincubated in the same waterbath. The reaction mixture was then divided into two. One portion was quickly transferred to a spectrophotometric cell with a 1-mm path length (monitoring cell) and the other to a conventional cell with a 1-cm path length (sampling cell). Both cells were maintained at 37 ± 0.1 °C in a thermostated cell holder equipped with a UV/Vis spectrophotometer (JASCO, Model V-560). While monitoring spectrophotometric changes over time from 450 nm to 650 nm in the monitoring cell, sample collection was made from the sampling cell at given intervals. These samples were then submitted to valency hybrid analyses as well as a measurement study for the detection of the oxidized ratio of the constituted chains.

Isoelectric-focusing electrophoresis was carried out using a flatbed apparatus (Model-LKB-Multiphor II, Pharmacia, Uppsala, Sweden). By use of sample application pieces, each 20 μL of sample was applied to a precast ampholine plate gel (ampholine PAG-plate, pH 5.5–8.5, Pharmacia) and thereafter an electrophoresis was carried out within 2.5 h under cooling conditions at 10 °C with constant current of 50 mA and constant voltage of 1,600 V. The ampholine plate gel was then fixed for 30 min with fixing solution containing 0.14 M sulfosalicylic acid, 0.7 M trichloroacetic acid, and 7 M methanol. After fixation, densitometric scanning was undertaken using an image scanner (Model AE-6905C; ATTO Co., Tokyo, Japan) allied with computer software.

Also, 7.5% polyacrylamide gel electrophoresis was carried out simultaneously to detect the oxidized ratio of the constituted chains just after chain separation using p-MB. With respect to chain separation, p-MB (100 mg) was dissolved in 2 mL of 0.1 M NaOH in the presence of 0.1 M NaCl and neutralized with 1 M CH_3COOH. Ten microliters of this solution were then mixed with each 100 μL of a series of collected Hb A samples. Chain separation was continued overnight (~16 h) at 4 °C in 30 mM phosphate buffer (pH 6.0) containing 0.1 M NaCl and 20% (v/v) glycerol. Thereafter, electrophoresis was then carried out for 6 h on a 7.5% polyacrylamide slab gel in Tris-glycine buffer (pH 8.6) at a constant current of 12 mA and constant voltage of 150 V. The buffer contained 25 mM Tris and 192 mM glycine. Fixation and staining were undertaken in 7.5% acetic acid containing 1% Coomassie blue. Densitometry was identical to that described for the ampholine plate gel.

The α_{SH} and β_{SH} chains were prepared by removal of p-MB with 2-mercaptoethanol from the $\alpha_{p\text{-}MB}$ and $\beta_{p\text{-}MB}$ chains. According to our specifications as described elsewhere (Tsuruga, *et al.*, 1998), the mixture with 15 mM 2-mercaptoethanol was applied on a CM-cellulose column for isolation of the α_{SH} chains, whereas it was on a DEAE-cellulose column for the β_{SH} chains. Each column was then washed with buffer solution containing 2-mercaptoethanol. Thereafter the mercaptoethanol was removed by washing the column with buffer alone. The buffers used were 10 mM piperazine-N, N'-bis(2-ethanesulfonic acid) (pH 6.5) for the α_{SH} chains and 10 mM HEPES (pH 8.2) for the β_{SH} chains.

Glycerol was unaffected not only with respect to spectrophotometric changes but also with regard to values of k_A^f and k_A^s. Similarly, there were no quantitative differences between the resulting isoelectric-focusing profiles in the presence or absence of glycerol, whereas the presence of glycerol had a good effect in preventing hemichrome formation during the time course of the experiment.

Figure 10 demonstrates some findings resulting from UV/Vis spectrophotometric, isoelectric-focusing electrophoretic and polyacrylamide gel electrophoretic measurements in which the reaction proceeded under high HbO_2 concentration (1.25 mM in heme content) in 0.05 M phosphate buffer (pH 5.0) at 37 °C in the presence of 20% (v/v) glycerol.

(a)

(b)   progress of the reaction in terms of decrease of [HbO₂] (%)

100	90	80	70	60	50	40	30	20	10	met

(c)   progress of the reaction in terms of decrease of [HbO₂] (%)

100	90	80	70	60	50	40	30	20	10	met

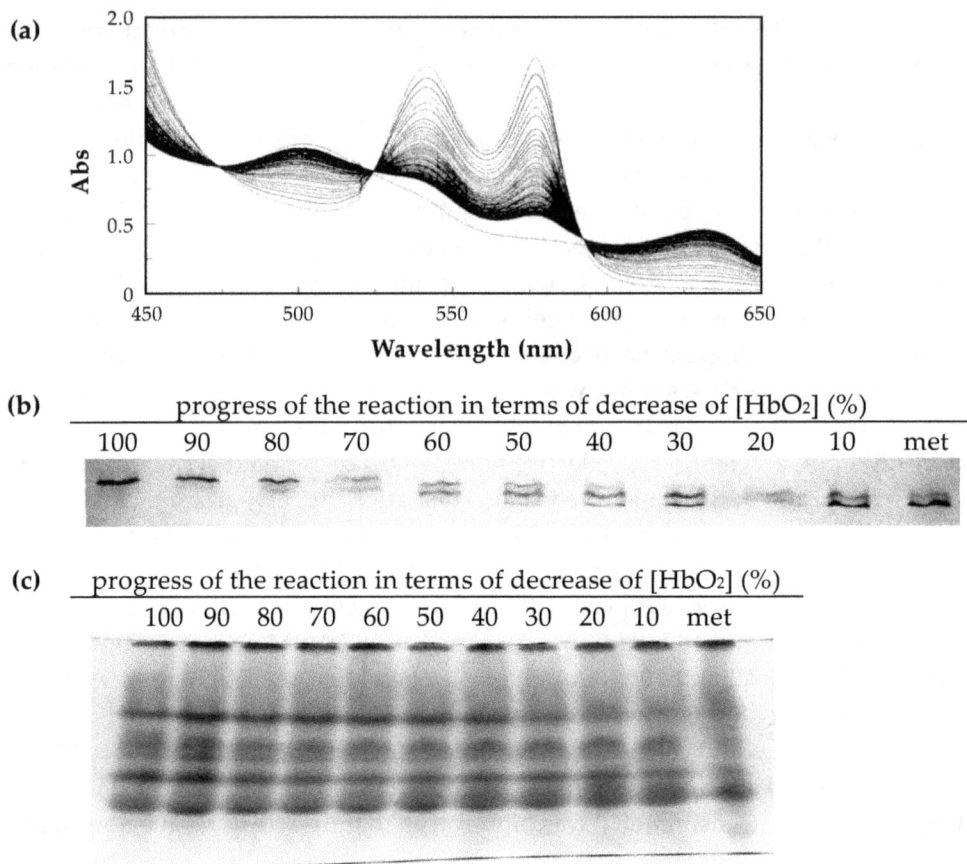

Figure 10: The available data resulting from UV/Vis spectrophotometric, isoelectric-focusing electrophoretic and polyacrylamide gel electrophoretic measurements for autoxidation of human HbO₂, redrawn from Sugawara *et al.* (2011). The reaction proceeded in the presence of 20% (*v/v*) glycerol in 0.05 M phosphate buffer (pH 5.0) at 37 °C. (a) Spectrophotometric changes with scanning interval = 10 min; (b) isoelectric-focusing electrophoretic profiles; and (c) polyacrylamide gel electrophoretic profiles.

Figure 10(a) shows the spectrophotometric changes every 10 min from 450 nm to 650 nm in the monitoring cell. Simultaneously, sample collection was carried out from the sampling cell at 0, 1.2, 2.5, 4.5, 7, 10.5, 16, 25, 42.5, and 76 h. In terms of percentage decrease of HbO₂ concentration in the reaction mixture, the sample picked up at time (*t*) = 0 h corresponded to 100% [HbO₂], and that at: *t* = 1.2 h to 90%; *t* = 2.5 h to 80%; *t* = 4.5 h to 70%; *t* = 7 h to 60%; *t* = 10.5 h to 50%; *t* = 16 h to 40%; *t* = 25 h to 30%; *t* = 42.5 h to 20%; *t* = 76 h to 10%. As mentioned above, these were used for valency hybrid analyses (Figure 10(b)) as well as detection of the oxidized ratio of the constituted chains (Figure 10(c)).

Figure 11 describes the densitometric profiles of the ampholine plate gel shown in Figure 10(b). Four components appeared during the entire reaction process. These had satisfactory-to-good consistency with those reported by Tomoda *et al.* (1978b; 1978c; 1979a; 1979b; 1980a; 1980b; 1981). On the basis of the arguments and assignments of Tomoda *et al.* (1978b; 1978c; 1979a; 1979b; 1980a; 1980b; 1981), the first peak must be $(\alpha^{2+}\beta^{2+})_2$, the second can be $(\alpha^{3+}\beta^{2+})_2$, the third can be $(\alpha^{2+}\beta^{3+})_2$, whereas the fourth must be $(\alpha^{3+}\beta^{3+})_2$ as an endpoint. In theory, the following seven species of valency hybrids can be in existence during the entire process: $(\alpha^{2+}\alpha^{2+}\beta^{3+}\beta^{2+})$, $(\alpha^{3+}\alpha^{2+}\beta^{2+}\beta^{2+})$, $(\alpha^{2+}\beta^{3+})_2$, $(\alpha^{3+}\beta^{2+})_2$, $(\alpha^{2+}\alpha^{3+}\beta^{2+}\beta^{3+})$, $(\alpha^{2+}\alpha^{3+}\beta^{3+}\beta^{3+})$ and $(\alpha^{3+}\alpha^{3+}\beta^{3+}\beta^{2+})$. Among these, however, it was evident that only two valency hybrids, *i.e.*, $(\alpha^{3+}\beta^{2+})_2$ and $(\alpha^{2+}\beta^{3+})_2$, emerged in the human HbO_2 autoxidation as demonstrated by Tomoda *et al.* (1978b; 1978c; 1980a; 1980b; 1981). It was also shown that the appearance (or disappearance) of $(\alpha^{3+}\beta^{2+})_2$ (the second peak) seemed to be preceded by $(\alpha^{2+}\beta^{3+})_2$ (the third peak).

Figure 12 illustrates the densitometric changes of the 7.5% polyacrylamide slab gel (Figure 10(c)) resulting from oxidized ratio analyses of the constituted chains. In contrast to the ampholine plate gel, the obtained electrophoretic migration profiles were complex. Hence, the initial sample (HbO_2) and partially (50%) oxidized sample just after the chain separation using *p*-MB were applied on a 7.5% polyacrylamide slab gel as well as the isolated chains (α_{SH} and β_{SH}) as an endpoint species. These were completely converted to the ferric met form by addition of potassium ferricyanide and thereafter the chain separation procedure was carried out. The resulting densitometric profiles are shown in Figure 13. Even under these qualified conditions, the profiles were complex. However, it was shown that two bands reflecting fast mobility could be attributed to the α chain, whereas those with medium mobility seemed to be unreacted Hbs with *p*-MB. Two bands found to have relatively slower mobility could have originated from the β chain. From this point of view, designation was made in Figures 12 and 13 as follows: I and II originated from the α chains, III and IV were attributed to unreacted Hbs with *p*-MB, and V and VI derived from the β chains. We could not ascertain which band corresponded to α_{O2} and α_{met} or β_{O2} and β_{met}. However, we made an attempt by plotting the ratios of II/I and VI/V against time (Figure 14). It was obvious that a decrease in II/I (as a reflection of α-chain oxidation) was much faster than a decrease in VI/V (as a reflection due to β-chain oxidation). On the basis of these findings, the reaction can be written as follows:

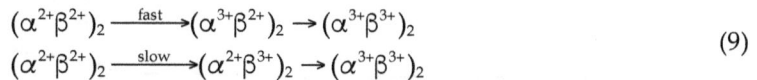

$$(\alpha^{2+}\beta^{2+})_2 \xrightarrow{\text{fast}} (\alpha^{3+}\beta^{2+})_2 \rightarrow (\alpha^{3+}\beta^{3+})_2$$
$$(\alpha^{2+}\beta^{2+})_2 \xrightarrow{\text{slow}} (\alpha^{2+}\beta^{3+})_2 \rightarrow (\alpha^{3+}\beta^{3+})_2 \tag{9}$$

7 Is Protein Allostery Involved? Mechanistic Details of Autoxidation of Human HbO_2 by Computer Simulations

To not only shed light on the mechanistic details of human HbO_2 autoxidation but also to clarify whether or not protein allostery is involved in the reaction and its inseparably related instability (degradation) of the Hb molecule to hemichrome (hemichrome for-

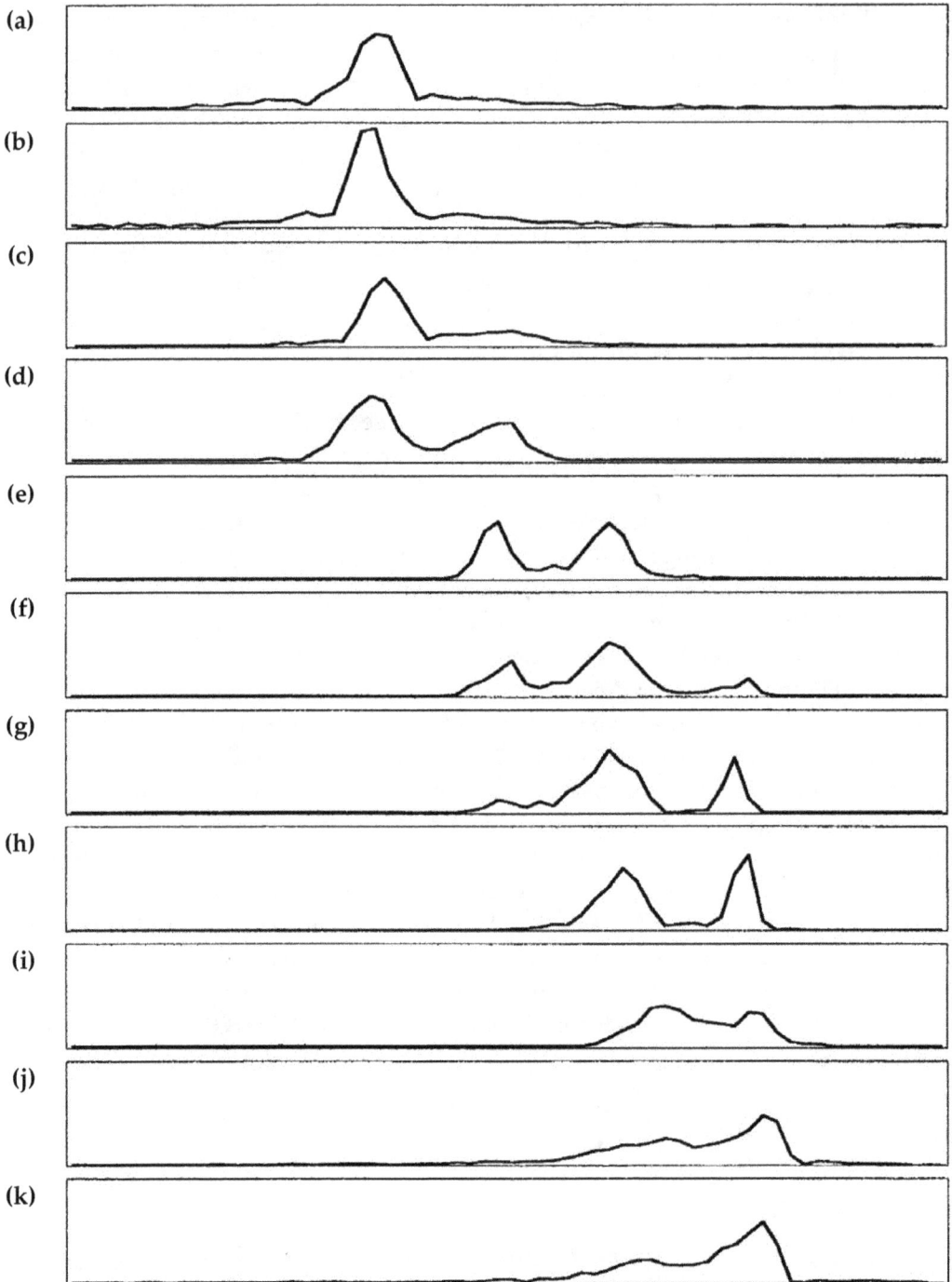

Figure 11: Densitometric profiles resulting from isoelectric-focusing electrophoresis by use of an image scanner, redrawn from Sugawara *et al.* (2011). Each curve corresponds to the relevant column shown in Figure 10(b).

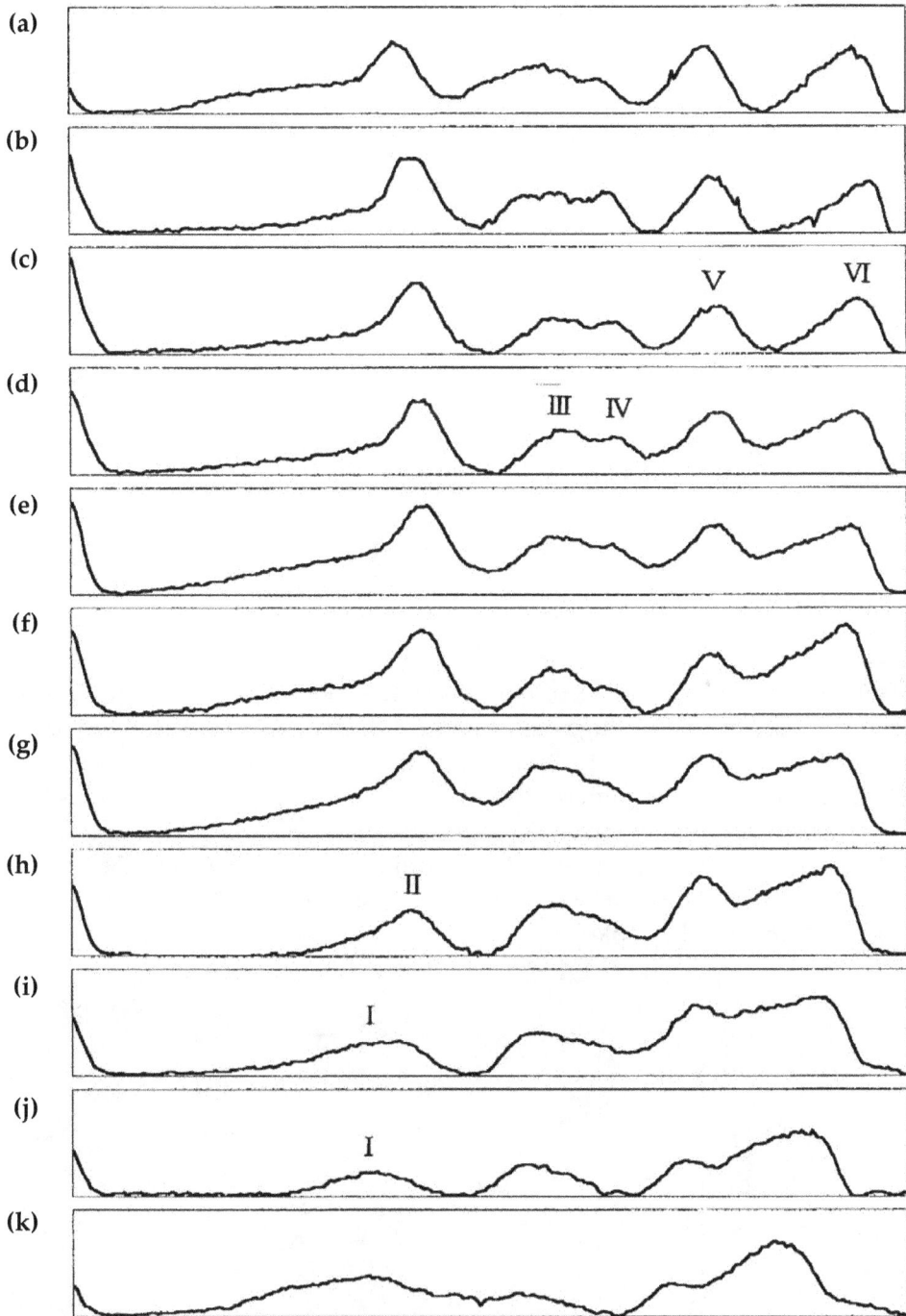

Figure 12: Densitometric profiles resulting from polyacrylamide gel electrophoresis by use of an image scanner, redrawn from Sugawara *et al.* (2011). Each curve corresponds to the relevant column shown in Figure 10(c).

(a)

(b)

(c)

(d)

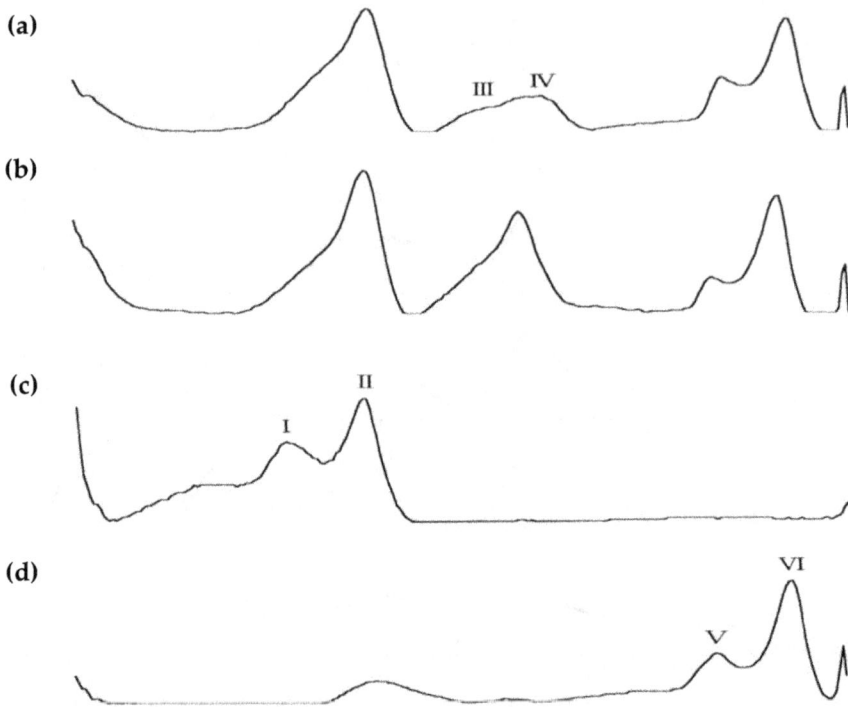

Figure 13: Densitometric profiles of polyacrylamide gel electrophoresis for quali-fied samples, redrawn from Sugawara *et al.* (2011). Densitometric changes corre-spond to: (a) initial HbO_2 sample, (b) partially (50%) oxidized sample, (c) isolated αSH chain sample as an endpoint product and (d) isolated βSH chain sample as the other endpoint species. The isolated chains (αSH and βSH) were completely con-verted to the ferric met form by addition of potassium ferricyanide. Thereafter, the chain-separation procedure was carried out for the initial HbO_2 sample and partially (50%) oxidized sample.

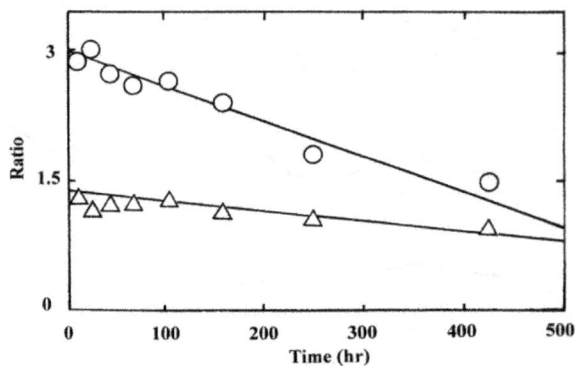

Figure 14: Peak-height ratios of II/I and VI/V versus time plots, redrawn from Sugawara *et al.* (2011). Peak-height ratios of II/I (○) and VI/V (◉) in each column shown in Figure 12 were plotted against time.

mation), we here propose two tentative models and make a kinetic formulation. Curve fittings were made against the data obtained by UV/Vis spectrophotometric, isoelectric-focusing electrophoretic and polyacrylamide gel electrophoretic measurements (Sugawara *et al.*, 2011). According to our specifications (Sugawara, *et al.*, 1995) to solve differential equations numerically using the Runge-Kutta method by setting a tentative reaction model, concentration progress curves for species assumed in a given model can be displayed on a personal computer at a given time. The first tentative model can be written as follows:

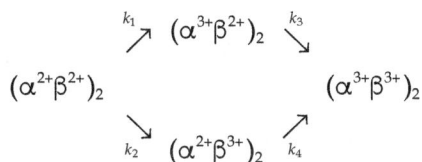

$$\begin{array}{ccc} & \overset{k_1}{\nearrow} (\alpha^{3+}\beta^{2+})_2 \overset{k_3}{\searrow} & \\ (\alpha^{2+}\beta^{2+})_2 & & (\alpha^{3+}\beta^{3+})_2 \\ & \underset{k_2}{\searrow} (\alpha^{2+}\beta^{3+})_2 \overset{}{\underset{k_4}{\nearrow}} & \end{array}$$

In this scheme, it is assumed that the reaction can proceed via two valency hybrid intermediates, *i.e.*, $(\alpha^{3+}\beta^{2+})_2$ and $(\alpha^{3+}\beta^{2+})_2$, leading to the oxidation of Hb $((\alpha^{2+}\beta^{2+})_2)$ to metHb $([(\alpha^{2+}\beta^{3+})_2)$ with the rate constants of k_1, k_2, k_3 and k_4, respectively.

For numerical analysis of the reaction steps deduced from the reaction model shown above, we may write the following rate equations in differential calculus:

$$d[(\alpha^{2+}\beta^{2+})_2]/dt = -(k_1 + k_2) \times [(\alpha^{2+}\beta^{2+})_2], \tag{10}$$

$$d[(\alpha^{3+}\beta^{2+})_2]/dt = k_1 \times [(\alpha^{2+}\beta^{2+})_2] - k_3 \times [(\alpha^{3+}\beta^{2+})_2], \tag{11}$$

$$d[(\alpha^{2+}\beta^{3+})_2]/dt = k_2 \times [(\alpha^{2+}\beta^{2+})_2] - k_4 \times [(\alpha^{2+}\beta^{3+})_2], \tag{12}$$

$$[(\alpha^{3+}\beta^{3+})_2]_t = [(\alpha^{2+}\beta^{2+})_2]_{t=0} - [(\alpha^{2+}\beta^{2+})_2]_t - [(\alpha^{3+}\beta^{2+})_2]_t - [(\alpha^{2+}\beta^{3+})_2]_t. \tag{13}$$

Here the total concentration of Hb $(= [(\alpha^{2+}\beta^{2+})_2]_{t=0})$ is given by the following equation:

$$[(\alpha^{2+}\beta^{2+})_2]_{t=0} = [(\alpha^{2+}\beta^{2+})_2]_t + [(\alpha^{3+}\beta^{2+})_2]_t + [(\alpha^{2+}\beta^{3+})_2]_t + [(\alpha^{3+}\beta^{3+})_2]_t. \tag{14}$$

By solving differential equations 10–13 employing the Euler and Runge-Kutta methods, we can constitute the consecutive concentration progress curves of the species as a function of time (t) at Δt (*i.e.*, setting intervals of time) while displaying these curves on screen of a personal computer. The numerical successive approximation using the Euler method is represented by the following equations, as Δt is setting intervals of time:

$$[(\alpha^{2+}\beta^{2+})_2](t + \Delta t) = [(\alpha^{2+}\beta^{2+})_2](t) - (k_1 + k_2) \times [(\alpha^{2+}\beta^{2+})_2](t) \times \Delta t, \tag{15}$$

$$[(\alpha^{3+}\beta^{2+})_2](t + \Delta t) = [(\alpha^{3+}\beta^{2+})_2](t) + k_1 \times [(\alpha^{2+}\beta^{2+})_2](t) \times \Delta t - k_3 \times [(\alpha^{3+}\beta^{2+})_2](t) \times \Delta t, \tag{16}$$

$$[(\alpha^{2+}\beta^{3+})_2](t + \Delta t) = [(\alpha^{2+}\beta^{3+})_2](t) + k_2 \times [(\alpha^{2+}\beta^{2+})_2](t) \times \Delta t - k_4 \times [(\alpha^{2+}\beta^{3+})_2](t) \times \Delta t, \tag{17}$$

$$[(\alpha^{3+}\beta^{3+})_2](t + \Delta t) = [(\alpha^{2+}\beta^{2+})_2]_{t=0} - [(\alpha^{2+}\beta^{2+})_2](t + \Delta t) - [(\alpha^{3+}\beta^{2+})_2](t + \Delta t) - [(\alpha^{2+}\beta^{3+})_2](t + \Delta t). \tag{18}$$

On the other hand, numerical successive calculation utilizing the Runge–Kutta method can be achieved by stepping up one-by-one along with the steps shown below. Note: each and all of O, P, Q and R seen in the following steps was representative of dummy argument for numerical successive calculation utilizing the Runge–Kutta method.

Step 1:

$\text{O}\Delta[(\alpha^{2+}\beta^{2+})_2] = -[(\alpha^{2+}\beta^{2+})_2](t) \times (k_1 + k_2).$

$\text{P}\Delta[(\alpha^{2+}\beta^{2+})_2] = -\{[(\alpha^{2+}\beta^{2+})_2](t) + 1/2 \times \Delta t \times \text{O}\Delta[(\alpha^{2+}\beta^{2+})_2]\} \times (k_1 + k_2).$

$\text{Q}\Delta[(\alpha^{2+}\beta^{2+})_2] = -\{[(\alpha^{2+}\beta^{2+})_2](t) + 1/2 \times \Delta t \times \text{P}\Delta[(\alpha^{2+}\beta^{2+})_2]\} \times (k_1 + k_2).$

$\text{R}\Delta[(\alpha^{2+}\beta^{2+})_2] = -\{[(\alpha^{2+}\beta^{2+})_2](t) + \Delta t \times \text{Q}\Delta[(\alpha^{2+}\beta^{2+})_2]\} \times (k_1 + k_2).$

Step 2:

$\text{O}\Delta[(\alpha^{3+}\beta^{2+})_2] = [(\alpha^{2+}\beta^{2+})_2](t) \times k_1 - [(\alpha^{3+}\beta^{2+})_2](t) \times k_3.$

$\text{P}\Delta[(\alpha^{3+}\beta^{2+})_2] = [(\alpha^{2+}\beta^{2+})_2](t) \times k_1 - \{[(\alpha^{3+}\beta^{2+})_2](t) + 1/2 \times \Delta t \times \text{O}\Delta[(\alpha^{3+}\beta^{2+})_2]\} \times k_3.$

$\text{Q}\Delta[(\alpha^{3+}\beta^{2+})_2] = [(\alpha^{2+}\beta^{2+})_2](t) \times k_1 - \{[(\alpha^{3+}\beta^{2+})_2](t) + 1/2 \times \Delta t \times \text{P}\Delta[(\alpha^{3+}\beta^{2+})_2]\} \times k_3.$

$\text{R}\Delta[(\alpha^{3+}\beta^{2+})_2] = [(\alpha^{2+}\beta^{2+})_2](t) \times k_1 - \{[(\alpha^{3+}\beta^{2+})_2](t) + \Delta t \times \text{Q}\Delta[(\alpha^{3+}\beta^{2+})_2]\} \times k_3.$

Step 3:

$\text{O}\Delta[(\alpha^{2+}\beta^{3+})_2] = [(\alpha^{2+}\beta^{2+})_2](t) \times k_2 - [(\alpha^{2+}\beta^{3+})_2](t) \times k_4.$

$\text{P}\Delta[(\alpha^{2+}\beta^{3+})_2] = [(\alpha^{2+}\beta^{2+})_2](t) \times k_2 - \{[(\alpha^{2+}\beta^{3+})_2](t) + 1/2 \times \Delta t \times \text{O}\Delta [(\alpha^{2+}\beta^{3+})_2]\} \times k_4.$

$\text{Q}\Delta[(\alpha^{2+}\beta^{3+})_2] = [(\alpha^{2+}\beta^{2+})_2] (t) \times k_2 - \{[(\alpha^{2+}\beta^{3+})_2](t) + 1/2 \times \Delta t \times \text{P}\Delta[(\alpha^{2+}\beta^{3+})_2]\} \times k_4.$

$\text{R}\Delta[(\alpha^{2+}\beta^{3+})_2] = [(\alpha^{2+}\beta^{2+})_2] (t) \times k_2 - \{[(\alpha^{2+}\beta^{3+})_2](t) + \Delta t \times \text{Q}\Delta [(\alpha^{2+}\beta^{3+})_2]\} \times k_4.$

Step 4:

$\Delta[(\alpha^{2+}\beta^{2+})_2] = \Delta t \times 1/6 \times (\text{O}\Delta[(\alpha^{2+}\beta^{2+})_2] + 2 \times \text{P}\Delta[(\alpha^{2+}\beta^{2+})_2] + 2 \times \text{Q}\Delta[(\alpha^{2+}\beta^{2+})_2] + \text{R}\Delta[(\alpha^{2+}\beta^{2+})_2]).$

$\Delta[(\alpha^{3+}\beta^{2+})_2] = \Delta t \times 1/6 \times (\text{O}\Delta[(\alpha^{3+}\beta^{2+})_2)] + 2 \times \text{P}\Delta[(\alpha^{3+}\beta^{2}_2)] + 2 \times \text{Q}\Delta[(\alpha^{3+}\beta^{2+})_2)] + \text{R}\Delta[(\alpha^{3+}\beta^{2+})_2)]).$

$\Delta[(\alpha^{2+}\beta^{3+})_2] = \Delta t \times 1/6 \times (\text{O}\Delta[(\alpha^{2+}\beta^{3+})_2] + 2 \times \text{P}\Delta[(\alpha^{2+}\beta^{3+})_2] + 2 \times \text{Q}\Delta[(\alpha^{2+}\beta^{3+})_2] + \text{R}\Delta[(\alpha^{2+}\beta^{3+})_2]).$

Step 5:

$[(\alpha^{2+}\beta^{2+})_2](t + \Delta t) = [(\alpha^{2+}\beta^{2+})_2](t) + \Delta[(\alpha^{2+}\beta^{2+})_2].$ (19)

$[(\alpha^{3+}\beta^{2+})_2](t + \Delta t) = [(\alpha^{3+}\beta^{2+})_2](t) + \Delta[(\alpha^{3+}\beta^{2+})_2].$ (20)

$[(\alpha^{2+}\beta^{3+})_2](t + \Delta t) = [(\alpha^{2+}\beta^{3+})_2](t) + \Delta[(\alpha^{2+}\beta^{3+})_2].$ (21)

$[(\alpha^{3+}\beta^{3+})_2] (t + \Delta t) = [\alpha^{2+}\beta^{2+})_2]_{t=0} - [(\alpha^{2+}\beta^{2+})_2](t + \Delta t) - [(\alpha^{3+}\beta^{2+})_2](t + \Delta t) - [(\alpha^{2+}\beta^{3+})_2](t + \Delta t).$ (22)

As a pilot study, curve fittings were made against the data obtained by isoelectric-focusing electrophoresis using equations 15–18 as for the Euler method and equations 19–22 as with the Runge-Kutta method. The resulting fittings attained by both methods showed a mutually good consistency, although the Runge-Kutta method was superior to the Euler method in terms of the precision of successive approximation; this was estimated by a degree of around $(\Delta t)^4$ for the Runge-Kutta method and Δt for the Euler method.

Figure 15(a) illustrates the best-suited fitting attained by the Runge-Kutta method for the consecutive changes of the components attained by isoelectric-focusing electrophoresis while setting $\Delta t = 0.1$ h. In Figure 15(a), the first ($\bigcirc$; $[\alpha^{2+}\beta^{2+}]_2$), second ($\triangle$; $[\alpha^{3+}\beta^{2+}]_2$), third ($\blacktriangle$; $[\alpha^{2+}\beta^{3+}]_2$) and fourth ($\bullet$; $[\alpha^{3+}\beta^{3+}]_2$) components were plotted against time in terms of peak area calculated from the diagrams shown in Figure 11. Each solid line was achieved by non-linear least-squares fitting when setting the kinetic constants as follows: $k_1 = 0.009$ (h^{-1}), $k_2 = 0.002$ (h^{-1}), $k_3 = 0.005$ (h^{-1}), and $k_4 = 0.00008$ (h^{-1}). The resulting curve fittings show mutually good consistency for the aspects resulting from the isoelectric-focusing electrophoretic study. However, it was evident that the obtained concen-

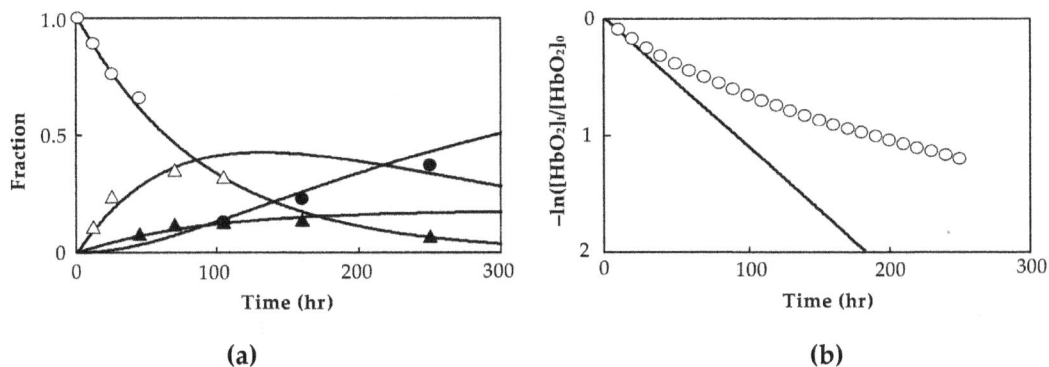

(a)

(b)

Figure 15: Outcomes achieved by a computer simulation using the consecutive reaction model with k_1, k_2, k_3, and k_4 for human HbO$_2$ autoxidation, redrawn from Sugawara *et al.* (2011). (a) Isoelectric-focusing electrophoretic changes of the 1st (O), 2nd ($\triangle$), 3rd ($\blacktriangle$) and 4th peaks ($\bullet$), respectively; and (b) the $-\ln([HbO_2]_t/[HbO_2]_0)$ versus time plot (first-order plot). Solid lines represent the curves derived from the Runge–Kutta method while setting the following constants: $k_1 = 0.009$ (h^{-1}), $k_2 = 0.002$ (h^{-1}), $k_3 = 0.005$ (h^{-1}), $k_4 = 0.00008$ (h^{-1}) and $\Delta t = 0.1$ h.

tration progress curves derived from this model did not fully explain the aspects of spectrophotometric and polyacrylamide gel electrophoretic profiles. Figure 15(b) shows such an example.

Here k_A^f and k_A^s represent the first-order rate constants calculated from the least-squares fittings against $-\ln([HbO_2]_t/[HbO_2]_0)$ *versus* time plot that was monitored in 0.05 M phosphate buffer (pH 5.0) at 37 °C in the presence of 20% (*v/v*) glycerol (Figure 10(a)). By these least-squares fittings, the following kinetic constants and molar fraction of the initial fast component (*P*) were established: $k_A^f = 0.148$ h^{-1} (4.7 h for $t_{1/2}$), $k_A^s = 0.0208$ h^{-1} (1.4 d for $t_{1/2}$), and $P = 0.51$. Thus, by setting the values of k_A^f and k_A^s at 0.148 h^{-1} and 0.0208 h^{-1}, respectively, and $\Delta t = 0.1$ h, the relevant concentration progress curves were displayed on a personal computer for the possible species assumed in this model. Figure 16 illustrates the outcomes: Figure 16(a) shows aspects of the spectrophotometric changes in terms of the $-\ln([HbO_2]_t/[HbO_2]_0)$ *versus* time plot, whereas Figure 16(b,c) describe aspects of the associated isoelectric-focusing electropho retic profiles (Figure 16(b)) and polyacrylamide gel electrophoretic profiles (Figure 16(c)), respectively. In Figure 16, each computed curve (solid line) showed satisfactory-to-good agreements with the experimental data. These demonstrated that almost all of the reaction aspects could be fully explained by the consecutive changes of the species supposed in this model. Thus, the β chain was seen to carry delayed autoxidation in the tetrameric protein architecture. The rate of the initial rapid phase (k_A^f) characterized with the HbO$_2$ autoxidation represented the intrinsic α-chain oxidation, whereas the rate of the second slower phase (k_A^s) reflected the intrinsic β-chain oxidation. These findings led us to conclude that the β chain manifests delayed autoxidation in the human HbO$_2$, which could be much more evident in acidic solutions.

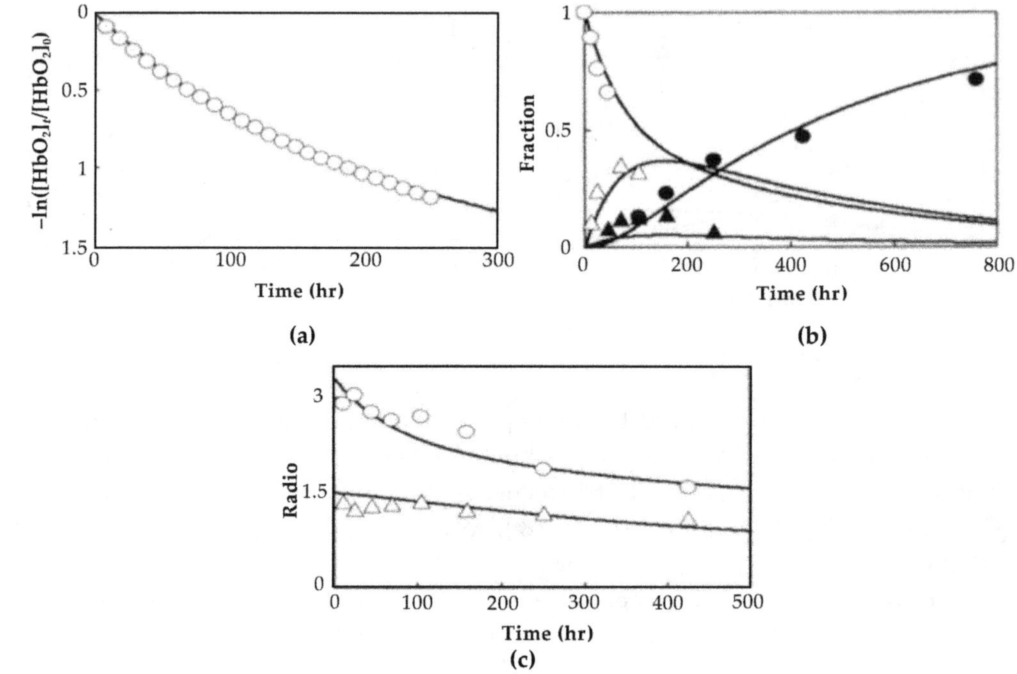

Figure 16: Outcomes achieved by a computer simulation using the consecutive reaction model with k_A^f and k_A^s for human HbO_2 autoxidation, redrawn from Sugawara *et al.* (2011). (a) The $-\ln([HbO_2]_t/[HbO_2]_0)$ versus time plot; (b) isoelectric-focusing electrophoretic profiles; and (c) polyacrylamide gel electrophoretic profiles. Solid lines represent the curves derived from the Runge–Kutta method with setting of the following constants: $k_A{}^f$= 0.148 h^{-1}, $k_A{}^s$ = 0.0208 $h^{-1}$and Δt = 0.1 h. For (b), the symbols are designated as follows: the 1st (○), 2nd (△), 3rd (▲) and 4th peaks (●), respectively.

The following second tentative model was thus taken for assessment:

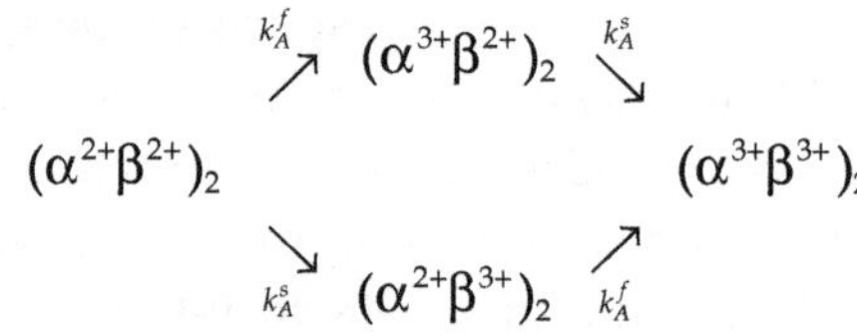

$$(\alpha^{2+}\beta^{2+})_2 \quad \overset{k_A^f}{\nearrow} \quad (\alpha^{3+}\beta^{2+})_2 \quad \overset{k_A^s}{\searrow} \quad (\alpha^{3+}\beta^{3+})_2$$
$$\searrow_{k_A^s} \quad (\alpha^{2+}\beta^{3+})_2 \quad \nearrow_{k_A^f}$$

On the basis of these findings and taking into account the results that were gained through a series of studies described in the preceding sections, we proposed a new function assigned to the α_1–β_1 (and α_2–β_2) interface for stabilizing the HbO_2 tetramer against acidic autoxidation as reported in 1998 (Tsuruga *et al.*, 1998) and in 2002 (Yasuda, *et al.*, 2002). That is, the α_1–β_1 (and α_2–β_2) interface produces a conformational constraint in the β chain whereby the distal (E7) His at position 63 is tilted slightly away from the bound O_2 so as to prevent the proton-catalyzed displacement of O_2^- from the

Fe(II)O$_2$ center by entrance of a water molecule. The β chain thus acquires a remarkably delayed oxidation rate in the HbO$_2$ tetramer.

Regarding to this issue, we will demonstrate in the following sections that the α$_1$–β$_1$ (and α$_2$–β$_2$) interface of the Hb molecule may exert delicate control over the intrinsic tilting capability of the distal (E7) His residues (*i.e.*, α58His (E7) in the α chain and β63His (E7) in the β chain), and be in charge of removal of erythrocytes from the blood circulation by triggering degradation of the molecule to hemichrome, and subsequent clustering of Heinz bodies within the erythrocytes depending on the internal and extraneous conditions of the erythrocyte.

8   Discussion

Cellular life is reliant upon rapid and efficient responses to internal and external conditions. The basic molecular events associated with these processes are the structural transitions of the proteins involved (Vitagliano, *et al.*, 2008). The human Hb molecule (α$_2$β$_2$; alternatively, a dimer of αβ protomers), which has two types of αβ interface (*i.e.*, α$_1$β$_1$ [and α$_2$β$_2$] and α$_1$β$_2$ [and α$_2$β$_1$]) and whose α and β chains contain 141 and 146 amino-acid residues, respectively, holds a special position in these structural transitions. This is due to the achievements of Perutz, whose pioneering studies led to the identification of two distinct Hb structures, the T (tense) and the R (relaxed) state, which are associated with the deoxygenated and oxygenated form of the protein, respectively (Perutz, 1970; 1972; Perutz, *et al.*, 1986).

Regarding human HbO$_2$, a representative set of successive O$_2$-binding constants is given in terms of mmHg^{-1} as follows: $K_1 = 0.0188$, $K_2 = 0.0566$, $K_3 = 0.407$, $K_4 = 4.28$ in 0.1 M buffer (pH 7.4) containing 0.1 M KCl at 25 °C (Imai, 1994). In this reaction, by comparing their X-ray crystal structures, major differences have been defined between the deoxygenated and oxygenated forms. These include: movement of the iron atom into the heme plane with simultaneous change in the orientation of the proximal (F8) His; rotation of the α$_1$β$_1$ dimer relative to the other α$_2$β$_2$ dimer about an axis *P* by 12–15 °; and a translation of one dimer relative to the other along the *P* axis by ~1 Å (10^{-1} nm). These changes are accompanied with sequential breaking of "salt bridges" by C-terminal residues (Baldwin & Chothia, 1979; Fermi & Perutz, 1981; Dickerson, 1983; Perutz, 1990; Perutz, *et al.*, 1998). When HbO$_2$ goes from the deoxygenated to the oxygenated quaternary structure, the α$_1$–β$_2$ (and α$_2$–β$_1$) interface undergoes the principal changes associated with the cooperative oxygen binding, so it is named as the "sliding contact" that involves 19 residues, including mainly helices C and H and the FG corner (Dickerson, 1983; Borgstahl, *et al.*, 1994).

Conversely, negligible changes are found with respect to the crystal structure examined for the α$_1$–β$_1$ (and α$_2$–β$_2$) interface that associates 35 residues including B, G, and H helices as well as the GH corner. As mentioned, understanding of subunit interactions between the four Hb chains (and how these explain cooperative O$_2$ binding) has been the primary focus in Hb research. This has been coupled with a tendency for structural analyses to focus on the changes at the proximal side of the heme and at the α$_1$–β$_2$

(and $\alpha 2$–$\beta 1$) interface. This is despite the fact that the configuration of the residues lining the distal side of the heme pocket (where molecular O_2 binds) are also altered by oxygenation, and are thought to have a role in controlling access of the ligand to the heme pocket (Levy, *et al.*, 1992). Hence, the possibility of subunit interactions originating from or being transmitted via distal effects has, for the most part, been neglected.

In this chapter, we deliberately aimed to deal with useful and basic methods in protein purification and analysis that led us to grasp new roles assigned to the $\alpha 1$–$\beta 2$ (and $\alpha 2$–$\beta 1$) interface of the human hemoglobin molecule. By good use of these methods, we drew seven main conclusions. First, autoxidation of human HbO_2 (the reaction of which is inevitable in nature for all O_2–binding proteins and which has been dealt with in the periphery of Hb research) seemed to be inseparably related to the instability of the Hb molecule and its degradation to hemichrome. Second, in terms of pH-dependent biphasic autoxidation (k_A^f for the initial fast oxidation and k_A^s for the second oxidation) seen in acidic solutions, participation of a single dissociation group of an amino-acid residue (probably a His residue) with $pK_a = 7.4$ (at 37 °C) appeared to have a key role in how the Hb molecule can prompt the range of fast (k_A^f) and slow (k_A^s) components against the pH values of the solutions. Third, the isolated α and β chains were oxidized much more readily over the measured pH range (5–10.5) when compared with the respective rates of the parent molecules used as a reference. Fourth, in terms of pH- and temperature-dependent hemichrome emergence observed by UV/Vis spectroscopy, HbO_2 was supposed to be highly susceptible to hemichrome formation (even under physiological pH and temperature). Fifth, in contrast to the tetrameric human HbO_2 as O_2^- carrying protein in the blood, the monomeric bovine heart Mb (MbO_2) did not show any propensity for hemichrome formation over a wide pH range of 4.5 to 10.5 and over a wide temperature range from physiological to temperatures just before thermal unfolding. Sixth, UV/Vis spectrophotometric, isoelectric-focusing electrophoretic and polyacrylamide gel electrophoretic measurements following human HbO_2 autoxidation demonstrated that the intrinsic α-chain oxidation seemed to be much faster than the intrinsic β-chain oxidation among the HbO_2 tetramer, *i.e.*, $(\alpha^{2+}\beta^{2+})_2$, and the reaction would follow the scheme:

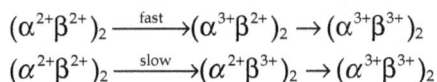

$$(\alpha^{2+}\beta^{2+})_2 \xrightarrow{\text{fast}} (\alpha^{3+}\beta^{2+})_2 \rightarrow (\alpha^{3+}\beta^{3+})_2$$
$$(\alpha^{2+}\beta^{2+})_2 \xrightarrow{\text{slow}} (\alpha^{2+}\beta^{3+})_2 \rightarrow (\alpha^{3+}\beta^{3+})_2$$

Finally, by means of computer simulations on the basis of data obtained from measurements (UV/Vis spectrophotometry, isoelectric-focusing electrophoresis, and polyacrylamide gel electrophoresis), k_A^f represented intrinsic α-chain oxidation whereas k_A^s reflected intrinsic β-chain oxidation, and the β chain manifested delayed autoxidation in human HbO_2 (which could be much more evident in acidic solutions).

On the basis of these findings, in the following, two major subjects will be discussed and interpreted in terms of the $\alpha 1$–$\beta 1$ (and $\alpha 2$–$\beta 2$) interface. The first subject is the pH-dependent delayed autoxidation of β (O_2) subunits when compared with α (O_2) subunits in the tetrameric architecture. The second subject is the inherent tilting capability of the distal (E7) His residues (*i.e.*, $\alpha 58$His (E7) in the α chain and $\beta 63$His (E7) in the β chain) to hemichrome formation or Hb degradation. In the latter mechanism, the $\alpha 1$–$\beta 1$

(and α_2–β_2) interface play a key role as an equipped (inherent) molecular sensor to control the fate of the own erythrocyte via tilting of the distal (E7) His (*i.e.*, α58His (E7) in the α chain and β63His (E7) in the β chain) that can be triggered degradation of the Hb molecule to hemichrome, and subsequent clustering of Heinz bodies within the erythrocyte depending on the internal and extraneous conditions of the erythrocyte, including pH and temperature. In the spleen (which is responsible for the removal of aged and damaged red cells from the blood circulation), rigid intra-erythrocytic hemichrome inclusions (Heinz bodies) are known to act as "sticking points," hence Heinz body-containing red cells become trapped and undergo hemolysis (Jacob, 1970).

In our discussion, we start with the oxidative behavior (autoxidation; oxidation of ferrous heme iron by bound O_2) of the human HbO_2 molecule. This is because autoxidation is inseparably related to the instability of the molecule and its degradation to hemichrome, relying upon the intrinsic tilting capability of the distal (E7) His residues and their bis-histidyl coordination proficiency to the heme iron. Relatively little attention has been paid to the autoxidation of HbO_2, even though autoxidation is inevitable in nature for all O_2-binding heme proteins. It has been customary to deal with the "periphery" in Hb research.

As with autoxidation, Shikama (1985; 1988; 1990; 1998; 2006) evaluated various mechanisms proposed for autoxidation involving MbO_2 and HbO_2. He clearly demonstrated that the autoxidation reaction does not simply involve the dissociative loss of O_2^- from HbO_2, but is instead caused by the nucleophilic displacement of O_2^- from HbO_2 by a water molecule or a hydroxyl ion that enters the heme pocket from the surrounding solvent. The iron is thus converted to the ferric met form, and the water molecule or hydroxyl ion remains bound to Fe(III) at the sixth coordinate position to form the aqua- or hydroxide-met species. A generalized pathway for this S_N2 mechanism can be written using Mb (MbO_2) as an example:

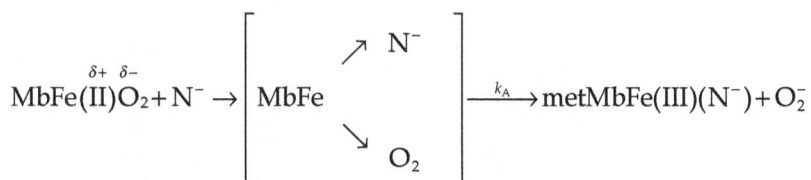

$$\text{MbFe(II)}\overset{\delta+}{O_2}\overset{\delta-}{}+N^- \rightarrow \left[\text{MbFe}\begin{array}{c}\nearrow N^- \\ \searrow \\ O_2\end{array}\right]\xrightarrow{k_A}\text{metMbFe(III)}(N^-)+O_2^-$$

Here k_A represents the rate constant of anion-induced autoxidation with nucleophilic anion displacement and N^- can be SCN^-, F^-, OCN^-, N_3^-, or CN^- and, *in vivo*, it can be H_2O or OH^-. Anion-induced autoxidation with nucleophilic anion displacement of O_2 results in an intermediate ferrous heme/anion complex that acts as an electron donor to displace oxygen. Shikama (1985; 1998) also demonstrated that, *in vacua*, oxyheme is inherently stable and unlikely to dissociate O_2^- spontaneously. Because O_2 is a rather poor one-electron acceptor, a considerable thermodynamic barrier exists for such an electron transfer. In aqueous media (*i.e.*, in contrast to *in vacua*), oxyheme is always subject to the nucleophilic attack of an entering water molecule (with or without proton catalysis) and to the attack of an entering hydroxide anion. These can cause irreversible oxidation of oxyheme to met-species with generation of O_2^-. Mb and Hb have therefore evolved with a globin moiety that can protect the Fe(II) O_2 center from the easy access of a water molecule, including its conjugate ions OH⁻ and H⁺.

In an aqueous protein-free system, Kao & Wang (1965) reported the oxidation of dipyridine-ferrohemochrome by O_2 using a stopped-flow technique. The main pathway was interpreted to involve one O_2 molecule replacing one of the pyridine molecules in dipyridine-ferrohemochrome to form an oxyheme and then undergoing decomposition to ferrihemochrome and O_2^-. Unfortunately, the rate constant for this oxidation reaction could not be obtained because the concentration term of pyridine was always involved in its rate equation in a complicated manner. By numerical calculations, however, it follows that oxyheme autoxidation can proceed with a rate constant that is much higher than 1 s⁻¹ in 0.1 M buffer, pH 8.5, at 25 °C (Figure 17). If such an oxyheme is placed in a protein matrix, it would be protected against the nucleophilic attack of the solvent water molecule or hydroxyl ion so as to reduce its autoxidation by a factor of approximately 10^3. This was the case in our study with denatured MbO_2 in 8 M urea (the details of which can be referred to in Sugawara *et al.*, 1995). A globin moiety can act as a "breakwater" in aqueous media even in denatured conditions with 8 M urea. Furthermore, if an oxyheme is embedded in the native Mb architecture, MbO_2 acquires remarkable stability against oxyheme autoxidation by a factor of approximately 10^6 (Figure 17).

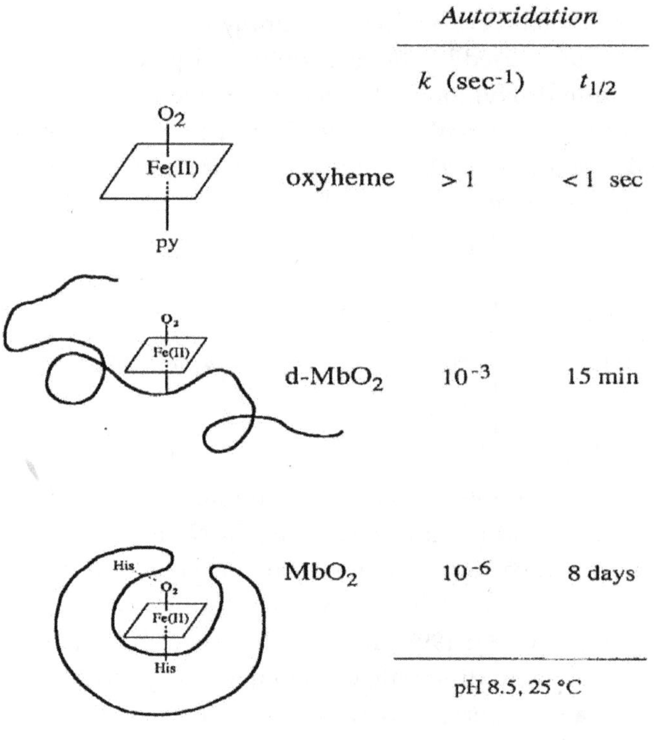

Figure 17: Roles of a globin moiety in Mb or Hb molecules, redrawn from Sugawara *et al.* (2011).

With regard to oxyheme stability in human HbO_2, the half-life ($t_{1/2}$) was only 1.5 d in 0.1 M buffer and at physiological pH and temperature (Sugawara *et al.*, 1993) even though the content of metHb in normal red cells *in situ* (Paul & Kemp, 1944; Bodansky, 1951) has been maintained to be less than or equal to 1% as a consequence of a NADH-dependent reducing system that can reduce the ferric-metHb resulting from autoxidation to deoxy-ferrous Hb (Scott, *et al.*, 1965; Hultquist & Passon, 1971; Sugita, *et al.*, 1971). However, as compared with the rates of monomeric mammalian Mbs, human HbO_2 seemed to be 2.2–3.6 times more stable against autoxidation (probably due to its tetrameric architecture). Even though the autoxidation rate is a function of pH and temperature, the observed first-order rate constant was 0.0023 h^{-1} (12.6 d for $t_{1/2}$) for the human HbO_2 autoxidation under the conditions of 0.1 M buffer at pH 7.2 and 25 °C in our study (Sugawara *et al.*, 1993), because this value was calculated from the first rapid phase. Conversely, the relevant values of the monomeric mammalian Mbs were 0.0082 h^{-1} (3.5 d for $t_{1/2}$) for human MbO_2, 0.0072 h^{-1} (4.0 d for $t_{1/2}$) for bovine MbO_2, and 0.0050 h^{-1} (5.8 d for $t_{1/2}$) for sperm whale MbO_2 under the same conditions of human HbO_2.

In our experiments, tetrameric human $HbO2$ showed a biphasic autoxidation curve in acidic solutions in terms of the $-\ln([HbO2]t/[HbO2]0)$ versus time plot (Figure 3(a)); an initial rapid reaction (k_A^f) could be followed with a slower second phase (k_A^s). The difference in the rates between k_A^f and k_A^s decreased with increasing pH values of solutions, and finally disappeared (i.e., k_A^f equal to k_A^s) if the pH of the solutions was more than 8 and became k_A^f equal to k_A^s (Figure 3(b)). This finding leads to certain questions: how does the Hb molecule prompt the the range of fast (k_A^f) and slow (k_A^s) components in acidic solutions? How does the molecule provoke k_A^f equal to k_A^s, if the pH of solutions is more than 8? Does the biphasic autoxidation seen in acidic pH regions reflect a different rate owing to the individual Hb chains or the presence of valency hybrid intermediates such as $(\alpha^{2+}\beta^{3+})_2$ and $(\alpha^{3+}\beta^{2+})_2$?

A plot for the obtained values of k_A^f / k_A^s *versus* pH indicated that the reaction involves a single dissociation group of amino-acid residue with $pK_a = 7.4$ (at 37 °C) (Figure 4), probably a His residue. In addition, study of rate measurement for the isolated $\alpha_{p\text{-MB}}$ and $\beta_{p\text{-MB}}$ chains (and α_{SH} and β_{SH} chains) disclosed that once the constituted chains were isolated from the parent molecule, both separated chains could be oxidized much more rapidly to the ferric met-form over the measured pH range (5–10) when compared with the respective rates (k_A^f and k_A^s) of the parent molecules calculated from biphasic autoxidation curves as a reference (Figure 5). Also, there were no practical differences regarding the rate between the isolated individual chains (Figure 5). These findings may indicate that the individual chains have acquired considerable resistance to oxyheme autoxidation in their tetrameric protein architecture. It was also suggested that human HbO_2 seems to have acquired a "pH-sensitive molecular device" as a consequence of development of the tetrameric protein architecture. Hence, the molecule shows remarkable stability against oxyheme autoxidation more than in cases of isolated individual chains from the parent molecules and monomeric mammalian Mbs.

Moreover, our UV/Vis spectrophotometric, isoelectric-focusing electrophoretic and polyacrylamide gel electrophoretic measurements for autoxidation of human HbO_2 revealed that only two valency hybrids, *i.e.*, $(\alpha^{3+}\beta^{2+})_2$ and $(\alpha^{2+}\beta^{3+})_2$, emerged in the tetrameric HbO$_2$ autoxidation (figures 10(b), 11), even though, in theory, seven species of valency hybrids can be in existence during the reaction time course. These species are $(\alpha^{2+}\alpha^{2+}\beta^{3+}\beta^{2+})$, $(\alpha^{3+}\alpha^{2+}\beta^{2+}\beta^{2+})$, $(\alpha^{2+}\beta^{3+})_2$, $(\alpha^{3+}\beta^{2+})_2$, $(\alpha^{2+}\alpha^{3+}\beta^{2+}\beta^{3+})$, $(\alpha^{2+}\alpha^{3+}\beta^{3+}\beta^{3+})$ and $(\alpha^{3+}\alpha^{3+}\beta^{3+}\beta^{2+})$. These had satisfactory-to-good consistency with those reported by Tomoda *et al.*(1978b; 1978c; 1980a; 1980b; 1981). Computer simulations on the basis of these measurements (UV/Vis spectrophotometry, isoelectric-focusing electrophoresis, and polyacrylamide gel electrophoresis) indicated that the relevant concentration progress curves derived from the subsequent tentative model could explain not only aspects of the spectrophotometric changes in terms of the $-\ln([HbO_2]_t/[HbO_2]_0)$ *versus* time plot, but also aspects of the associated isoelectric-focusing electrophoretic profiles and polyacrylamide gel electrophoretic profiles, respectively, as shown below (Figure 16):

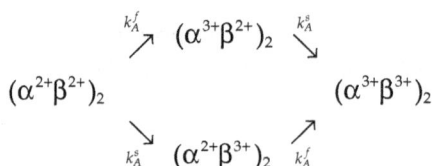

$$(\alpha^{2+}\beta^{2+})_2 \quad \overset{k_A^f}{\nearrow} (\alpha^{3+}\beta^{2+})_2 \overset{k_A^s}{\searrow} \quad (\alpha^{3+}\beta^{3+})_2$$
$$\overset{}{\searrow} \underset{k_A^s}{} (\alpha^{2+}\beta^{3+})_2 \underset{k_A^f}{\nearrow}$$

In an autoxidation reaction monitored in 0.05 M phosphate buffer (pH 5.0) at 37 °C in the presence of 20% (*v/v*) glycerol, the following kinetic constants and molar fraction of the initial fast component (*P*) were established by least-squares fitting: k_A^f = 0.148 h^{-1} (4.7 h for $t_{1/2}$), k_A^s = 0.0208 h^{-1} (1.4 d for $t_{1/2}$), and *P* = 0.51. These findings led us to conclude that k_A^f represents intrinsic α-chain oxidation and k_A^s reflects intrinsic β-chain oxidation, and that the β chain manifests delayed autoxidation in human HbO$_2$, which could be much more evident in acidic solutions.

Figure 18(a) shows our proposal with respect to this issue as reported in 1998 (Tsuruga *et al.*) and 2002 (Yasuda *et al.*) in which we suggested a new function to the α1–β1 (and α2–β2) interface for stabilizing the HbO$_2$ tetramer against acidic autoxidation. That is, the α1–β1 (and α2–β2) interface produces a conformational constraint in the β chain whereby the distal (E7) His at position 63 is tilted slightly away from the bound O$_2$ so as to prevent the proton-catalyzed displacement of O$_2^-$ from the Fe(II)O$_2$ center by entrance of a water molecule. The β chain thus acquires a remarkably delayed oxidation rate in the HbO$_2$ tetramer. This is the origin of the chain heterogeneity seen in acidic solutions of HbO$_2$ autoxidation.

In fact, the most recent refinement of the crystallographic structure of human HbO$_2$ (where the O$_2$ molecule is clearly visible in the high-resolution electron density maps) not only demonstrated that the hydrogen bond made by His E7β (*i.e.*, β63His) is much weaker than that made by His E7α (*i.e.*, α58His), but also substantiated that the geometry of the ligand and distal histidine is slightly different in the two subunits, with the O$_2$ atom lying 2.7 ± 0.1 Å (10^{-1} nm) from the N$\cdot$ atom of the distal histidine in the α subunits, and 3.0 Å away in the β subunits (Park, *et al.*, 2006). However, it is an unavoidable fact that negligible changes are found for the α1–β1 (and α2–β2) interface with respect to examination of the crystal structure.

Similar phenomena suggesting participation of the α1–β1 (and α2–β2) interface (*i.e.*, participation of the inherent tilting capability of the distal (E7) His residues of the

Hb molecule) garnered our interest. As shown in Figures 6 and 7, our UV/Vis spectroscopic study suggested that human HbO_2 was highly susceptible to hemichrome formation even under physiological pH and temperature and, once isolated from the tetrameric parent molecule, the α ($\alpha_{p\text{-MB}}$) and β ($\beta_{p\text{-MB}}$) chains showed much higher susceptibilities to hemichrome when compared with the parent molecule.

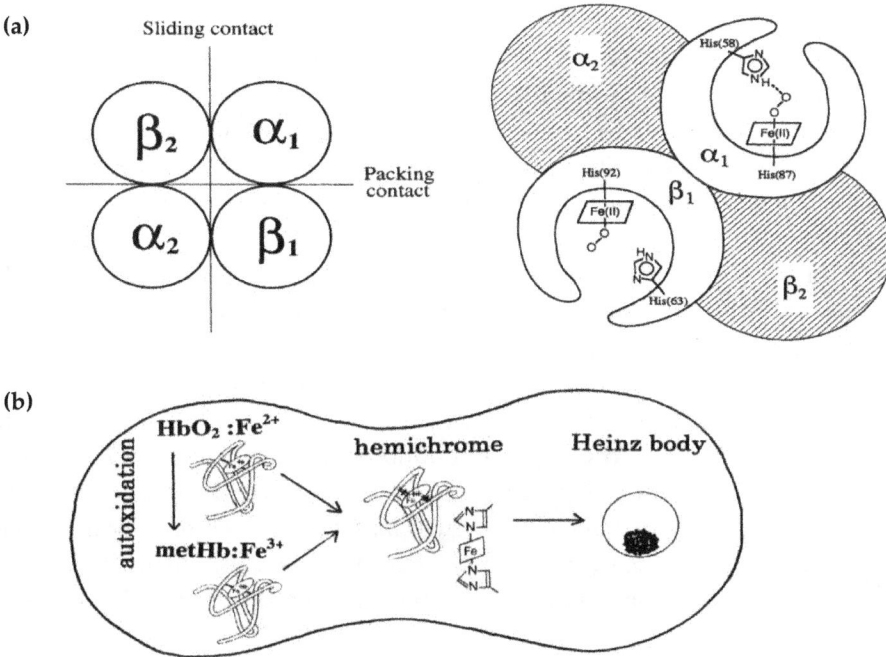

Figure 18: Schematic representation of the role of the α_1–β_1 (and α_2–β_2) interface in human HbO_2, redrawn from Sugawara *et al.* (2013). (a) The left figure shows a molecular dyad axis of Hb tetramer (which is perpendicular to the plane of the figure) relating the $\alpha_1\beta_1$ dimer to the $\alpha_2\beta_2$ dimer and consisting of the two different types of $\alpha\beta$ contacts: one is the α_1–β_1 (and α_2–β_2) (packing contact); and the other is the α_1–β_2 (and α_2–β_1) (sliding contact). The right figure illustrates that the α_1–β_1 (and α_2–β_2) produces in the β chain a tilting of the distal (E7) His residue, thereby preventing the proton-catalyzed displacement of O_2^- by a solvent water molecule. (b) The figure demonstrates that depending on internal and extraneous circumstances of the erythrocyte including pH and temperature, the α_1–β_1 (and α_2–β_2) interface produces a conformational constraint in the constituted chains *via* tilting of the distal His (E7) residues so as to cause degradation of the Hb molecule to hemichrome, and subsequent Heinz-body clustering within the erythrocyte. In the spleen, Heinz body-containing red cells become trapped and hence undergo hemolysis.

Heinz bodies are intra-erythrocytic inclusions of hemichrome formed as a result of Hb oxidation. They have been detected and characterized in drug-induced hemolytic anemia, defects in the intra-erythrocytic reducing system (e.g., G-6-PD deficiency) and in unstable Hb disease (Winslow & Anderson, 1978; Weatherall *et al.*, 1995). Using unstable Hb disease as an example, quite a large number of unstable Hbs have been reported. Regarding the molecular pathogenesis of unstable Hbs, it is known that the instability of labile Hb variants in patients can be attributed to amino-acid substitutions (or deletions), which disrupt and perturb the Hb structure via interference with α-helix formation, disruption of heme binding, or altered α_1–β_1 (and α_2–β_2) or α_1–β_2 (and α_2–β_1) contacts (Winslow & Anderson, 1978). The consequent changes in circulating red cells in patients with unstable Hb disease include: an inherent tendency towards irreversible denaturation of Hb or globin due to a defect in the amino-acid composition of labile Hb molecules; a continuous tendency toward hemichrome formation; precipitation or aggregation of Hb molecules resulting in buildup of the molecules to form Heinz bodies; and hemolysis.

Exposure of red cells to acetylphenylhydrazine and subsequent staining with crystal violet also revealed a greater abundance of Heinz bodies within G-6-PD-deficient cells compared with that in normal cells (Jandel, *et al.*, 1960; Peisach, *et al.*, 1975). In addition, Sear *et al.* (1975) and Campwala & Desforges (1982) reported that Heinz bodies often appeared in normal-aging red cells, and that this age-related appearance of Heinz bodies was particularly pronounced in splenectomized individuals (Selwyn, 1955). According to several authors (Weiss, 1962; 1963; Wennberg & Weiss, 1968), aged or damaged red cells affected by drugs may be "filtered off" by the spleen irrespective of whether or not they contain Heinz bodies in a similar manner to the filtering off of red blood cells in patients with unstable Hb caused by unstable Hb hemolytic anemia.

Using freshly drawn venous blood from healthy donors, we found that the number of Heinz bodies formed in red cells increased with increasing temperature when blood samples were subjected to mild heating at temperatures greater than 37 °C for 30 min (Sugawara, *et al.*, 2009; 2010; 2011; 2013). Under identical conditions of mild heating, we measured blood fluidity using a micro-channel array flow analyzer (MC-FAN) (Sugawara, *et al.*, 2010; 2011; 2013) because it involves a characteristic V-shaped groove array with micro flow paths (width, 7 μm; length, 30 μm; depth, 4.5 μm) engraved on a single-crystal silicon substrate in an integral circuit. When red cells passing through individual micro-channel arrays were monitored using an inverted metallographic microscope, images revealed good erythrocyte deformability when temperature-untreated samples were subjected to MC-FAN. Conversely, a marked decline in erythrocyte deformability was observed in blood samples treated at temperatures more than 37 °C for 30 min. Temperature-treated samples also demonstrated an increased transit time for low transit sample volumes. We therefore concluded that erythrocyte deformability decreased with increasing temperature of blood samples at above 37 °C. The combination of our experimental findings and *in situ* observations suggests that instability leading to hemichrome formation is not only a peculiarity of labile Hb variants, but is also an innate characteristic of physiologically normal Hb molecules. In this regard, one must note that monomeric bovine heart MbO_2 did not show a propensity for hemichrome formation over a wide range of pH (4.5–10.5) and temperature from physiological to temperatures just before thermal unfolding (Figure 8).

In our experiments, the occurrence of hemichrome can be described as shown in equation (6). Taking into account the accepted framework of the S_N2 mechanism for autoxidation (Shikama: 1985; 1988; 1990; 1998; 2006) and the accepted framework for hemichrome formation (Rifkind, *et al.*, 1994) in physiologically conditions, hemichrome can form as follows:

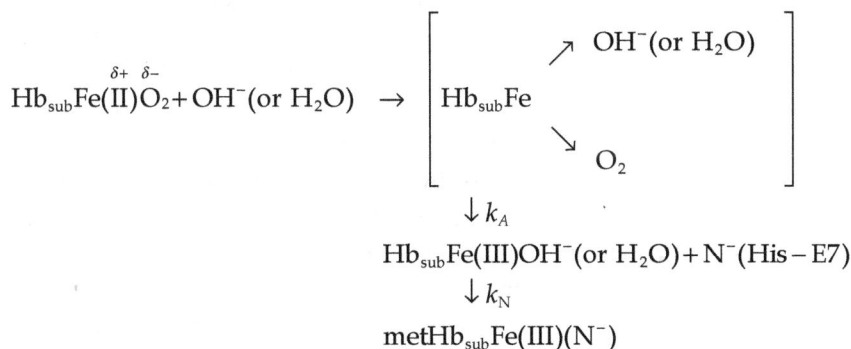

$$Hb_{sub}\overset{\delta+}{Fe}(II)\overset{\delta-}{O_2} + OH^- (or\ H_2O) \rightarrow \begin{bmatrix} Hb_{sub}Fe \overset{\nearrow\ OH^- (or\ H_2O)}{\searrow\ O_2} \end{bmatrix}$$

$$\downarrow k_A$$

$$Hb_{sub}Fe(III)OH^- (or\ H_2O) + N^- (His-E7)$$

$$\downarrow k_N$$

$$metHb_{sub}Fe(III)(N^-)$$

In this scheme, Hb_{sub} represents each subunit of the Hb molecule. Nucleophilic displacement of O_2^- by entry of a water molecule or a hydroxyl ion should be the rate-limiting step, and the subsequent conversion of the met form into hemichrome by a heme ligand (N^-) endogenous to the protein must proceed very quickly with the kinetic relationship $k_N \gg k_A$. The most probable candidate for N^- in the HbA molecule is the N^ε-nitrogen of the distal His (E7) (the only amino-acid side chain in the ligand pocket) of each subunit because N^ε-nitrogen is located more than 4 Å (10^{-1} nm) from the iron in Hb, and is therefore not expected to coordinate in native Hb (Phillips, 1978; Rifkind, *et al.*, 1994).

The content of metHb in normal erythrocytes (Paul, 1944; Bodansky, 1951) has been reported to be less than or equal to 1% by a NADH-dependent enzyme system (Scott, *et al.*, 1965; Hultquist & Passon, 1971; Sugita, *et al.*, 1971). This fact poses the question of how erythrocytes can elicit the range of responses to hemichrome with such a small amount of metHb. We suggest that this can be achieved by intramolecular anion-induced nucleophilic displacement of molecular dioxygen via an intermediate ferrous heme/anion complex (a low-spin hemichrome) (Sugawara, *et al.*, 2003). Such a reaction would follow the scheme:

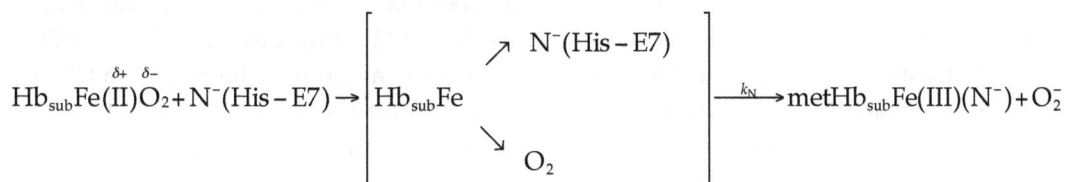

$$Hb_{sub}\overset{\delta+}{Fe}(II)\overset{\delta-}{O_2} + N^- (His-E7) \rightarrow \begin{bmatrix} Hb_{sub}Fe \overset{\nearrow\ N^- (His-E7)}{\searrow\ O_2} \end{bmatrix} \xrightarrow{k_N} metHb_{sub}Fe(III)(N^-) + O_2^-$$

In this reaction, nucleophilic displacement can be caused within the heme pocket by the N^ε-nitrogen of the distal His (E7) instead of nucleophilic incursion of the water molecule or the hydroxyl ion from outside the molecule. As indicated above, hemi-chrome formation occurs at every stage during the autoxidation reaction of HbO_2 (*i.e.*, at the initial, intermediate, and final stages) as a function of the pH and temperature of the solution. While the reaction proceeds along this scheme, hemichromes may be derived not only from HbO_2 species, but also from deoxyHb and metHb (Figure 18(b)). Vital hemichromes in erythrocytes *in situ* might arise from this intramolecular anion-induced nucleophilic displacement of O_2 via an intermediate ferrous heme/anion complex.

Our electron paramagnetic resonance (EPR) measurement study (Tsuruga, *et al.*, 1998) showed a low-spin spectrum for the resulting oxidation products of isolated β chains with values of $g_1 = 2.77$, $g_2 = 2.27$, and $g_3 = 1.68$, in addition to the usual aquo-met species with g values of 5.86 and 1.99 under a magnetic field of 0–500 mT at 8.0 K in 10 mM maleate buffer (pH 6.2) and in the presence of 50% (*v/v*) glycerol. According to Rifkind *et al.* (1994), such low-spin complexes characterized by the highest g values in the range 2.83–2.75 and the lowest g values in the range 1.69–1.63 have been designated as "complex B", indicating the crystal field parameters of the reversible hemichrome (*i.e.*, a water-retained bis-histidine complex). The molar fraction of the hemichrome (complex B) in the oxidized β chains was estimated to be 85% at pH 6.2 because a low-spin species was in equilibrium with a high-spin species corresponding to the usual aquo-met species.

Interestingly, recent crystallographic and EPR spectroscopic studies concerning tetrameric Hbs isolated from the Antarctic fish species *Trematomus bernacchii*, *Trematomus newnesi*, and *Gymnodraco acuticep* show that endogenous coordination at the sixth coordination site of the heme iron could be the bis-histidyl adducts in the ferric state in the solid and solution state (Vitagliano, *et al.*, 2004; Vergara, *et al.*, 2007; Vitagliano, *et al.*, 2008; Vergara, *et al.*, 2009). In Antarctic fish, isolated Hbs are readily oxidized at room temperature to a partial hemichrome state in which only the iron of the β chain is bonded to the distal His. Such bis-histidyl coordination was also discovered in the crystals of horse metHb exposed to acidic pH (where the proximal His [His87(F8)α] and a water molecule are the axial heme ligands) to the hemichrome (bis-histidine) form (in which the proximal His and the distal His [His58(E7)α] are the axial heme ligands) (Robinson, *et al.*, 2003). In the case of horse metHb, the bis-histidyl coordination was seen in α chains, and not in β chains. These crystal structures suggest a different binding state of α and β chains as well as a different pathway to hemichrome.

As described above, the α_1–β_1 (and α_2–β_2) interface seemed to have dual faces. One is for stabilizing the HbO_2 tetramer against the acidic autoxidation and the other is for controlling the fate (removal) of its own erythrocyte from the blood circulation. The α_1–β_1 (and α_2–β_2) interface produces a conformational constraint in the constructed chains of the Hb molecule via tilting of the distal (E7) His residues, *i.e.*, α58His (E7) in the α chain and β63His (E7) in the β chain. It was also shown that the α_1–β_1 (and α_2–β_2) interface appears to have a pH-sensor and a temperature-sensor. By virtue of these en-dowments, it seemed that Hb molecules can accomplish their roles not only as particu-larly suitable O_2 carriers between the lungs and tissues but also as equipped "molecular sensors" within the erythrocyte to control the fate (removal) of their own erythrocytes from the blood circulation depending on internal and extraneous circumstances, including pH and temperature (Figure 18).

Regarding the latter issue, normal erythrocytes develop Heinz bodies late in their lifespan. A wide variety of biochemical changes have been reported to accompany the aging of red cells (Clark, 1988). These include carboxymethylation of proteins, activation of proteases, glycosylation of proteins, loss of membrane area, decline in changes in the ratio of bands 4.1a to 4.1b, increases in oxidized lipids and proteins, changes in the rheology and fragility of cells, changes in the exposure of cell-surface sugars, and gradual accumulation of Ca^{2+}. Low (1991) demonstrated that band-3 clustering might warrant closer scrutiny as a possible transducer of distress signals from the cytoplasm to the external surface of the cell because it can be caused by hemichrome binding, ATP depletion, malondialdehyde formation, Ca^{2+} accumulation, oxidative crosslinking, or weakening of the skeletal membrane. It is known that hemichromes formed within erythrocytes bind to the cytoplasmic portion of band 3 in the membrane, then rapidly copolymerize with the soluble cytoplasmic domain of membrane band 3, forming an insoluble copolymer, followed by other changes involved in the pathogenesis of red-cell destruction (Walder, *et al.*, 1984; Waugh & low, 1985; Low and Waugh, 1985; Schlueter & Drenckhahn, 1986; Waugh, *et al.*, 1987). The dominant role of band-3 clustering suggests that hemichrome formation-induced band-3 clustering could also provide a key to the control of the fate of senescent and damaged red cells in the blood circulation.

9   Discussion (Additional): To Seek New *Vistas* for Understanding of Clinical Aspects of Drug-Induced Hemolytic Anemia and the Like

Human red blood corpuscles survive in the circulation for an average of 120 days. Red cells are formed in the bone marrow in adults and can be found in the peripheral blood ever after. Erythrocytes in the circulation adopt a biconcave disk shape, 7.8 x 1.8 μm, 1 μm thin in the middle. They lack a nucleus, endoplasmic reticulum, mitochondria, and ribosomes, and are essentially a bag of Hb with relatively few other proteins. Erythrocytes function to transport oxygen (O_2) from the lungs to the tissues, and transport carbon dioxide from the tissues back to the lungs. The average normal red cell counts are 5.4×10^6/μL in men and 4.8×10^6/μL in women, and each cell contains approximately 29 pg of Hb. There are therefore about 3×10^{13} red blood cells and about 900 g of Hb in the circulating blood in an adult man. Moreover, the mean corpuscular Hb concentration (MCHC) in human erythrocytes is up to 34 % (g/dL) for male and female.

Erythrocytes possess unique deformability (Braasch, 1971; Huang *et al.*, 2011), thus being able to squeeze through capillaries as narrow as 2 μm in diameter of the microcirculation. During the ~240 km journey in their life span (~120 days) (Huang *et al.*, 2011), they incessantly traverse through narrow capillaries. However, aged or deformed red cells are less flexible, and become trapped in the spleen while traversing small apertures in the basement membranes separating the cords from the sinusoids (where the spaces are sufficiently small to require extreme deformation of red cells) (Jacob, 1971), and lysed (ingested) by macrophages.

Red blood cells can be lysed as a result of exposure to drugs and infections (Winslow & Anderson, 1978; Weatherall *et al.*, 1995). The susceptibility of red cells to hemolysis by these agents is increased by a deficiency of the enzyme glucose 6-phosphate dehydrogenase (G-6-PD), which catalyzes the initial step in the oxidation of glucose via the hexose monophosphate pathway. This pathway generates dihydronicotinamide adenine dinucleotide phosphate (NADPH), which is needed for the maintenance of normal red cell fragility. Congenital deficiency of G-6-PD activity in red cells as a result of the presence of enzyme variants is common; indeed, G-6-PD deficiency is the commonest known genetically-determined human enzyme abnormality. More than 80 genetic variants of G-6-PD have been described; 40 of these cause no appreciable reduction in enzyme activity, but others reduce G-6-PD activity, and increase sensitivity to hemolytic agents and the risk of hemolytic anemia.

Removal of aged and damaged red cells from the blood circulation is thus essential for homeostasis, and the mechanisms whereby human erythrocytes register their aging and determine their lifespan is a key factor in erythrocyte physiology. In this chapter, we detailed necessary basic methods in protein purification and analysis that led us to grasp new roles assigned to the α_1–β_2 (and α_2–β_1) interface of the human hemoglobin molecule, so far: one is for stabilizing the HbO$_2$ tetramer against acidic autoxidation; and the other is for controlling the fate (removal) of its own erythrocyte from the blood circulation. In this section, focusing on the latter, whereby the involvement of intrinsic tilting capability of distal (E7) His residues (their bis-histidyl coordination proficiency to the heme iron) as well as the participation of the α_1–β_1 (and α_2–β_2) interface of the Hb molecule thus far examined concerning the oxidative behavior of human Hb molecules, pH- and temperature-dependent hemichrome emergence (*i.e.*, degradation of the Hb molecule to hemichrome inseparably related to autoxidation), and subsequent accumulation of soluble and insoluble hemichromes.

Heinz bodies, that are intra-erythrocytic inclusions of hemichrome formed from oxidized or denatured Hb, are commonly seen by phase contrast microscopy as dark spots free in the cytoplasm or attached to the cytoplasmic surface of the erythrocyte membrane. Heinz bodies occur in red cells naturally under three distinct conditions. First, erythrocytes containing unstable Hbs, especially Hbs with mutations near the heme site in the β subunits, show elevated levels of Heinz bodies (Winslow & Anderson, 1978; Weatherall *et al.*, 1995). Second, Heinz bodies are seen in normal cells (containing normal Hb) under conditions of oxidant stress. The oxidant stress can arise either in cells suffering from a diminished capacity to maintain intracellular reducing power, e.g., in G-6-PD and glutathione peroxidase deficiency diseases (Jandel, *et al.*, 1960; Peisach, *et al.*, 1975). Third, Heinz bodies often appear in normal cells as they age (Sears, *et al.*, 1975; Campwala & Desforges, 1982). This age-related appearance of Heinz bodies is especially pronounced in splenoectomized individuals where a major organ of senescent cell removal has been excised (Selwyn, 1955). Heinz body formation, however, whether natural or drug induced or oxidant stress promoted or unstable Hb disease produced, has considered to be occurred by a similar mechanism.

From this point of view, the sequential changes occurring within red corpuscles upon the removal of non-functional erythrocytes, in our proposal, (whether natural or drug induced or oxidant stress promoted or unstable Hb disease produced), include: 1) receipt for internal and external stimuli around the erythrocyte (e.g., pH, temperature, oxidative stress) via the α_1–β_1 (and α_2–β_2) interface of the molecule; 2) an invocation to distal-side perturbations of the heme pocket as the end result of the receipt of incoming stimuli; 3) temporal bis-histidyl coordination of the distal (E7) His residues to the heme iron that lead to hemichrome (degradation of the Hb molecule); 4) hemichrome emergence and subsequent hemichrome precipitation and aggregation of the Hb molecules that lead to formation of Heinz bodies within the erythrocyte; and 5) hemolysis of Heinz body-containing red cell in the spleen.

Granting this new mode (molecular-sensing) of Heinz body formation mechanisms to be basic premise, we hereinafter make an attempt to examine how this new epitome can serve as a basis not only for understanding how human erythrocytes appreciate aging and determine their lifespan but also for deeper understanding of clinical aspects of drug-induced hemolytic anemia, defects in the intra-erythrocytic reducing system and unstable Hb disease, on the basis of the finding and arguments appeared in *J. Bioanal. Biomed.* 2013:5:36-56 (Sugawara *et al.*).

First of all, we take up unstable Hb disease, as over 90 different unstable Hbs have been reported so far (Winslow & Anderson, 1978; Weatherall *et al.*, 1995). In establishing a diagnosis of unstable Hb disease, the heat denaturation test is considered to be the single most important procedure, in which a fresh hemolysate is diluted into 50 volumes of buffer solution and heated at 60 °C; at intervals the precipitates are removed from samples by centrifugation, and the optical density of the supernatant is measured. The reason of such instability even on mild heating (*i.e.*, inclination toward accelerated degradation of Hb molecule to hemichrome resulting hemichrome precipitation and subsequent formation of Heinz bodies within the erythrocytes) is quite well understood at the molecular level, but there is still a lack of knowledge of the changes occurring during precipitation and ultimate cause of hemolysis.

Addition to this, the similarity to events observed in the oxidative hemolytic anemia suggests that the precipitation of unstable Hbs is accompanied by oxidative changes (Winslow & Anderson, 1978; Weatherall *et al.*, 1995). The oxidative hemolytic anemia arise either from formation of excess oxidizing products (as with acetylphenylhydrazine administration) or from breakdown of protective mechanisms against oxidants (as in G-6-PD deficiency). In either case, the end result is the same as with unstable Hbs; the precipitation of Hb, the formation of Heinz bodies, and hemolysis.

In our hypothesis, incoming stimuli of the erythrocyte (e.g., pH, temperature, oxidative stress), whether natural or drug induced or oxidant stress promoted or unstable Hb disease produced, can be transmitted ultimately to the distal-side perturbations of residues lining the distal side of the heme pocket *via* the α_1–β_1 (and α_2–β_2) interface, so that they let the distal (E7) His residues coordinate at the sixth coordination position of the heme iron to form a bis-histidyl complex. This temporal bis-histidyl coordination by virtue of the inherent tilting capability of the distal (E7) His residues (*i.e.*, hemichrome emergence) in turn triggers a series of irreversible chemical reactions (including hemichrome formation-induced band-3 clustering and subsequent formation of Heinz bodies) that lead to the removal of non-functional erythrocytes from the blood circulation. Our hypothesis definitely demonstrates that there is positive correlation between the oxidative behavior of human Hb, its inseparably related instability (accelerated inclination toward degradation of Hb molecule to hemichrome), the subsequent formation of Heinz bodies within the erythrocyte and its ultimate fate (hemolysis) even on mild conditions at close-to-physiological temperatures and pH.

The defect in unstable Hbs involves important internal bonding amino acids, particularly those forming bonds with the heme group. Many of the mutants that occur at the $\alpha 1-\beta 2$ (and $\alpha 2-\beta 1$) interface have altered oxygen affinity, but the bulk of evidence suggests that the $\alpha 1-\beta 1$ (and $\alpha 2-\beta 2$) interface is much more important in maintaining the molecular stability of Hb than the $\alpha 1-\beta 2$ (and $\alpha 2-\beta 1$) interface. Hemolytic anemia results from substitutions affecting the $\alpha 1-\beta 1$ (and $\alpha 2-\beta 2$) interface or the heme pocket. If such mutations occur, the heme iron will be oxidized more readily, and a sequence of events leads to hemichrome formation and subsequent Heinz-body clustering in red cells that causes hemolytic anemia. Typical examples of such variants are summarized in Table 2.

• E [β26(B8)Glu → Lys]	• Volga [β27(B9)Ala → Asp]
• Genova [β28(B10)Leu → Pro]	• St. Louis [β28(B10)Leu → Gln]
• Tacoma [β30(B12)Arg → Ser]	• Abraham Lincoln [β32(B14)Leu → Pro]
• Castilla [β32(B14)Leu → Arg]	• Philly [β35(C1)Tyr → Phe]
• Rush [β101(G3)Glu → Gln]	• Peterborough [β111(G13)Val → Phe]
• Madrid [β115(G17)Ala → Pro]	• Khartoum [β124(H2)Pro → Arg]
• J. Guantanamo [β128(H6)Ala → Asp]	• Wien [β130(H8)Tyr → Asp]
• Leslie [β131(H9)Gln → deleted]	• Torino [α43(CD1)Phe → Val]
• L. Ferrara [α47(CD5)Asp → Gly]	• Setif [α94(G1)Asp → Tyr]
• St. Lukes [α95(G2)Pro → Arg]	

Table 2: Unstable hemoglobin variants, showing sites of amino acid substitutions (or deletions), redrawn from Sugawara *et al.* (2011). Each individual row illustrates variant's name, the residue concerned (chain; number; position), and replacement (from → to), respectively.

Surprisingly, almost all of these pathological mutations are found on the β chain, especially in the $\alpha 1-\beta 1$ (and $\alpha 2-\beta 2$) contact region: Tacoma [β30(B12)Arg → Ser], Abraham Lincoln [β32(B14)Leu → Pro], Castilla [β32(B14)Leu → Arg], Peterborough [β111(G13)Val → Phe], Madrid [β115(G17)Ala → Pro], Khartoum [β124(H2)Pro → Arg], J. Guantanamo [β128(H6)Ala → Asp] and Leslie [β131(H9)Gln → deleted]. In these Hbs, the $\alpha 1-\beta 1$ (and $\alpha 2-\beta 2$) interface would become loose or disruptive due to many different causes including: the insertion of proline (Abraham Lincoln, Madrid), the substitution with a too-small amino acid side chain (Tacoma) or a too-large side chain (Peterborough), the introduction of a charged or very polar group (Castilla, Khartoum, J. Guantanamo), and the deletion of amino acid residue (Leslie).

The situation in patients with G-6-PD deficiency (Winslow & Anderson, 1978; Weatherall *et al.*, 1995) can serve as another example. Red cells are known to be vulnerable to injury by endogenous and exogenous oxidants. Oxidants can be inactivated by reduced glutathione in erythrocytes with normal G-6-PD activity because the pentose phosphate shunt supplies NADPH (which is required for glutathione recycling). In G-6-PD-deficient erythrocytes, however, the reduced glutathione cannot be restored, and the cells sustain irreversible oxidative damage. However, G-6-PD deficiency produces symptoms only if the patient is exposed to an environmental factor that results in increased oxidative stress. Such stress includes antimalarials (e.g., primaquine, pamaquine, dapsone), sulfonamides, nitrofurantoin and phenacetin. The resulting crisis can lead to hemolysis of up to 25–30% of red cells within hours. However, the crisis is self-limited, and only the older population of red cells is destroyed. The mechanisms responsible for such an acute hemolytic crisis in patients taking these drugs cannot be explained on the basis of conventional views. Figure 18 suggests that this crisis could be triggered by fluctuations in endogenous and exogenous oxidative stress under the fragile pentose phosphate shunt.

Malaria provides the other example. This is a protozoal disease transmitted by the bite of female *Anopheles* mosquitoes (*Plasmodium falciparum, P. malariae, P. vivax, and P. ovale*). Blackwater fever syndrome is caused by infection with *P. falciparum*, and is characterized by repeated bouts of chills and fevers, severe intravascular hemolysis and anemia, jaundice, hemoglobinuria (black urine) and splenic enlargement (Ende, *et al.*, 1998; White, 2003; Hue *et al.*, 2009). Patients often develop fevers above 40 °C. A feature of this syndrome is that symptoms can be exacerbated in patients with G-6-PD deficiency as a result of taking quinine. In these patients, massive destruction of red cells infected by the parasite occurs, but similar numbers of normal erythrocytes are also ruptured, resulting in characteristic hemoglobinuria. The reason for the massive hemolysis of non-infected red cells is unclear. However, the possibility of a relationship between quinine ingestion and the associated massive hemolysis, as well as the relevance of G-6-PD deficiency, is addressed in Figure 18. Fevers above 40 °C, endogenous G-6-PD deficiency, and exogenous quinine ingestion represent conditions that induce acute hemolysis, thereby leading to massive blood loss and hemoglobinuria.

10   Conclusions

Cellular life is reliant upon rapid and efficient responses to internal and external conditions whereby basic molecular events associated with these processes are the structural transitions of the proteins (structural protein allostery) involved. The human hemoglobin (Hb) molecule ($\alpha_2\beta_2$) holds a special position in these structural transitions. Hb has two types of α–β interface (*i.e.*, α_1–β_1 [and α_2–β_2] and α_1–β_2 [and α_2–β_1]). The latter α_1–β_2 (and α_2–β_1) interface is associated with cooperative O_2 binding, and exhibits principal roles if the molecule goes from its deoxygenated to oxygenated quaternary structure.

However, the role of the former α_1–β_1 (and α_2–β_2) interface has been unclear for a long time. In this regard, important and intriguing observations have been accumulating, so that a new gaze can be focused on the α_1–β_1 (and α_2–β_2) interface.

In this chapter, we aimed to detail necessary basic methods in protein purification and analysis that led us to grasp new roles assigned to the α_1–β_2 (and α_2–β_1) interface of the human hemoglobin molecule: one is for stabilizing the HbO_2 tetramer against acidic autoxidation; and the other is for controlling the fate (removal) of its own erythrocyte from the blood circulation.

First of all, we demonstrated that the following seven main conclusions could be drawn by good use of these methods. First, autoxidation of human HbO_2 seemed to be inseparably related to the instability of the Hb molecule and its degradation to hemichrome. Second, in terms of pH-dependent biphasic autoxidation (k_A^f for the initial fast oxidation and k_A^s for the second oxidation) seen in acidic solutions, participation of a single dissociation group of an amino-acid residue (probably a His residue) with pK_a = 7.4 (at 37 °C) appeared to have a key role in how the Hb molecule can prompt the range of fast (k_A^f) and slow (k_A^s) components against the pH values of the solutions. Third, the isolated α and β chains were oxidized much more readily over the measured pH range (5–10.5) when compared with the respective rates of the parent molecules used as a reference. Fourth, in terms of pH- and temperature-dependent hemichrome emergence observed by UV/Vis spectroscopy, HbO_2 was supposed to be highly susceptible to hemichrome formation (even under physiological pH and temperature). Fifth, in contrast to the tetrameric human HbO_2 as O_2^- carrying protein in the blood, the monomeric bovine heart Mb (MbO_2) did not show any propensity for hemichrome formation over a wide pH range of 4.5 to 10.5 and over a wide temperature range from physiological to temperatures just before thermal unfolding. Sixth, UV/Vis spectrophotometric, isoelectric-focusing electrophoretic and polyacrylamide gel electrophoretic measurements following human HbO_2 autoxidation demonstrated that the intrinsic α-chain oxidation seemed to be much faster than the intrinsic β-chain oxidation among the HbO_2 tetramer. Finally, by means of computer simulations on the basis of data obtained from measurements (spectrophotometry, isoelectric-focusing electrophoresis, and polyacrylamide gel electrophoresis), k_A^f represented intrinsic α-chain oxidation whereas k_A^s reflected intrinsic β-chain oxidation, and the β chain manifested delayed autoxidation in human HbO_2 (which could be much more evident in acidic solutions).

Next, on the basis of these findings, two major subjects were discussed and interpreted in terms of the α_1–β_1 (and α_2–β_2) interface. The first subject was the pH-dependent delayed autoxidation of β (O_2) subunits when compared with α (O_2) subunits in the tetrameric architecture. The second subject was the inherent tilting capability of the distal (E7) His residues (*i.e.*, α58His (E7) in the α chain and β63His (E7) in the β chain) to hemichrome formation or Hb degradation. In the latter mechanism, the α_1–β_1 (and α_2–β_2) interface play a key role as an equipped (inherent) molecular sensor to control the fate of the own erythrocyte via tilting of the distal (E7) His (*i.e.*, α58His (E7) in the α chain and β63His (E7) in the β chain) that can be triggered degradation of the Hb molecule to hemichrome, and subsequent clustering of Heinz bodies within the erythrocyte depending on the internal and extraneous conditions of the erythrocyte, including pH and temperature.

Later on, focusing on the latter, and taken together with the previous findings accomplished by our search for similar phenomena in normal human erythrocyte during mild heating (Sugawara *et al.*, 2009; 2010; 2011; 2013) and the related current interpretations and arguments, we made an attempt to propose a new mode of Heinz body formation mechanisms, wherein the inherent tilting capability of the distal (E7) His residues (*i.e.*, α58His (E7) in the α chain and β63His (E7) in the β chain) of the Hb molecule plays a major role as well as involvement of the α_1–β_1 (and α_2–β_2) interface. Specifically, the suggested sequential changes occurring within the erythrocyte upon the removal of non-functional erythrocytes, whether natural or drug induced or oxidant stress promoted or unstable Hb disease produced, include: 1) receipt for internal and external stimuli around the erythrocyte (e.g., pH, temperature, oxidative stress) via the α_1–β_1 (and α_2–β_2) interface of the molecule; 2) an invocation to distal-side perturbations of the heme pocket as the end result of the receipt of incoming stimuli; 3) temporal bis-histidyl coordination of the distal (E7) His residues to the heme iron that lead to hemichrome (degradation of the Hb molecule); 4) hemichrome emergence and subsequent hemichrome precipitation and aggregation of the Hb molecules that lead to formation of Heinz bodies within the erythrocyte; and 5) hemolysis of Heinz body-containing red cell in the spleen.

Granting this new mode (molecular-sensing) of Heinz body formation mechanisms to be basic premise, we also made an attempt to examine how this new epitome can serve as a basis not only for understanding how human erythrocytes appreciate aging and determine their lifespan but also for deeper understanding of clinical aspects of drug-induced hemolytic anemia, defects in the intra-erythrocytic reducing system and unstable Hb disease, in which the mechanisms for acute hemolytic crisis cannot be explained on the basis of conventional views.

With respect to the latter issue, the followings were shown:

1. Almost all of pathological mutations of unstable Hbs are found on the β chain, especially in the α_1–β_1 (and α_2–β_2) contact region: Tacoma [β30(B12)Arg → Ser], Abraham Lincoln [β32(B14)Leu → Pro], Castilla [β32(B14)Leu → Arg], Peterborough [β111(G13)Val → Phe], Madrid [β115(G17)Ala → Pro], Khartoum [β124(H2)Pro → Arg], J. Guantanamo [β128(H6)Ala → Asp] and Leslie [β131(H9)Gln → deleted].

2. Acute hemolytic crisis observed in patients of G-6-PD deficiency while taking drugs such as antimalarials (e.g., primaquine, pamaquine, dapsone), sulfonamides, nitrofurantoin and phenacetin can be explained by increased oxidative stress against inadequate reduced glutathione levels in erythrocytes of the patients.

3. Acute hemolytic crisis associated with blackwater fever syndrome of malarial patients caused by infection with *Plasmodium falciparum* can be also explained by fevers above 40 °C, endogenous G-6-PD deficiency, and exogenous quinine ingestion.

References

Baldwin, J. & Chothia, C. (1979). Haemoglobin. The structural changes related to ligand binding and its allosteric mechanism. J. Mol. Biol., 129, 175–220.

Bodansky, O. (1951). Methemoglobinemia and methemoglobin-producing compounds. Pharmacol. Rev., 3, 144–196.

Borgstahl, G. E. O., Rogers, P.H. & Arnone, A. (1994). The 1.8 Å structure of carbonmonoxy-β4 hemoglobin. J. Mol. Biol., 236, 817–830.

Boyer, P. D. (1954). Spectrophotometric study of the reaction of protein sulfhydryl groups with organic mercurials. J. Am. Chem. Soc., 76, 7331–4337.

Braasch, D. (1971). Red cell deformability and capillary blood flow. Physiol. Rev., 51, 679–701.

Brooks, J. (1931) The oxidation of haemoglobin to methaemoglobin by oxygen. Proc. Roy. Soc. London Ser. B, 109, 35–50.

Brooks, J. (1935) The oxidation of haemoglobin to methaemoglobin by oxygen II – The relation between the rate of oxidation and the partial pressure of oxygen. Proc. Roy. Soc. London Ser. B, 118, 560–570.

Brunori, M., Falcioni, G., Fioretti, E., Giardina, B. & Rotilio, G. (1975). Formation of superoxide in the autoxidation of the isolated α and β chains of human hemoglobin and its involvement in hemichrome precipitation. Eur. J. Biochem., 53, 99–104.

Campwala, H. Q. & Desforges, J. F. (1982). Membrane-bound hemichrome in density-separated cohorts of normal (AA) and sickled (SS) cells. J. Lab. Clin. Med., 99, 25–28.

Clark, M. R. (1988). Senescence of red blood cells: Progress and problems. Physiol. Rev., 68, 503–554.

Dickerson, R. E. & Geis, I. (1983). Hemoglobin: Structure, Function, Evolution and Pathology, The Benjamin/Cummings Publishing Co., Inc., Menlo Park, CA, USA.

Ende, J. V. D., Coppena, G., Verstraeten, T., Haegenborgh, T. V., Depraetere, K., Gompel, A. V., Enden, E. V. D., Clerinx, J., Colebunders, R., Peetermans, W.E., & et al. (1998). Recurrence of blackwater fever: triggering relapses by different antimararials. Trop. Med. Inter. Health., 3, 632–639.

Fermi, G. & Perutz, M. F. (1981). Haemoglobin and Myoglobin. In Atlas of Molecular Structure in Biology (Eds.: Phillips, D. C. & Richards, F. M.,), Clarendon Press, Oxford, UK, Volume 2.

Fasman, G.D. (1976) Physical and chemical data. In Handbook of Biochemistry and Molecular Biology, 3rd ed., CRC Press, Cleveland, OH, USA, p. 220.

Gotoh, T. & Shikama, K. (1974) Autoxidation of native oxymyoglobin from bovine heart muscle. Arch. Biochem. Biophys., 163, 476–481.

Hermans, J., Jr. & Rialdi, G. (1965). Heat of ionization and denaturation of sperm-whale myoglobin determined with a microcalorimeter. Biochemistry, 4, 1277–1281.

Huang, Y-X, Wu, Z-J, Mrhrishi, J., Huang B-T, Chen X-Y, Zheng, X-J, Liu, W-J. & Luo, M.

(2011). *Human red blood cell aging: correlative changes in surface charge and cell properties. J. Cell Mol. Med., 15, 2634–2642.*

Hue, N. T., Charlieu, J. P., Chau, T. T. H., Day, N., Farra, J. J., Hien, T. T. & Dunstan, S. J. (2009). *Glucose-6-phosphate dehydrogenase (G6PD) mutations and Haemoglobinuria syndrome in the Vietnamese population. Malaria J., 8, 152–160.*

Hultquist, D. E. & Passon, P. G. (1971). *Catalysis of methemoglobin reduction by erythrocyte cytochrome b5 and cytochrome b5 reductase. Nature, 229, 252–254.*

Imai, K. (1994). *Adair fitting to oxygen equilibrium curves of hemoglobin. Methods Enzymol., 232, 559–576.*

Jacob, H. S. (1970). *Mechanisms of Heinz body formation and attachment red cell membrane. Semin. Hematol., 7, 341–353.*

Jandel, J. H., Engle, L. K. & Allen, D. W. (1960). *Oxidative hemolysis and precipitation of hemoglobin. I. Heinz body anemias as an acceleration of red cell aging. J. Clin. Invest., 39, 1818–1836.*

Kao, O. H. W. & Wang, J. H. (1965). *Kinetic study of the oxidation of ferrohemochrome by molecular oxygen. Biochemistry, 4, 342–347.*

Levy, A., Sharma, V. S., Zhang, L. & Rifkind, J. M. (1992). *A new mode for heme-heme interaction in hemoglobin associated with distal perturbations. Biophys. J., 61, 750–755.*

Low, P. S. (1991). *Role of Hemoglobin Denaturation and Band 3 Clustering in Initiating Red Cell Removal. In Red Blood Cell Aging (Eds.: Magnani, M. & De Flora, A.), Plenum Press: New York, NY, USA, pp. 173–183.*

Low, P. S. & Waugh, S. M. (1985). *The role of hemoglobin denaturation and band 3 clustering in red blood cell aging. Science, 227, 531–533.*

Macdonald, V. W. (1994). *Measuring relative rates of hemoglobin oxidation and denaturation. Methods Enzymol., 231, 480–490.*

Mansouri, A. & Winterhalter, K. H. (1973). *Nonequivalence of chains in hemoglobin oxidation. Biochemistry, 12, 4946–4949.*

McDonald, M. J., Turci, S. M., Mrabet, N. T., Himelstein, B. P. & Bunn, H. F. (1987). *The kinetics of assembly of normal and variant human oxyhemoglobin. J. Biol. Chem., 262, 5951–5956.*

Park, S. -Y., Yokoyama, T., Shibayama, N., Shiro, Y. & Tame, J. R. H. (2006). *1.25 Å resolution crystal structure of human haemoglobin in the oxy, deoxy and carbonmonooxy forms. J. Mol. Biol., 360, 690–701.*

Paul, W. D. & Kemp, C. R. (1944). *Methemoglobin: A normal constituent of blood. Proc. Soc. Exp. Biol. Med., 56, 55–56.*

Peisach, J., Blumberg, W. E. & Rachmilewitz, E. A. (1975). *Detection of formation, and relevance of hemichromes and hemochromes. Biochim. Biophys. Acta, 393, 404–418.*

Perutz, M. F. (1970). *Stereochemistry of cooperative effects in haemoglobin. Nature, 228, 726–*

739.

Perutz, M. F. (1972). Nature of haem-haem interaction. Nature, 237, 495–499.

Perutz, M. F. (1990). Mechanisms of Cooperativity and Allosteric Regulation in Proteins, Cambridge University Press, Cambridge, UK.

Perutz, M. F, Fermi, G., Abraham, D.J., Poyart, C. & Bursaux, E. (1986). Hemoglobin as a receptor of drugs and peptides: X-ray studies of the stereochemistry of binding. J. Am. Chem. Soc., 108, 1064–1078.

Perutz, M. F., Wilkinson, A. J., Paoli, M. & Dodson, G. G. (1998). The stereochemical mechanism of the cooperative effects in hemoglobin revisited. Annu. Rev. Biophys. Biomol. Struct., 27, 1–34.

Phillips, S. E. V. (1978). Structure of oxymyoglobin. Nature, 273, 247–248.

Rachmilewitz, E.A. (1974). Denaturation of the normal and abnormal hemoglobin molecule. Semin. Hematol., 11, 441–462.

Rachmilewitz, E. A., Peisach, J., Bradley, T. B. & Blumberg, W. E. (1969). Role of haemichromes in the formation of inclusion bodies in haemoglobin H disease. Nature, 222, 248–250.

Rachmilewitz, E. A., Peisach, J. & Blumberg, W.E. (1971). Studies on the stability of oxyhemoglobin A and its constituent chains and their derivatives. J. Biol. Chem., 246, 3356–3366.

Rifkind, J. M., Abugo, O., Levy, A. & Heim, J. (1994). Detection, formation, and relevance of hemichromes and hemochromes. Methods Enzymol., 231, 449–480.

Robinson, V. L., Smith, B. B. & Arnone, A. (2003). A pH-dependent aquomet-to-hemichrome transition in crystalline horse methemoglobin. Biochemistry, 42, 10113–10125.

Schlueter, K. & Drenckhahn, D. (1986). Co-clustering of denatured hemoglobin with band 3: Its role in binding of autoantibodies against band 3 to abnormal and aged erythrocytes. Proc. Natl. Acad. Sci. USA, 83, 6137–6141.

Scott, E. M., Duncan, I. W. & Ekstrand, V. (1965). The reduced pyridine nucleotide dehydrogenases of human erythrocytes. J. Biol. Chem., 240, 481–485.

Sears, D. A., Friedman, J. M. & White, D. R. (1975). Binding of intracellular protein to the erythrocyte membrane during incubation: The production of Heinz bodies. J. Lab. Clin. Med., 86, 722–732.

Selwyn, J. G. (1955). Heinz bodies in red cells after splenectomy and after phenacetin administration. Br. J. Hematol., 1, 173–183.

Shikama, K. (1985). Nature of the FeO2 bonding in myoglobin: An overview from physical to clinical. Experientia, 41, 701–706.

Shikama, K. (1988). Stability properties of dioxygen-iron (II) porphyrins: An overview from simple complexes to myoglobin. Coord. Chem. Rev., 83, 73–91.

Shikama, K. (1990). Autoxidation of oxymyoglobin: A meeting point of the stabilixation and the activation of molecular oxygen. Biol. Rev., 65, 517–527.

Shikama, K. (1998). *The molecular mechanism of autoxidation for myoglobin and hemoglobin: A venerable puzzle. Chem. Rev., 98, 1357–1373.*

Shikama, K. (2006). *Nature of the FeO₂ bonding in myoglobin and hemoglobin: A new molecular paradigm. Prog. Biophys. Mol. Biol., 91, 83–162.*

Shikama, K. & Sugawara, Y. (1978) *Autoxidation of native oxymyoglobin: Kinetic analysis of the pH profile. Eur. J. Biochem., 91, 404–413.*

Sugawara, Y. & Shikama, K. (1979) *Autoxidation of native oxymyoglobin: Effect of pH on autoxidation rate. Sci. Rep. Tohoku Univ. Ser. IV (Biol.), 37, 253–262.*

Sugawara, Y., Sakoda, M., Shibata, N. & Sakamoto, H. (1993). *Autoxidation of human hemoglobin: Kinetic analysis of the pH-profile. Jpn. J. Phys., 43, 21–34.*

Sugawara, Y., Matsuoka A., Kaino, A. & Shikama, K. (1995). *Roles of globin moiety in the autoxidation reaction of oxymyoglobin: Effect of 8 M urea. Biophys. J., 69, 583–592.*

Sugawara, Y., Kadono, E., Suzuki, A., Yukuta, Y., Shibasaki, Y., Nishimura, N., Kameyama, Y., Hirota, M., Ishida, C., Higuchi, N., Haramoto, K., Sakai, Y. & Soda, H. (2003). *Hemichrome formation observed in human haemoglobin A under various buffer conditions. Acta. Physiol. Scand., 179, 49–59.*

Sugawara, Y., Abe, Y., Ohgushi, I., Ueno, E. & Shimamoto, F. (2009). *Roles of innate instability characteristic of hemoglobin molecule to hemichrome and subsequent Heinz body formation within normal human erythrocytes. Res. Rev. Biosci., 3, 204–215.*

Sugawara, Y., Hayashi, Y., Shigemasa, Y., Abe, Y., Ohgushi, I., Ueno, E. & Shimamoto, F. (2010). *Molecular biosensing mechanisms in the spleen for the removal of aged and damaged red cells from the blood circulation. Sensors, 3, 7099–7121.*

Sugawara, Y., Yamada, M., Ueno, E., Abe, Y., Okazaki, M., Okamoto, A., Miyake, M., Fukami, F. & Yano, A. (2011). *New roles assigned to the α₁–β₁ (and α₂–β₂) interface of the human hemoglobin molecule from physiological to cellular. Appl. Sci., 1, 13–55.*

Sugawara, Y., Shigemasa, Y., Hayashi, Y., Abe, Y., Ohgushi, I. & Ueno, E. (2013) *New mode (molecular-sensing) of Heinz body formation mechanisms inherent in human erythrocytes: Basis for understanding of clinical aspects of drug-induced hemolytic anemia and the like. J. Bioanal. Biomed., 5, 36–56.*

Sugita, Y., Nomura, S. & Yoneyama, Y. (1971). *Purification of reduced pyridine nucleotide dehydrogenase from human erythrocytes and methemoglobin reduction by the enzyme. J. Biol. Chem., 246, 6072–6078.*

Tomoda, A., Sugimoto, K., Suhara, M., Takeshita, M. & Yoneyama, Y. (1978a). *Haemichrome formation from haemoglobin subunits by hydrogen peroxide. Biochem. J., 171, 329–335.*

Tomoda, A., Takeshita, M. & Yoneyama, Y. (1978b) *Characterization of intermediate hemoglobin produced during methemoglobin reduction by ascorbic acid. J. Biol. Chem., 253, 7415–7419.*

Tomoda, A., Tsuji, A., Matsukawa, S., Takeshita, M. & Yoneyama, Y. (1978c) *Mechanism of methemoglobin reduction by ascorbic acid under anaerobic conditions. J. Biol. Chem., 253, 7420–7423.*

Tomoda, A., Yubisui, T., Tsuji, A. & Yoneyama, Y. (1979a). *Kinetic studies on methemoglobin reduction by human red cell NADH cytochrome b_5 reductase. J. Biol. Chem., 254, 3119–3123.*

Tomoda, A., Yubisui, T., Tsuji, A. & Yoneyama, Y. (1979b). *Analysis of met–form haemoglobin in human erythrocytes of normal adults and of a patient with hereditary methaemoglobi-naemia due to deficiency of NADH-cytochrome b_5 reductase. Biochem. J., 181, 505–507.*

Tomoda, A., Tsuji, A. & Yoneyama, Y. (1980a). *Mechanism of hemoglobin oxidation by ferricy-tochrome c under aerobic and anaerobic conditions. J. Biol. Chem., 255, 7978–7983.*

Tomoda, A., Ida, M., Tsuji, A. & Yoneyama, Y. (1980b). *Mechanism of methemoglobin reduc-tion by human erythrocytes. Biochem. J., 188, 535–540.*

Tomoda, A., Yoneyama, Y. & Tsuji, A. (1981). *Changes in intermediate haemoglobins during autoxidation of haemoglobin. Biochem. J., 195, 485–492.*

Tsuruga, M., Matsuoka, A., Hachimori, A., Sugawara, Y. & Shikama, K. (1998). *The molecular mechanism of autoxidation for human oxyhemoglobin: Tilting of the distal histidine causes nonequivalent oxidation in the β chain. J. Biol. Chem., 273, 8607–8615.*

Vergara, A., Franzese, M., Merlino, A., Vitagliano, L., Verde C., Prisco, G. D., Lee, H. C., Pei-sach, J. & Mazzarella, L. (2007). *Structural characterization of ferric hemoglobins from three Antarctic fish species of the suborder notothenioidei. Biophys. J., 93, 2822–2829.*

Vergara, A., Franzese, M., Merlino, A., Bonomi, G., Verde, C., Giordano, D., Prisco, G. D., Lee, H. C., Peisach, J. & Mazzarella, L. (2009). *Correlation between hemichrome stability and the root effect in tetrameric hemoglobins. Biophys. J., 97, 866–874.*

Vitagliano, L., Bonomi, G., Riccio, A., Prisco, G. D., Smulevich, G. & Mazzarella, L. (2004). *The oxidation process of Antarctic fish hemoglobins. Eur. J. Biochem., 271, 1651–1659.*

Vitagliano, L., Vergara, A., Bonomi, G., Merlino, A., Verde, C., Prisco, G. D., Howes, B. D., Smulevich, G. & Mazzarella, L. (2008). *Spectroscopic and crystallographic characterization of a tetrameric hemoglobin oxidation reveals structural features of the functional intermedi-ate relaxed/tense state. J. Am. Chem. Soc., 130, 10527–10535.*

Walder, J. A., Chatterjee, R., Steck, T. L., Low, P. S., Musso, G. F., Kaiser, E. T., Rogers, P. H. & Arnone, A. (1984). *The interaction of hemoglobin with the cytoplasmic domain of band 3 of the human erythrocyte membrane. J. Biol. Chem., 259, 10238–10246.*

Waugh, S. M. & Low, P. S (1985). *Hemichrome binding to band 3: Nucleation of Heinz bodies on the erythrocyte membrane. Biochemistry, 24, 34–39.*

Waugh, S. M., Walder, J. A. & Low, P. S. (1987). *Partial characterization of the copolymeriza-tion reaction of erythrocyte membrane band 3 with hemichromes. Biochemistry, 26, 1777–1783.*

Weiss, L. (1962). *The structure of fine splenic arterial vessels in relation to hemoconcentration and red cell destruction. Am. J. Anat., 111, 131–179.*

Weiss, L. (1963). *The structure of intermediate vascular pathways in the spleen of rabbits. Am. J. Anat., 113, 51–59.*

Wennberg, E. & Weiss, L. (1968). *Splenic erythroclasia: An electron microscopic study of hemo-*

globin H disease. Blood, 31, 778–790.

Weatherall, D. J., Clegg, J. B., Higgs, D. R. & Wood, W.G. (1995). The Hemoglobinopathies. In The Metabolic and Molecular Basis of Inherited Disease (Eds.: Scriver, C.R., Beaudet, A.L., William, S.S. & Valle, D.), McGraw-Hill Inc., New York, NY, USA, Volume, III, pp. 3413–3484.

White, J. M. (2003). Mararia. In Manson's Tropical Diseases (Eds.: Cook, G. C. & Zumura, A. I.), W.B. Saunders, Philadelphia, PA, USA, pp. 1205–1295.

Winterboun, C. C. & Carrell, R. W. (1974). Studies of hemoglobin denaturation and Heinz body formation in the unstable hemoglobin. J. Clin. Invest., 54, 678–689.

Winslow, R. M. & Anderson, W. F. (1978). The Hemoglobinopathies. In The Metabolic Basis of Inherited Disease (Eds.: Stanbury, J. B., Wyngaarden, J. B. & Fredricks, D. S.), McGraw-Hill Book Company, New York, NY, USA, pp. 1465–1507.

Yasuda, J. -P., Ichikawa T., Tsuruga, M., Matuoka, A., Sugawara, Y. & Shikama, K. (2002). The α1β1 contact of human hemoglobin plays a key role in stabilizing the bound dioxygen: Further evidence from the iron valency hybrids. Eur. J. Biochem., 269, 202–211.

Chapter 7

Cholesterol and Liver Inflammation: from Mice to Human

Sofie M.A. Walenbergh[1], Tim Hendrikx[1] and Ronit Shiri-Sverdlov[1]

1   Introduction

Nowadays, obesity is seen as one of the leading health concerns worldwide. The dramatically increasing occurrence of obesity in Western countries is accompanied with the development of the metabolic syndrome. This syndrome refers to a cluster of multiple metabolic abnormalities, the so-called "deadly quartet", which increases the susceptibility for the development of atherosclerotic cardiovascular disease and has rapidly evolved as the leading cause of death in the developed world (Roger *et al.*, 2011).

The metabolic syndrome is a significant predictor of atherosclerosis; a chronic inflammatory cardiovascular disease that starts developing from a young age and slowly leads to formation of lesions (made of excess fat deposits) and narrowing of the arteries over the years. Rupture of these atherosclerotic lesions is the cause of severe cardiovascular manifestations that appear later in life, such as stroke and myocardial infarction (Weber & Noels, 2011). Apart from atherosclerosis, the metabolic syndrome is also a strong predictor for disease development in the liver, termed non-alcoholic fatty liver disease (NAFLD). NAFLD involves a cluster of liver disease pathologies starting with the simplest form, termed hepatic steatosis, whereby excessive fat is stored and accumulates inside the liver. While steatosis is a reversible liver condition, it is the presence of hepatic inflammation, or non-alcoholic steatohepatitis (NASH) that precedes and sets the stage for more advanced stages of the disease, including fibrosis, cirrhosis and hepatocellular carcinoma. By then, patients await liver transplantation as the only curative treatment option left (Kopec & Burns, 2011).

---

[1] Department of Molecular Genetics, Faculty of Health, Medicine and Life Sciences, Maastricht University, The Netherlands

Altogether, the presence of inflammation in different tissues, such as the arteries during atherosclerosis and the liver during NASH, are both common features of adult and pediatric obesity. As these patients have a clearly increased mortality risk, there is a critical need for treatment options against these inflammatory obesity-related diseases. In order to develop such treatment options, the etiology of these diseases needs to be clarified first.

2   Cholesterol as a Consistent Risk Factor

The disease spectrum of the metabolic syndrome is strongly associated with a disturbed lipid profile. Individuals with the metabolic syndrome often demonstrate decreased levels of high-density lipoproteins (HDL) in plasma, while levels of triglycerides (TGs) and low-density lipoprotein (LDL)-cholesterol are increased (Grundy *et al.*, 2004). Therefore, cholesterol may play an important role in inflammatory diseases related to the metabolic syndrome.

Due to mutations in the LDL receptor (*LDLR*) gene, the main characteristic of patients with familial hypercholesterolemia is the presence of extremely high LDL-cholesterol levels in plasma. As expected, these patients demonstrate high morbidity and mortality rates due to the development of coronary heart disease early in life. Application of a lipid-lowering therapy reduced the amount of plasma LDL-cholesterol and contributed to a prolonged lifespan of these patients, suggesting that LDL-cholesterol is the main lipid involved in cardiovascular disease (Raal *et al.*, 2011). Additional human research demonstrated increased cholesterol deposition in livers of NASH patients compared to control subjects, and in line, a clear elevation of total cholesterol levels in plasma (Caballero *et al.*, 2009; Puri *et al.*, 2007). Despite the common association between obesity and NAFLD, non-obese patients with NAFLD had a greater intake of dietary cholesterol compared to their control group (Musso *et al.*, 2003; Yasutake *et al.*, 2009), strengthening the role of cholesterol during the pathogenesis of NAFLD even outside the scope of the metabolic syndrome.

Data from numerous mouse experiments confirm the role of cholesterol as found in human cardiovascular disease and NAFLD and can be summarized as follows. First, similar to the genetic cause of cardiovascular disease during familial hypercholesterolemia, transgenic mouse models have been developed that lack the *LDLR* gene. When fed a high-fat, high-cholesterol (HFC) diet, these mice fully mimic a human-like lipoprotein profile with typical hypercholesterolemia. As a result, the LDLR knockout (LDLR-/-) mouse model has been established as an excellent animal model to study the development of atherosclerosis and NASH (Bieghs, Van Gorp, Wouters, *et al.*, 2012; Ishibashi *et al.*, 1993; Ishibashi *et al.*, 1994). Secondly, elimination of dietary cholesterol to LDLR-/- mice prevented the development of steatohepatitis compared to mice fed a cholesterol-supplemented diet, suggesting that cholesterol is the main trigger for NASH (Wouters *et al.*, 2008). Thirdly, it was found that dietary cholesterol demonstrated an induction of genes involved in the inflammatory response, especially acute inflammation in the context of atherosclerosis in mice. These data were confirmed by biochemical measurements of representative proteins for the acute inflammatory response (Vergnes *et al.*, 2003). Consistently, the administration of increasing loads of dietary cholesterol to AP-OE*3-Leiden mice for 10 weeks displayed a marked systemic inflammatory response and the formation of early atherosclerotic lesions. Micro-array analysis in the livers of these mice demonstrated an upregulation of several inflammatory pathways, suggesting that high dietary cholesterol is correlated with liver inflammation (Kleemann *et al.*, 2007). In line, increased dietary cholesterol intake also exacerbated inflammation in the livers of LDLR$^{-/-}$ mice (Subramanian *et al.*, 2011).

In conclusion, the derived observations from mouse and human research, consistently point towards nutritional cholesterol as the best documented risk factor for atherogenesis (Steinberg, 2002). Increasing evidence now demonstrates that, similar to atherosclerosis, dietary cholesterol can also be viewed as the initiating factor for the development of NASH.

3   Inflammatory Mechanisms Triggered by Cholesterol

Macrophages are a certain type of immune cells that play a central role in the initiation, maintenance and resolution of inflammation within different tissues. Depending on the activation signals, tissue resident macrophages can be either classically activated (pro-inflammatory) or alternatively activated (anti-inflammatory) (Martinez & Gordon, 2014). During inflammation, macrophages initiate three important processes; antigen presentation, phagocytosis (= ingestion of cells, bacteria or particles), and production of several cytokines and chemokines (Bhargava & Lee, 2012; Fujiwara & Kobayashi, 2005). Since macrophages are the body's first line of defense and are therefore the most crucial immune cells during inflammation, we will in particular focus on the role of macrophages during atherosclerosis and NASH.

3.1   Foam Cell Formation

As described above, LDL-cholesterol levels are elevated in the circulation during metabolic inflammation and cause injury to the endothelium and underlying smooth muscle cells. In order to protect the body against these harmful effects of excess plasma LDL-cholesterol, macrophages are recruited into the vascular wall where they bind and take up LDL particles via the so-called scavenger receptors. Consequently, LDL starts to accumulate inside the macrophages leading to a 'foamy' macrophage phenotype. While this process is initially intended to be protective, it is now shifted towards inflammation as the foamy appearance causes the macrophage to activate the inflammatory response through the secretion of pro-inflammatory mediators and matrix-degrading proteases (Moore *et al.*, 2013). Macrophage-derived foam cells are the main characteristic of fatty streaks, one of the hallmarks of early-stage atherosclerosis in mice and humans and promote disease progression (Ross, 1999). The prolonged presence of these foamy macrophages inside the atherosclerotic plaque creates a cytotoxic environment due to endoplasmic reticulum and oxidative stress. These aberrations cause the foamy macrophages to go into apoptosis, release their lipid contents and attract even more macrophages and other immune cells for phagocytic clearance, thus further propagating inflammation. These events lead to the formation and expansion of the pro-thrombotic necrotic core, hereby triggering plaque disruption and thrombosis (Moore *et al.*, 2013). Similar to foam cell formation during atherosclerosis, LDLR$^{-/-}$ mice also displayed foamy Kupffer cells (KCs), the resident macrophage population in the liver, which correlated with hepatic inflammation (Wouters *et al.*, 2008). These fat-laden KCs predominantly contained cholesterol and displayed a pro-inflammatory phenotype (Leroux *et al.*, 2012). Additionally, by using agents that mimic cholesterol accumulation in macrophages, tumor necrosis factor-α production was induced *in vitro* (Iftakhar *et al.*, 2009). In line, feeding the same mice a high-fat diet without cholesterol demonstrated reduced hepatic inflammation without swollen KCs (Wouters *et al.*, 2008). Recent evidence in patients is consistent with the data obtained from cell culture and mice; whereas steatotic patients have normal KCs, in NASH patients the KCs transformed into foam cells (Ioannou *et al.*, 2013). Inflammation triggered by cholesterol-rich foam cells, is a well-established mechanism in the field of cardiovascular disease and has been recognized as a significant parameter during atherosclerotic plaque formation. Increasing evidence now shows similar observations in mice and patients with NASH, suggesting a shared disease mechanism between NASH and atherosclerosis (Bieghs, Rensen, *et al.*, 2012).

Altogether, accumulation of LDL-cholesterol inside macrophages and the subsequent formation of foam cells is a trigger for both atherosclerosis and NASH.

3.2 Cholesterol Uptake via LDL- and Scavenger Receptors

Foam cell formation has been shown to depend on the route of cholesterol uptake and therefore, a separation must be addressed between non-modified LDL and modified LDL cholesterol. Non-modified LDL is taken up by cells via receptor-mediated endocytosis, a mechanism by which cells recognize extracellular ligands by the LDLR and subsequently internalize these ligands by inward budding of the plasma membrane (Goldstein & Brown, 2009). Upon binding to the LDLR, LDL is internalized as clathrin coated vesicles that are then converted into endosomes. Here, a more acidic pH (4.5 to 5) exists, which leads to the dissociation of the ligand-receptor complex. The LDLR is recycled to the surface of the cell, and the endosomes combine with lysosomes, which contain acid hydrolases that can easily degrade all components of LDL. After hydrolysis, cholesterol is transferred into the cytoplasm via Niemann-Pick type C proteins where it can be further degraded to bile acids or secreted via cholesterol efflux transporters (Rosenbaum & Maxfield, 2011). The cholesterol derived from LDL in the lysosome was found to be responsible for the regulation of processes that are aimed at stabilizing the cholesterol content of the cell (Goldstein & Brown, 2009). First of all, transport of sterol-regulated membrane-bound transcription factors, called SREBPs, to the Golgi complex is blocked. As a result, genes encoding for enzymes involved in cholesterol synthesis are suppressed (Horton *et al.*, 2002). One of these enzymes includes 3-hydroxy-3methylglutaryl coenzyme A reductase (HMG-CoA), the rate-limiting enzyme of cholesterol production (Brown & Goldstein, 1999). Next to that, LDL-derived cholesterol is able to activate a cholesterol-esterifying enzyme, acyl CoA: cholesterol acyl-transferase (ACAT), thereby storing excess cholesterol as cholesteryl droplets in the cytoplasm (Brown *et al.*, 1975). Most importantly, the LDLR is subject of negative feedback regulation in the presence of marked elevations of cholesterol, as cholesterol suppresses the transcription of the LDLR gene (Brown & Goldstein, 1999). Taken together, non-modified LDL uptake via the LDLR activates several intracellular processes that are aimed at lowering the cholesterol content, i.e. by decreasing LDL internalization, by transportation of cholesterol out of the lysosome into the cytoplasm and by inhibition of cholesterol production. These intracellular mechanisms give rise to the concept that in case of LDLR-mediated cholesterol uptake, cells are protected from cholesterol accumulation and subsequent foam cell formation.

Unlike the uptake of non-modified LDL, *in vitro* studies have shown that the uptake of oxidative modified LDL by macrophages can contribute to cholesterol accumulation and subsequent formation of foam cells (Griffin *et al.*, 2005b; Jerome *et al.*, 1998). These oxidized LDL (oxLDL) fractions are taken up by scavenger receptors (SRs), present on macrophages. In contrast to the LDLR, SRs are *not* downregulated in response to an increase in cellular cholesterol content. These results suggest that SR-mediated LDL uptake is the main cause for foam cell formation (Kunjathoor *et al.*, 2002b). The two main SRs responsible for the uptake of modified LDL by macrophages are scavenger receptor A (SR-A) and CD36 (Kunjathoor *et al.*, 2002b). Unlike LDL and acetylated LDL (acLDL), treatment with modified LDL elevated gene expression and protein levels of SR-A and CD36 in macrophages (Yimin *et al.*, 2011; Yoshida *et al.*, 1998). Literature describes distinct affinity for binding of oxLDL between these two SRs. In contrast to CD36, SR-A binds and mediates uptake of oxLDL to a lesser extent. Next to SR-mediated uptake of modified LDL, but to a much lesser extent, the phagocytic uptake of aggregated LDL by macrophages is an additional proposed mechanism that contributes to foam cell formation (Khoo *et al.*, 1988).

In summary, whereas the processes involved in non-modified LDL uptake are tightly regulated and protect cells from becoming foam cells, the SR-mediated uptake of modified LDL was found to be responsible for the development of macrophage foam cell formation. Rather than non-modified cholesterol, these data suggest that modified cholesterol in particular is the substantial risk factor for foam cell formation. Since foam cells are a major source of pro-inflammatory cytokine production (Libby, 2002), modified LDL could drive inflammatory responses.

3.3   Oxidized LDL and Its Implications in Atherosclerosis and NASH

The most common form of cholesterol modification described in literature, is oxidation. Minimally oxidized forms of LDL contain lipid oxidation products without extensive protein modification. These oxLDL particles stay longer in the plasma and are therefore more prone for further oxidation. As modification proceeds, the highly oxLDL particle now turns into a structure similar to pathogen-related epitopes and therefore will be removed from plasma through binding to SRs and uptake by macrophages (Itabe *et al.*, 2011). Recent studies show that oxLDL contributes to inflammatory processes through interaction with immune cells and disturbed intracellular cholesterol trafficking. To date, an increasing amount of evidence implicates an important role for oxLDL in obesity-related inflammatory disorders, such as atherosclerosis (Li & Mehta, 2005; Nishi et al., 2002) and cardiovascular disease (Fraley & Tsimikas, 2006; Holvoet et al., 2001). In this paragraph, we will evaluate current data that supports the view of oxLDL as the inflammatory trigger for atherosclerosis and NASH.

Oxidatively modified LDL has been implicated in the pathogenesis of atherosclerotic disease as it has been observed within atherosclerotic lesions (Yla-Herttuala et al., 1989). A mouse model for atherosclerosis lacking either CD36 or SR-A is protected from atherosclerotic development (Febbraio et al., 2000; Makinen et al., 2010; H. Suzuki et al., 1997) and demonstrates defective foam cell formation in vitro (Febbraio et al., 2000). In line, oxLDL is associated with increased intima-media thickness in the carotid arteries of clinically healthy men (Hulthe & Fagerberg, 2002). Moreover, a study of patients undergoing angiography 6 months following coronary angioplasty indicated that levels of antibodies against oxidatively modified LDL may predict progression and regression of atherosclerotic lesions (Hulthe, 2004). It has been suggested that circulating oxLDL may be considered a biochemical risk marker for coronary heart disease (Toshima et al., 2000) and an increase in the ratio of oxLDL to LDL has been independently associated with the severity of coronary atherosclerosis in humans (Vasankari et al., 2001).

Similar to atherosclerosis, oxLDL was shown to be involved in the development of NASH. Recently, a novel mouse model for NASH has been developed by using a combination of oxLDL and a high-fat diet. Administration of oxLDL to wildtype high-fat diet-fed mice displayed the entire pathology of NASH, i.e. steatosis, hepatic inflammation, fibrosis, and also lipid-laden macrophages, dyslipidemia and aggravated hepatic lipid peroxidation (Yimin et al., 2011). Like typical macrophages, KCs also express these SRs (Naito et al., 1991) and are thus capable of taking up modified cholesterol (Kunjathoor et al., 2002a). Haematopoietic deletion of SR-A and/or CD36 in hyperlipidemic mice resulted in decreased hepatic inflammation, indicating that SR-mediated uptake of modified cholesterol by KCs is the trigger for the development of steatohepatitis (Bieghs, Verheyen, et al., 2012; Bieghs et al., 2010). By specifically inactivating one of the two predominant SRs on macrophages, research has shown that contribution of each one of these two receptors to hepatic inflammation is similar.

Altogether, internalization of modified lipids by SR-A and CD36 plays an important role during atherosclerosis and NASH. In line, loading bone marrow-derived macrophages of LDLR−/− mice with oxLDL, hereby mimicking foam cell formation, showed to be more inflammatory than macrophages without oxLDL loading (Bieghs, Van Gorp, Wouters, et al., 2012). Taken together, these data demonstrate the causal role of oxLDL as a driver of the inflammatory response.

3.4   Disturbed Intracellular Cholesterol Trafficking

From the data described above it is clear that SR-mediated macrophage uptake of oxLDL is the leading trigger for foam cell formation and inflammation, however, the subsequent intracellular pathway has not been established. One proposed theory is a defective intrinsic mechanism of lipid trafficking inside macrophages, which is described as follows: Once internalized, oxLDL is transported to the lysosomal compartment where it is poorly degraded or hydrolyzed and therefore accumulates in lysosomes. This is in contrast to native or acLDL, which are normally degraded by lysosomal enzymes followed by relocation into the cytoplasm for further processing (Jerome *et al.*, 2008b). Lysosomal trapping of oxLDL, probably due to impaired cholesteryl ester hydrolysis or an alteration in lysosomal pH (Schmitz & Grandl, 2009), has the potential to damage and disrupt the lysosomal membrane. Since lysosomes are involved in a wide variety of biological processes, cholesterol-induced lysosomal damage can lead to inflammation by several mechanisms. Evidence showed that intracellular cholesterol crystals were formed by CD36-mediated uptake of oxLDL. In turn, these crystals triggered the release of proteases and reactive oxygen species and induced lysosomal disruption, hereby activating the NLRP3 inflammasome and subsequent pro-inflammatory interleukin-1 production (Duewell *et al.*, 2010; Hornung *et al.*, 2008; Moore *et al.*, 2013; Sheedy *et al.*, 2013). A process closely connected to the inflammasome is a process called autophagy, a pathway whereby proteins are targeted to the lysosome for disposal. On the one hand evidence supports the view that autophagy controls inflammasome activation, on the other hand it has been demonstrated that components of the inflammasome itself can mediate autophagy (Byrne *et al.*, 2013; Harris *et al.*, 2011). Impairments in the autophagic pathway have been strongly associated with lysosomal storage disorders (Nixon, 2013). Moreover, mice deficient for macrophage-specific caspase-1 and -11, two essential inflammasome components, were protected from lysosomal cholesterol crystallization, autophagy and hepatic inflammation (Hendrikx *et al.*, 2013). These data suggest that autophagy and the inflammasome play an important role in cholesterol-induced inflammation. Additional to inflammasome activation and autophagy, the toll-like receptor (TLR) signaling pathway has also been proposed to promote a cholesterol-induced inflammatory response. In Niemann-Pick type C1 (NPC1) cells, a model for lysosomal cholesterol accumulation, the TLR4 level was shown to be increased, particularly in the intracellular endosomal fraction. In turn, this could lead to enhanced cytokine secretion that contributes to the inflammatory phenotype present in NPC1 disease (M. Suzuki *et al.*, 2007). Additional studies demonstrated that, depending on its extent of oxidation, oxLDL is recognized by different TLRs, hereby leading to NF-κB activation as well as chemokine and cytokine production (Bae *et al.*, 2009; Stewart *et al.*, 2010).

Macrophage-derived foam cells, as those present during atherosclerosis, predominantly contain enlarged lysosomes filled with cholesterol and cholesterol crystals, instead of cholesterol ester storage into the cytoplasm (Duewell *et al.*, 2010; Griffin *et al.*, 2005a). In accordance with atherosclerosis, accumulation of cholesterol and cholesterol crystals inside lysosomes of KCs were also observed in a mouse model representing NASH (Figure 1) (Bieghs, van Gorp, Walenbergh, *et al.*, 2012; Bieghs, Verheyen, *et al.*, 2012). In line with these data, hepatic inflammation was found to be associated with increased cholesterol storage inside lysosomes of KCs, providing evidence that lysosomal cholesterol accumulation in KCs is crucial for inflammation in the context of NASH (Bieghs, van Gorp, Walenbergh, *et al.*, 2012; Bieghs, Verheyen, *et al.*, 2012).

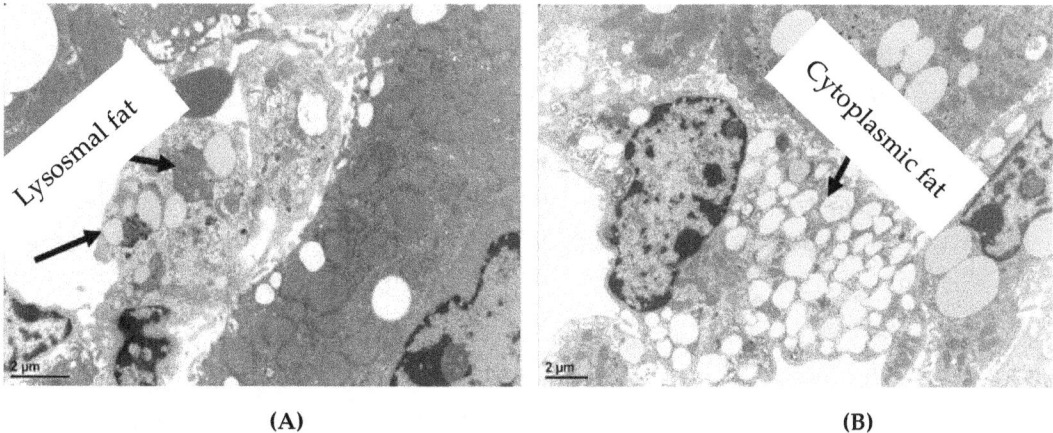

(A)   (B)

Figure 1: Electron microscopy pictures of KCs from mice showing that lysosomal cholesterol accumulation is correlated with hepatic inflammation. Pictures of KCs were taken of LDLR$^{-/-}$ mice on an HFC diet for 3 weeks, i.e. these mice develop hepatic inflammation (A). The LDLR$^{-/-}$ mice on chow for 3 weeks do not develop hepatic inflammation (B).

Altogether, mounting evidence demonstrate that NASH exhibits similar characteristics to atherosclerosis, including foam cell formation and cholesterol-filled lysosomes. Regarding the latter observation, it has been proposed that advanced stages of atherosclerosis are analogous to a modified form of lysosomal storage disorders (Jerome, 2006). Therefore, these results indicate that NASH can be considered as a modified form of a lysosomal storage disorder as well.

In conclusion, unlike acLDL or native LDL, oxLDL is trapped inside lysosomes and is able to trigger inflammation during atherosclerosis and NASH. Remarkably, the observed lysosomal cholesterol trapping during these inflammatory diseases is similar to the pathogenesis of the so-called lysosomal storage disorders, whereby excessive amounts of cholesterol are stored inside lysosomes. One of the lysosomal storage disorders is the NPC1 disease, whereby dysfunctional NPC1 proteins are not able to transport cholesterol out of the lysosome into the cytoplasm (Frolov *et al.*, 2013).

3.5   Intercellular Communication in the Liver during Cholesterol-induced Inflammation

Besides KCs as the initial trigger for cholesterol-induced hepatic inflammation, other liver cells play an important role in mediating liver inflammation. Once KCs are activated, for example by uptake of modified cholesterol (Bieghs, Van Gorp, Wouters, *et al.*, 2012), a wide range of inflammatory mediators and signaling molecules such as cytokines, reactive oxygen species, proteases and lipid mediators are released rapidly (Roberts *et al.*, 2007). These mediators are important for further amplifying the inflammatory response through direct cell-cell communication either between KCs themselves or between KCs and neighbouring hepatocytes (Hoebe *et al.*, 2001), sinusoidial endothelial cells and hepatic stellate cells. KC-derived tumor necrosis factor-α and CC-chemokine receptor 2 contribute to the elevated secretion of other cyto- and chemokines, facilitating activation and infiltration of neutrophils and macrophages into the liver (Miura *et al.*, 2012; Roberts *et al.*, 2007). In short, cholesterol-induced KC activation and concomitant inflammation enhances cytokine-driven hepatocellular signaling pathways, hereby rendering KCs to further augment inflammation through interaction with other cell types in the liver. Thus, cellular interactions between cells in the liver are crucial for hepatic inflammation.

Interestingly, NPC1 might have an impact on hepatic intercellular communication. In the absence of tumor necrosis factor-α, a crucial cytokine that recruits macrophages, NPC1 mice demonstrated less foamy macrophages and hepatocyte apoptosis (Rimkunas *et al.*, 2009). Moreover, NPC1 mice showed disrupted features of intercellular communication (Saez *et al.*, 2013), which is known to play a role under inflammatory conditions in KCs (Eugenin *et al.*, 2007) and hepatocytes (Gonzalez *et al.*, 2002). On the other hand, NPC1 has been proven to be atheroprotective by contributing to intracellular cholesterol trafficking in macrophages (Zhang *et al.*, 2008). Interestingly, besides that Cx43 protein expression, one of the main proteins involved in intercellular communication, is affected by cholesterol (Elmes *et al.*, 2011; Zwijsen *et al.*, 1992), it also has been shown to contribute to interleukin-1 release and inflammasome activation in macrophages (Ali *et al.*, 2011). These data suggest that NPC1-mediated intercellular communication could also play an important role in cholesterol-induced liver inflammation.

4   Treatment Options against Cholesterol-induced Inflammation

Simple lifestyle modifications, such as body weight management and appropriate nutritional counseling (with or without regular physical exercise and cognitive-behavior programs), are currently recommended to reduce risk for cardiovascular diseases and were proven to be, so far, the most effective therapy for NASH. Body weight reduction leads to a loss of adipose tissue as well as liver TGs, which further leads to improvements in peripheral and hepatic insulin sensitivity, and prevention of hepatic injury (Hammer *et al.*, 2008; Satapathy & Sanyal, 2010). In addition to lifestyle changes, current therapies utilized weight loss drugs and possibly bariatric surgery (Hammer *et al.*, 2008; Satapathy & Sanyal, 2010). Moreover, we will describe specific therapy options for cholesterol-induced inflammation that are currently used or are subject of further research to improve treatment options.

4.1   Lipid-lowering Therapies

Given the fact that dyslipidemia, or high cholesterol levels, is a defining element of the metabolic syndrome, lipid-lowering agents are potential candidates for treatment options in the atherosclerosis field and for NASH. These lipid-lowering drugs include polyunsaturated fatty acids (PUFAs), peroxisome proliferator-activated receptor (PPAR) agonists, statins and niacin. These drugs all possess anti-inflammatory properties and regulate metabolism (Bieghs, Van Gorp, Wouters, *et al.*, 2012; Fu *et al.*, 2001; Knopp, 1999; Lukasova *et al.*, 2011; Wang *et al.*, 2002; Zambon & Cusi, 2007). It was previously reported that PUFAs have a blood cholesterol-lowering effect and thereby reduce the risk of heart disease. Recent work reported a positive effect of PUFAs on lobular inflammation and ballooning of the liver in mice, as well as in human NASH, although the human study lacked a control group (Ishii *et al.*, 2009; Tanaka *et al.*, 2008). Therefore, it has been proposed that randomized controlled trials of adequate size are needed in the future to propose such PUFA treatment to NASH patients (Musso *et al.*, 2010).

Another widely used class of lipid-modifying agents are fibrates. Treatment with fibrates resulted in a substantial decrease in plasma TGs and is usually associated with a moderate decrease in LDL cholesterol and an increase in HDL cholesterol concentrations. Mechanistically, it was shown that fibrates are ligands for PPAR, thereby modifying lipid metabolism. However, the use of fibrates is still controversial. Fenofibrate administered to mice has been shown to ameliorate hepatic inflammation, while human studies demonstrated no difference in plasma liver enzymes or without changes in histological endpoints for NASH (Basaranoglu *et al.*, 1999; Laurin *et al.*, 1996; Shiri-Sverdlov *et al.*, 2006). Although PPARα activation has been shown to improve metabolic syndrome parameters and liver tests in humans, it did not improve steatosis and effects on liver histology remained minimal and unclear (Fernandez-Miranda *et al.*, 2008). Activation of the other members of the PPAR family (PPARβ/δ) should also be tested in long-term studies in humans, to confirm efficacy for the attenuation of the metabolic syndrome (Bensinger & Tontonoz, 2008; Karpe & Ehrenborg, 2009; Reilly & Lee, 2008). Besides fibrates, statins are widely known to be used as lipid-lowering drugs. Statins lower cholesterol levels by inhibiting the enzyme HMG-CoA reductase, which plays a central role in the production of cholesterol in the liver. Recent studies using statins showed significant improvements or even normalization in serum aminotransferase and lipid/cholesterol levels, reduction in liver steatosis at follow-up, as well as improvements in hepatic inflammation in patients with NASH (Ekstedt *et al.*, 2007; Georgescu & Georgescu, 2007; Gomez-Dominguez *et al.*, 2006; Kiyici *et al.*, 2003). Interestingly, patients who received statins even demonstrated reduced oxLDL, which could be relevant for NASH patients with increased plasma oxLDL levels (Resch *et al.*, 2006). Still, statin-treated NAFLD patients developed advanced fibrosis based on liver histology after a long-term follow-up period (Ekstedt *et al.*, 2006; Hyogo *et al.*, 2008).

In conclusion, the beneficial effects of statins and fibrates on NASH are still debatable, due to clear limitations to monitor NASH. In atherosclerosis, current evidence suggests that statin and niacin therapy have pleiotropic effects on the vascular endothelium, plaque stability and inflammation and may benefit patients regardless of their cholesterol levels (Liao & Laufs, 2005; Ridker *et al.*, 2008; Wu *et al.*, 2010). It is important to note that the use of lipid-lowering drugs is controversial due to their potential hepatotoxicity in patients with underlying hepatic diseases (Ballantyne *et al.*, 2001; Pyorala *et al.*, 2004). Moreover, the combination of statins and fibrates may also raise the risk of myopathy and rhabdomyolysis (Jacobson & Zimmerman, 2006). The difference in beneficial outcome after statin therapy could be explained by the fact that statins are directed at lipid lowering in general and are not directly related to oxLDL. Therefore, future adequate and well-designed human intervention studies examining the effect of statins or fibrates on NAFLD/NASH should be conducted.

4.2   Anti-oxLDL Therapies

As evidence was provided for the relevant role of oxLDL in triggering inflammation, therapy options in which oxLDL are targeted directly are promising. Oxidation structurally modifies the LDL particle, whereby the phosphorylcholine (PC) headgroups, one of the so-called oxidation-specific epitopes, can be found on the outer surface (Shaw *et al.*, 2000). Oxidation-specific epitopes are viewed as damage associated molecular patterns (DAMPs) and therefore serve as ligands for immune recognition (Miller *et al.*, 2011). Since these PC epitopes are also present on the capsular polysaccharide cell wall of *Streptococcus pneumoniae* (Briles *et al.*, 1982), cross reactivity exists between PC epitopes from oxLDL and this bacterium. Therefore, a protective effect against atherosclerosis and NASH upon active immunization with heat-inactivated *S. pneumoniae* in LDLR$^{-/-}$ mice was found. Immunized mice fed an HFC diet showed less foamy KCs, decreased hepatic inflammation and a reduction in the development of atherosclerosis, compared to mice without immunization (Bieghs, van Gorp, Walenbergh, *et al.*, 2012; Binder *et al.*, 2003). More importantly, reduced inflammation was associated with lower cholesterol oxidation and an increase of IgM autoantibody levels against oxLDL in plasma (Bieghs *et al.*, 2010). Thus, anti-oxLDL antibodies of the IgM subtype are protective against atherosclerosis and steatohepatitis, supporting the view that oxLDL plays an important role in the development of obesity-related inflammatory diseases. Targeting oxLDL by using natural occurring antibodies could be further developed into a novel application to treat human NASH.

4.3   Intracellular Cholesterol Modulation Therapies

As the involvement of cholesterol trapping inside lysosomes of macrophages was described in triggering inflammation, the usage of lysosomal cholesterol accumulation as a potential target for novel therapy options in atherosclerosis and NASH is highlighted. A possible way to elucidate the effect of lysosomal cholesterol accumulation is stimulating the transport of cholesterol from lysosomes into the cytoplasm. However, this is a challenging issue as it was previously shown that lysosomal cholesterol derived from oxLDL is resistant to efflux (Dhaliwal & Steinbrecher, 2000; Lougheed *et al.*, 1991; Yancey & Jerome, 2001). Moreover, it was shown that even though acLDL-derived cholesteryl esters (CEs) are usually efficiently hydrolyzed and cleared, a 3-day pre-incubation of macrophages with oxLDL impaired the subsequent ability of lysosomes to hydrolyze acLDL-derived CEs (Jerome *et al.*, 2008a). Besides, studies in both arteries and cells in culture suggest that the cholesterol in lysosomes is trapped and cannot be decreased simply by inhibiting further uptake of lipoproteins or by increasing efflux of extra-lysosomal cholesterol stores (Jerome & Lewis, 1990; Yancey & Jerome, 2001; Yancey *et al.*, 2002). Thus, to therapeutically target lysosomal cholesterol accumulations, unique new methods must be investigated.

Potential mediators of intracellular cholesterol transport are liver X receptor (LXR) activating oxysterols such as 27-hydroxycholesterol (27HC). 27HC is an intermediate in bile acid synthesis and the major oxysterol present in the human circulation. In line with greatly reduced 27HC production in NPC1-deficient cells, incubation with 27HC was shown to dramatically reduce lysosomal cholesterol in NPC1$^{-/-}$ fibroblasts (Frolov *et al.*, 2003). Similarly, injecting LDLR$^{-/-}$ mice with 27HC during or after an HFC diet resulted in reduced lysosomal cholesterol accumulation in KCs and consequently reduced hepatic inflammation (Bieghs *et al.*, 2013). Recently also 25-hydroxycholesterol (25HC), another oxysterol, was shown to correct the transport defect in NPC1 mutant cells (Ohgane *et al.*, 2013). These data support the view that oxysterols can prevent and reduce lysosomal cholesterol accumulation in macrophages, thereby reducing the inflammatory response.

Finally, it was recently demonstrated that TGs delivered to cultured macrophages as part of TG-rich particles (TRPs), dramatically reduced lysosomal CE accumulation and improves lysosomal function, possibly by decreasing lysosomal pH and restoring lysosomal CE hydrolysis (Ullery-Ricewick *et al.*, 2009). Interestingly, it was shown that macrophages hydrolyze CE more efficiently when it is introduced into lysosomes of macrophages as a mixed CE and TG particle, compared to CE-containing particles alone (Mahlberg *et al.*, 1990). Knowing that TRPs can be taken up by macrophage foam cells, thereby influencing the ability of foam cells to metabolize the overload of lysosomal CE, make these TRPs an interesting therapeutic option for multiple related disorders. Collectively, these findings are promising, since so far lysosomal cholesterol has been shown to be highly resistant to removal (Dhaliwal & Steinbrecher, 2000; Lougheed *et al.*, 1991).

5   Conclusion

This book chapter summarizes mouse and human studies that provide mechanisms by which (modified) cholesterol could affect inflammation. Moreover, it offers an updated overview from basic research work concerning cholesterol and liver inflammation to potential therapeutic targets.

Appendix A   List of Abbreviations

25HC: 25-hydroxycholesterol
27HC: 27-hydroxycholesterol
ACAT: acyl CoA: cholesterol acyl-transferase
acLDL: acetylated LDL
CE: cholesteryl ester
DAMPs: damage associated molecular patterns

HDL: high-density lipoproteins
HFC: high-fat, high-cholesterol
HMG-CoA: 3-hydroxy-3methylglutaryl coenzyme A reductase
KC: Kupffer cell
LDL: low-density lipoprotein
LDLR: LDL receptor
LDLR$^{-/-}$: LDLR knockout
LXR: liver X receptor
NAFLD: non-alcoholic fatty liver disease
NASH: non-alcoholic steatohepatitis
NPC1: Niemann-Pick type C1
oxLDL: oxidized LDL
PC: phosphorylcholine
PPAR: peroxisome proliferator-activated receptor
PUFAs: polyunsaturated fatty acids
SR: scavenger receptor
SR-A: scavenger receptor A
TG(s): triglyceride(s)
TRPs: TG-rich particles

References

Ali, S. R., Timmer, A. M., Bilgrami, S., Park, E. J., Eckmann, L., Nizet, V., & Karin, M. (2011). Anthrax toxin induces macrophage death by p38 MAPK inhibition but leads to inflammasome activation via ATP leakage. Immunity, 35(1), 34–44. doi: 10.1016/j.immuni.2011.04.015

Bae, Y. S., Lee, J. H., Choi, S. H., Kim, S., Almazan, F., Witztum, J. L., & Miller, Y. I. (2009). Macrophages generate reactive oxygen species in response to minimally oxidized low-density lipoprotein: toll-like receptor 4- and spleen tyrosine kinase-dependent activation of NADPH oxidase 2. Circ Res, 104(2), 210–218, 221p following 218. doi: 10.1161/CIRCRESAHA.108.181040

Ballantyne, C. M., Olsson, A. G., Cook, T. J., Mercuri, M. F., Pedersen, T. R., & Kjekshus, J. (2001). Influence of low high-density lipoprotein cholesterol and elevated triglyceride on coronary heart disease events and response to simvastatin therapy in 4S. Circulation, 104(25), 3046–3051.

Basaranoglu, M., Acbay, O., & Sonsuz, A. (1999). A controlled trial of gemfibrozil in the treatment of patients with nonalcoholic steatohepatitis. J Hepatol, 31(2), 384.

Bensinger, S. J., & Tontonoz, P. (2008). Integration of metabolism and inflammation by lipid-activated nuclear receptors. Nature, 454(7203), 470–477.

Bhargava, P., & Lee, C. H. (2012). Role and function of macrophages in the metabolic syndrome. The Biochemical journal, 442(2), 253–262. doi: 10.1042/BJ20111708

Bieghs, V., Hendrikx, T., van Gorp, P. J., Verheyen, F., Guichot, Y. D., Walenbergh, S. M., . . . Shiri-Sverdlov, R. (2013). The cholesterol derivative 27-hydroxycholesterol reduces steatohepatitis in mice. Gastroenterology, 144(1), 167–178 e161.

Bieghs, V., Rensen, P. C., Hofker, M. H., & Shiri-Sverdlov, R. (2012). NASH and atherosclerosis are two aspects of a shared disease: central role for macrophages. Atherosclerosis, 220(2), 287–293. doi: 10.1016/j.atherosclerosis.2011.08.041

Bieghs, V., van Gorp, P. J., Walenbergh, S., Gijbels, M. J., Verheyen, F., Buurman, W. A., . . . Shiri-Sverdlov, R. (2012). Specific immunization strategies against oxidized LDL: A novel way to reduce non-alcoholic steatohepatitis in mice. Hepatology, 56(3), 894–903.

Bieghs, V., Van Gorp, P. J., Wouters, K., Hendrikx, T., Gijbels, M. J., van Bilsen, M., . . . Shiri-Sverdlov, R. (2012). LDL receptor knock-out mice are a physiological model particularly vulnerable to study the onset of inflammation in non-alcoholic fatty liver disease. PLoS One, 7(1), e30668.

Bieghs, V., Verheyen, F., van Gorp, P. J., Hendrikx, T., Wouters, K., Lutjohann, D., . . . Shiri-Sverdlov, R. (2012). Internalization of modified lipids by CD36 and SR-A leads to hepatic inflammation and lysosomal cholesterol storage in Kupffer cells. PLoS One, 7(3), e34378.

Bieghs, V., Wouters, K., van Gorp, P. J., Gijbels, M. J., de Winther, M. P., Binder, C. J., . . . Shiri-Sverdlov, R. (2010). Role of scavenger receptor A and CD36 in diet-induced nonalcoholic steatohepatitis in hyperlipidemic mice. Gastroenterology, 138(7), 2477–2486, 2486 e2471–2473.

Binder, C. J., Horkko, S., Dewan, A., Chang, M. K., Kieu, E. P., Goodyear, C. S., . . . Silverman, G. J. (2003). Pneumococcal vaccination decreases atherosclerotic lesion formation: molecular mimicry between Streptococcus pneumoniae and oxidized LDL. Nat Med, 9(6), 736–743.

Briles, D. E., Forman, C., Hudak, S., & Claflin, J. L. (1982). Anti-phosphorylcholine antibodies of the T15 idiotype are optimally protective against Streptococcus pneumoniae. J Exp Med, 156(4), 1177–1185.

Brown, M. S., Dana, S. E., & Goldstein, J. L. (1975). Cholesterol ester formation in cultured human fibroblasts. Stimulation by oxygenated sterols. The Journal of biological chemistry, 250(10), 4025–4027.

Brown, M. S., & Goldstein, J. L. (1999). A proteolytic pathway that controls the cholesterol content of membranes, cells, and blood. Proceedings of the National Academy of Sciences of the United States of America, 96(20), 11041–11048.

Byrne, B. G., Dubuisson, J. F., Joshi, A. D., Persson, J. J., & Swanson, M. S. (2013). Inflammasome components coordinate autophagy and pyroptosis as macrophage responses to infection. MBio, 4(1), e00620–00612. doi: 10.1128/mBio.00620–12

Caballero, F., Fernandez, A., De Lacy, A. M., Fernandez-Checa, J. C., Caballeria, J., & Garcia-Ruiz, C. (2009). Enhanced free cholesterol, SREBP-2 and StAR expression in human NASH. Journal of hepatology, 50(4), 789–796. doi: 10.1016/j.jhep.2008.12.016

Dhaliwal, B. S., & Steinbrecher, U. P. (2000). Cholesterol delivered to macrophages by oxidized low density lipoprotein is sequestered in lysosomes and fails to efflux normally. Journal of *lipid research, 41(10), 1658–1665.*

Duewell, P., Kono, H., Rayner, K. J., Sirois, C. M., Vladimer, G., Bauernfeind, F. G., . . . Latz, E. (2010). NLRP3 inflammasomes are required for atherogenesis and activated by cholesterol crystals. Nature, 464(7293), 1357–1361. doi: 10.1038/nature08938

Ekstedt, M., Franzen, L. E., Mathiesen, U. L., Holmqvist, M., Bodemar, G., & Kechagias, S. (2007). Statins in non-alcoholic fatty liver disease and chronically elevated liver enzymes: a histopathological follow-up study. J Hepatol, 47(1), 135–141.

Ekstedt, M., Franzen, L. E., Mathiesen, U. L., Thorelius, L., Holmqvist, M., Bodemar, G., & Kechagias, S. (2006). Long-term follow-up of patients with NAFLD and elevated liver enzymes. Hepatology, 44(4), 865–873.

Elmes, M. J., Tan, D. S., Cheng, Z., Wathes, D. C., & McMullen, S. (2011). The effects of a high-fat, high-cholesterol diet on markers of uterine contractility during parturition in the rat. Reproduction, 141(2), 283–290. doi: 10.1530/REP-10-0378

Eugenin, E. A., Gonzalez, H. E., Sanchez, H. A., Branes, M. C., & Saez, J. C. (2007). Inflammatory conditions induce gap junctional communication between rat Kupffer cells both in vivo and in vitro. Cell Immunol, 247(2), 103–110. doi: 10.1016/j.cellimm.2007.08.001

Febbraio, M., Podrez, E. A., Smith, J. D., Hajjar, D. P., Hazen, S. L., Hoff, H. F., . . . Silverstein, R. L. (2000). Targeted disruption of the class B scavenger receptor CD36 protects against atherosclerotic lesion development in mice. The Journal of clinical investigation, 105(8), 1049–1056. doi: 10.1172/JCI9259

Fernandez-Miranda, C., Perez-Carreras, M., Colina, F., Lopez-Alonso, G., Vargas, C., & Solis-Herruzo, J. A. (2008). A pilot trial of fenofibrate for the treatment of non-alcoholic fatty liver disease. Digestive and Liver Disease, 40(3), 200–205.

Fraley, A. E., & Tsimikas, S. (2006). Clinical applications of circulating oxidized low-density lipoprotein biomarkers in cardiovascular disease. Curr Opin Lipidol, 17(5), 502–509.

Frolov, A., Dong, H., Jiang, M., Yang, L., Cook, E. C., Matnani, R., . . . Crofford, L. J. (2013). Niemann-pick type C2 deficiency in human fibroblasts confers robust and selective activation of prostaglandin E2 biosynthesis. J Biol Chem, 288(33), 23696–23703. doi: 10.1074/jbc.M112.445916

Frolov, A., Zielinski, S. E., Crowley, J. R., Dudley-Rucker, N., Schaffer, J. E., & Ory, D. S. (2003). NPC1 and NPC2 regulate cellular cholesterol homeostasis through generation of low density lipoprotein cholesterol-derived oxysterols. The Journal of biological chemistry, 278(28), 25517–25525. doi: 10.1074/jbc.M302588200

Fu, X., Menke, J. G., Chen, Y., Zhou, G., MacNaul, K. L., Wright, S. D., . . . Lund, E. G. (2001). 27-hydroxycholesterol is an endogenous ligand for liver X receptor in cholesterol-loaded cells. J Biol Chem, 276(42), 38378–38387.

Fujiwara, N., & Kobayashi, K. (2005). Macrophages in inflammation. Curr Drug Targets Inflamm Allergy, 4(3), 281–286.*

Georgescu, E. F., & Georgescu, M. (2007). Therapeutic options in non-alcoholic steatohepatitis (NASH). Are all agents alike? Results of a preliminary study. J Gastrointestin Liver Dis, 16(1), 39–46.

Goldstein, J. L., & Brown, M. S. (2009). The LDL receptor. Arteriosclerosis, thrombosis, and vascular biology, 29(4), 431–438. doi: 10.1161/ATVBAHA.108.179564

Gomez-Dominguez, E., Gisbert, J. P., Moreno-Monteagudo, J. A., Garcia-Buey, L., & Moreno-Otero, R. (2006). A pilot study of atorvastatin treatment in dyslipemid, non-alcoholic fatty liver patients. Aliment Pharmacol Ther, 23(11), 1643–1647.

Gonzalez, H. E., Eugenin, E. A., Garces, G., Solis, N., Pizarro, M., Accatino, L., & Saez, J. C. (2002). Regulation of hepatic connexins in cholestasis: possible involvement of Kupffer cells and inflammatory mediators. Am J Physiol Gastrointest Liver Physiol, 282(6), G991–G1001. doi: 10.1152/ajpgi.00298.2001

Griffin, E. E., Ullery, J. C., Cox, B. E., & Jerome, W. G. (2005a). Aggregated LDL and lipid dispersions induce lysosomal cholesteryl ester accumulation in macrophage foam cells. J Lipid Res, 46(10), 2052–2060.

Griffin, E. E., Ullery, J. C., Cox, B. E., & Jerome, W. G. (2005b). Aggregated LDL and lipid dispersions induce lysosomal cholesteryl ester accumulation in macrophage foam cells. Journal of lipid research, 46(10), 2052–2060. doi: 10.1194/jlr.M500059-JLR200

Grundy, S. M., Brewer, H. B., Jr., Cleeman, J. I., Smith, S. C., Jr., Lenfant, C., American Heart, A., . . . Blood, I. (2004). Definition of metabolic syndrome: Report of the National Heart, Lung, and Blood Institute/American Heart Association conference on scientific issues related to definition. Circulation, 109(3), 433–438. doi: 10.1161/01.CIR.0000111245.75752.C6

Hammer, S., Snel, M., Lamb, H. J., Jazet, I. M., van der Meer, R. W., Pijl, H., . . . Smit, J. W. (2008). Prolonged caloric restriction in obese patients with type 2 diabetes mellitus decreases myocardial triglyceride content and improves myocardial function. J Am Coll Cardiol, 52(12), 1006–1012.

Harris, J., Hartman, M., Roche, C., Zeng, S. G., O'Shea, A., Sharp, F. A., . . . Lavelle, E. C. (2011). Autophagy controls IL-1beta secretion by targeting pro-IL-1beta for degradation. J Biol Chem, 286(11), 9587–9597. doi: 10.1074/jbc.M110.202911

Hendrikx, T., Bieghs, V., Walenbergh, S. M., van Gorp, P. J., Verheyen, F., Jeurissen, M. L., . . . Shiri-Sverdlov, R. (2013). Macrophage specific caspase-1/11 deficiency protects against cholesterol crystallization and hepatic inflammation in hyperlipidemic mice. PloS one, 8(12), e78792. doi: 10.1371/journal.pone.0078792

Hoebe, K. H., Witkamp, R. F., Fink-Gremmels, J., Van Miert, A. S., & Monshouwer, M. (2001). Direct cell-to-cell contact between Kupffer cells and hepatocytes augments endotoxin-induced hepatic injury. Am J Physiol Gastrointest Liver Physiol, 280(4), G720–728.

Holvoet, P., Mertens, A., Verhamme, P., Bogaerts, K., Beyens, G., Verhaeghe, R., . . . Van de Werf, F. (2001). Circulating oxidized LDL is a useful marker for identifying patients with coronary artery disease. Arterioscler Thromb Vasc Biol, 21(5), 844–848.

Hornung, V., Bauernfeind, F., Halle, A., Samstad, E. O., Kono, H., Rock, K. L., . . . Latz, E. (2008). Silica crystals and aluminum salts activate the NALP3 inflammasome through phagosomal destabilization. Nat Immunol, 9(8), 847–856. doi: 10.1038/ni.1631

Horton, J. D., Goldstein, J. L., & Brown, M. S. (2002). SREBPs: activators of the complete program of cholesterol and fatty acid synthesis in the liver. The Journal of clinical investigation, 109(9), 1125–1131. doi: 10.1172/JCI15593

Hulthe, J. (2004). Antibodies to oxidized LDL in atherosclerosis development–clinical and animal studies. Clinica chimica acta; international journal of clinical chemistry, 348(1–2), 1–8. doi: 10.1016/j.cccn.2004.05.021

Hulthe, J., & Fagerberg, B. (2002). Circulating oxidized LDL is associated with subclinical atherosclerosis development and inflammatory cytokines (AIR Study). Arteriosclerosis, thrombosis, and vascular biology, 22(7), 1162–1167.

Hyogo, H., Tazuma, S., Arihiro, K., Iwamoto, K., Nabeshima, Y., Inoue, M., . . . Chayama, K. (2008). Efficacy of atorvastatin for the treatment of nonalcoholic steatohepatitis with dyslipidemia. Metabolism, 57(12), 1711–1718.

Iftakhar, E. K. I., Koide, N., Hassan, F., Noman, A. S., Dagvadorj, J., Tumurkhuu, G., . . . Yokochi, T. (2009). Novel mechanism of U18666A-induced tumour necrosis factor-alpha production in RAW 264.7 macrophage cells. Clin Exp Immunol, 155(3), 552–558. doi: 10.1111/j.1365–2249.2008.03779.x

Ioannou, G. N., Haigh, W. G., Thorning, D., & Savard, C. (2013). Hepatic cholesterol crystals and crown-like structures distinguish NASH from simple steatosis. J Lipid Res, 54(5), 1326–1334.

Ishibashi, S., Brown, M. S., Goldstein, J. L., Gerard, R. D., Hammer, R. E., & Herz, J. (1993). Hypercholesterolemia in low density lipoprotein receptor knockout mice and its reversal by adenovirus-mediated gene delivery. The Journal of clinical investigation, 92(2), 883–893. doi: 10.1172/JCI116663

Ishibashi, S., Goldstein, J. L., Brown, M. S., Herz, J., & Burns, D. K. (1994). Massive xanthomatosis and atherosclerosis in cholesterol-fed low density lipoprotein receptor-negative mice. The Journal of clinical investigation, 93(5), 1885–1893. doi: 10.1172/JCI117179

Ishii, H., Horie, Y., Ohshima, S., Anezaki, Y., Kinoshita, N., Dohmen, T., . . . Ohnishi, H. (2009). Eicosapentaenoic acid ameliorates steatohepatitis and hepatocellular carcinoma in hepatocyte-specific Pten-deficient mice. J Hepatol, 50(3), 562–571.

Itabe, H., Obama, T., & Kato, R. (2011). The Dynamics of Oxidized LDL during Atherogenesis. J Lipids, 2011, 418313. doi: 10.1155/2011/418313

Jacobson, T. A., & Zimmerman, F. H. (2006). Fibrates in combination with statins in the management of dyslipidemia. J Clin Hypertens (Greenwich), 8(1), 35–41; quiz 42–33.

Jerome, W. G. (2006). Advanced atherosclerotic foam cell formation has features of an acquired lysosomal storage disorder. Rejuvenation Res, 9(2), 245–255.

Jerome, W. G., Cash, C., Webber, R., Horton, R., & Yancey, P. G. (1998). Lysosomal lipid accumulation from oxidized low density lipoprotein is correlated with hypertrophy of the Golgi apparatus and trans-Golgi network. Journal of lipid research, 39(7), 1362–1371.

Jerome, W. G., Cox, B. E., Griffin, E. E., & Ullery, J. C. (2008a). Lysosomal cholesterol accumulation inhibits subsequent hydrolysis of lipoprotein cholesteryl ester. Microscopy and microanalysis : the official journal of Microscopy Society of America, Microbeam Analysis Society, Microscopical Society of Canada, 14(2), 138–149. doi: 10.1017/S1431927608080069

Jerome, W. G., Cox, B. E., Griffin, E. E., & Ullery, J. C. (2008b). Lysosomal cholesterol accumulation inhibits subsequent hydrolysis of lipoprotein cholesteryl ester. Microsc Microanal, 14(2), 138–149.

Jerome, W. G., & Lewis, J. C. (1990). Early atherogenesis in White Carneau pigeons: effect of a short-term regression diet. Experimental and molecular pathology, 53(3), 223–238.

Karpe, F., & Ehrenborg, E. E. (2009). PPARdelta in humans: genetic and pharmacological evidence for a significant metabolic function. Curr Opin Lipidol, 20(4), 333–336.

Khoo, J. C., Miller, E., McLoughlin, P., & Steinberg, D. (1988). Enhanced macrophage uptake of low density lipoprotein after self–aggregation. Arteriosclerosis, 8(4), 348–358.

Kiyici, M., Gulten, M., Gurel, S., Nak, S. G., Dolar, E., Savci, G., . . . Memik, F. (2003). Ursodeoxycholic acid and atorvastatin in the treatment of nonalcoholic steatohepatitis. Can J Gastroenterol, 17(12), 713–718.

Kleemann, R., Verschuren, L., van Erk, M. J., Nikolsky, Y., Cnubben, N. H., Verheij, E. R., . . . Kooistra, T. (2007). Atherosclerosis and liver inflammation induced by increased dietary cholesterol intake: a combined transcriptomics and metabolomics analysis. Genome Biol, 8(9), R200. doi: 10.1186/gb-2007-8-9-r200

Knopp, R. H. (1999). Drug treatment of lipid disorders. N Engl J Med, 341(7), 498–511.

Kopec, K. L., & Burns, D. (2011). Nonalcoholic fatty liver disease: a review of the spectrum of disease, diagnosis, and therapy. Nutr Clin Pract, 26(5), 565–576.

Kunjathoor, V. V., Febbraio, M., Podrez, E. A., Moore, K. J., Andersson, L., Koehn, S., . . . Freeman, M. W. (2002a). Scavenger receptors class A-I/II and CD36 are the principal receptors responsible for the uptake of modified low density lipoprotein leading to lipid loading in macrophages. J Biol Chem, 277(51), 49982–49988. doi: 10.1074/jbc.M209649200

Kunjathoor, V. V., Febbraio, M., Podrez, E. A., Moore, K. J., Andersson, L., Koehn, S., . . . Freeman, M. W. (2002b). Scavenger receptors class A-I/II and CD36 are the principal receptors responsible for the uptake of modified low density lipoprotein leading to lipid loading in macrophages. The Journal of biological chemistry, 277(51), 49982–49988. doi: 10.1074/jbc.M209649200

Laurin, J., Lindor, K. D., Crippin, J. S., Gossard, A., Gores, G. J., Ludwig, J., . . . McGill, D. B. (1996). Ursodeoxycholic acid or clofibrate in the treatment of non-alcohol-induced steatohepatitis: a pilot study. Hepatology, 23(6), 1464–1467.

Leroux, A., Ferrere, G., Godie, V., Cailleux, F., Renoud, M. L., Gaudin, F., . . . Cassard-Doulcier, A. M. (2012). Toxic lipids stored by Kupffer cells correlates with their pro-inflammatory phenotype at an early stage of steatohepatitis. J Hepatol, 57(1), 141–149.

Li, D., & Mehta, J. L. (2005). Oxidized LDL, a critical factor in atherogenesis. Cardiovasc Res, 68(3), 353–354.

Liao, J. K., & Laufs, U. (2005). Pleiotropic effects of statins. Annu Rev Pharmacol Toxicol, 45, 89–118.

Libby, P. (2002). Inflammation in atherosclerosis. Nature, 420(6917), 868–874. doi: 10.1038/nature01323

Lougheed, M., Zhang, H. F., & Steinbrecher, U. P. (1991). Oxidized low density lipoprotein is resistant to cathepsins and accumulates within macrophages. The Journal of biological chemistry, 266(22), 14519–14525.

Lukasova, M., Malaval, C., Gille, A., Kero, J., & Offermanns, S. (2011). Nicotinic acid inhibits progression of atherosclerosis in mice through its receptor GPR109A expressed by immune cells. J Clin Invest, 121(3), 1163–1173.

Mahlberg, F. H., Glick, J. M., Jerome, W. G., & Rothblat, G. H. (1990). Metabolism of cholesteryl ester lipid droplets in a J774 macrophage foam cell model. Biochimica et biophysica acta, 1045(3), 291–298.

Makinen, P. I., Lappalainen, J. P., Heinonen, S. E., Leppanen, P., Lahteenvuo, M. T., Aarnio, J. V., . . . Yla-Herttuala, S. (2010). Silencing of either SR-A or CD36 reduces atherosclerosis in hyperlipidaemic mice and reveals reciprocal upregulation of these receptors. Cardiovasc Res, 88(3), 530–538. doi: 10.1093/cvr/cvq235

Martinez, F. O., & Gordon, S. (2014). The M1 and M2 paradigm of macrophage activation: time for reassessment. F1000Prime Rep, 6, 13. doi: 10.12703/P6-13

Miller, Y. I., Choi, S. H., Wiesner, P., Fang, L., Harkewicz, R., Hartvigsen, K., . . . Witztum, J. L. (2011). Oxidation-specific epitopes are danger-associated molecular patterns recognized by pattern recognition receptors of innate immunity. Circ Res, 108(2), 235–248.

Miura, K., Yang, L., van Rooijen, N., Ohnishi, H., & Seki, E. (2012). Hepatic recruitment of macrophages promotes nonalcoholic steatohepatitis through CCR2. Am J Physiol Gastrointest Liver Physiol, 302(11), G1310–1321. doi: 10.1152/ajpgi.00365.2011

Moore, K. J., Sheedy, F. J., & Fisher, E. A. (2013). Macrophages in atherosclerosis: a dynamic balance. Nat Rev Immunol, 13(10), 709–721. doi: 10.1038/nri3520

Musso, G., Gambino, R., Cassader, M., & Pagano, G. (2010). A meta-analysis of randomized trials for the treatment of nonalcoholic fatty liver disease. Hepatology, 52(1), 79–104.

Musso, G., Gambino, R., De Michieli, F., Cassader, M., Rizzetto, M., Durazzo, M., . . . Pagano, G. (2003). Dietary habits and their relations to insulin resistance and postprandial lipemia in nonalcoholic steatohepatitis. Hepatology, 37(4), 909–916. doi: 10.1053/jhep.2003.50132

Naito, M., Kodama, T., Matsumoto, A., Doi, T., & Takahashi, K. (1991). Tissue distribution, intracellular localization, and in vitro expression of bovine macrophage scavenger receptors.

The American journal of pathology, 139(6), 1411–1423.

Nishi, K., Itabe, H., Uno, M., Kitazato, K. T., Horiguchi, H., Shinno, K., & Nagahiro, S. (2002). Oxidized LDL in carotid plaques and plasma associates with plaque instability. *Arterioscler Thromb Vasc Biol, 22(10), 1649–1654.*

Nixon, R. A. (2013). The role of autophagy in neurodegenerative disease. *Nat Med, 19(8), 983–997. doi: 10.1038/nm.3232*

Ohgane, K., Karaki, F., Dodo, K., & Hashimoto, Y. (2013). Discovery of oxysterol-derived pharmacological chaperones for NPC1: implication for the existence of second sterol-binding site. *Chemistry & biology, 20(3), 391–402. doi: 10.1016/j.chembiol.2013.02.009*

Puri, P., Baillie, R. A., Wiest, M. M., Mirshahi, F., Choudhury, J., Cheung, O., . . . Sanyal, A. J. (2007). A lipidomic analysis of nonalcoholic fatty liver disease. *Hepatology, 46(4), 1081–1090. doi: 10.1002/hep.21763*

Pyorala, K., Ballantyne, C. M., Gumbiner, B., Lee, M. W., Shah, A., Davies, M. J., . . . Kjekshus, J. (2004). Reduction of cardiovascular events by simvastatin in nondiabetic coronary heart disease patients with and without the metabolic syndrome: subgroup analyses of the Scandinavian Simvastatin Survival Study (4S). *Diabetes Care, 27(7), 1735–1740.*

Raal, F. J., Pilcher, G. J., Panz, V. R., van Deventer, H. E., Brice, B. C., Blom, D. J., & Marais, A. D. (2011). Reduction in mortality in subjects with homozygous familial hypercholesterolemia associated with advances in lipid-lowering therapy. *Circulation, 124(20), 2202–2207. doi: 10.1161/CIRCULATIONAHA.111.042523*

Reilly, S. M., & Lee, C. H. (2008). PPAR delta as a therapeutic target in metabolic disease. *FEBS Lett, 582(1), 26–31.*

Resch, U., Tatzber, F., Budinsky, A., & Sinzinger, H. (2006). Reduction of oxidative stress and modulation of autoantibodies against modified low-density lipoprotein after rosuvastatin therapy. *Br J Clin Pharmacol, 61(3), 262–274.*

Ridker, P. M., Danielson, E., Fonseca, F. A., Genest, J., Gotto, A. M., Jr., Kastelein, J. J., . . . Glynn, R. J. (2008). Rosuvastatin to prevent vascular events in men and women with elevated C-reactive protein. *N Engl J Med, 359(21), 2195–2207.*

Rimkunas, V. M., Graham, M. J., Crooke, R. M., & Liscum, L. (2009). TNF-{alpha} plays a role in hepatocyte apoptosis in Niemann-Pick type C liver disease. *Journal of lipid research, 50(2), 327–333. doi: 10.1194/jlr.M800415-JLR200*

Roberts, R. A., Ganey, P. E., Ju, C., Kamendulis, L. M., Rusyn, I., & Klaunig, J. E. (2007). Role of the Kupffer cell in mediating hepatic toxicity and carcinogenesis. *Toxicol Sci, 96(1), 2–15. doi: 10.1093/toxsci/kfl173*

Roger, V. L., Go, A. S., Lloyd-Jones, D. M., Adams, R. J., Berry, J. D., Brown, T. M., . . . Stroke Statistics, S. (2011). Heart disease and stroke statistics–2011 update: a report from the American Heart Association. *Circulation, 123(4), e18–e209. doi: 10.1161/CIR.0b013e3182009701*

Rosenbaum, A. I., & Maxfield, F. R. (2011). Niemann-Pick type C disease: molecular mechanisms and potential therapeutic approaches. J Neurochem, 116(5), 789–795. doi: 10.1111/j.1471-4159.2010.06976.x

Ross, R. (1999). Atherosclerosis — an inflammatory disease. N Engl J Med, 340(2), 115–126. doi: 10.1056/NEJM199901143400207

Saez, P. J., Orellana, J. A., Vega-Riveros, N., Figueroa, V. A., Hernandez, D. E., Castro, J. F., . . . Saez, J. C. (2013). Disruption in connexin-based communication is associated with intracellular Ca(2)(+) signal alterations in astrocytes from Niemann-Pick type C mice. PloS one, 8(8), e71361. doi: 10.1371/journal.pone.0071361

Satapathy, S. K., & Sanyal, A. J. (2010). Novel treatment modalities for nonalcoholic steatohepatitis. Trends Endocrinol Metab, 21(11), 668–675.

Schmitz, G., & Grandl, M. (2009). Endolysosomal phospholipidosis and cytosolic lipid droplet storage and release in macrophages. Biochim Biophys Acta, 1791(6), 524–539.

Shaw, P. X., Horkko, S., Chang, M. K., Curtiss, L. K., Palinski, W., Silverman, G. J., & Witztum, J. L. (2000). Natural antibodies with the T15 idiotype may act in atherosclerosis, apoptotic clearance, and protective immunity. J Clin Invest, 105(12), 1731–1740.

Sheedy, F. J., Grebe, A., Rayner, K. J., Kalantari, P., Ramkhelawon, B., Carpenter, S. B., . . . Moore, K. J. (2013). CD36 coordinates NLRP3 inflammasome activation by facilitating intracellular nucleation of soluble ligands into particulate ligands in sterile inflammation. Nat Immunol, 14(8), 812–820. doi: 10.1038/ni.2639

Shiri-Sverdlov, R., Wouters, K., van Gorp, P. J., Gijbels, M. J., Noel, B., Buffat, L., . . . Hofker, M. H. (2006). Early diet-induced non-alcoholic steatohepatitis in APOE2 knock-in mice and its prevention by fibrates. J Hepatol, 44(4), 732–741. doi: 10.1016/j.jhep.2005.10.033

Steinberg, D. (2002). Atherogenesis in perspective: hypercholesterolemia and inflammation as partners in crime. Nat Med, 8(11), 1211–1217. doi: 10.1038/nm1102–1211

Stewart, C. R., Stuart, L. M., Wilkinson, K., van Gils, J. M., Deng, J., Halle, A., . . . Moore, K. J. (2010). CD36 ligands promote sterile inflammation through assembly of a Toll-like receptor 4 and 6 heterodimer. Nat Immunol, 11(2), 155–161. doi: 10.1038/ni.1836

Subramanian, S., Goodspeed, L., Wang, S., Kim, J., Zeng, L., Ioannou, G. N., . . . Chait, A. (2011). Dietary cholesterol exacerbates hepatic steatosis and inflammation in obese LDL receptor-deficient mice. Journal of lipid research, 52(9), 1626–1635. doi: 10.1194/jlr.M016246

Suzuki, H., Kurihara, Y., Takeya, M., Kamada, N., Kataoka, M., Jishage, K., . . . et al. (1997). A role for macrophage scavenger receptors in atherosclerosis and susceptibility to infection. Nature, 386(6622), 292–296. doi: 10.1038/386292a0

Suzuki, M., Sugimoto, Y., Ohsaki, Y., Ueno, M., Kato, S., Kitamura, Y., . . . Ninomiya, H. (2007). Endosomal accumulation of Toll-like receptor 4 causes constitutive secretion of cytokines and activation of signal transducers and activators of transcription in Niemann-Pick disease type C (NPC) fibroblasts: a potential basis for glial cell activation in the NPC brain. J Neurosci, 27(8), 1879–1891. doi: 10.1523/JNEUROSCI.5282-06.2007

Tanaka, N., Sano, K., Horiuchi, A., Tanaka, E., Kiyosawa, K., & Aoyama, T. (2008). Highly purified eicosapentaenoic acid treatment improves nonalcoholic steatohepatitis. J Clin Gastroenterol, 42(4), 413–418.

Toshima, S., Hasegawa, A., Kurabayashi, M., Itabe, H., Takano, T., Sugano, J., . . . Nagai, R. (2000). Circulating oxidized low density lipoprotein levels. A biochemical risk marker for coronary heart disease. Arteriosclerosis, thrombosis, and vascular biology, 20(10), 2243–2247.

Ullery-Ricewick, J. C., Cox, B. E., Griffin, E. E., & Jerome, W. G. (2009). Triglyceride alters lysosomal cholesterol ester metabolism in cholesteryl ester-laden macrophage foam cells. Journal of lipid research, 50(10), 2014–2026. doi: 10.1194/jlr.M800659-JLR200

Vasankari, T., Ahotupa, M., Toikka, J., Mikkola, J., Irjala, K., Pasanen, P., . . . Viikari, J. (2001). Oxidized LDL and thickness of carotid intima-media are associated with coronary atherosclerosis in middle-aged men: lower levels of oxidized LDL with statin therapy. Atherosclerosis, 155(2), 403–412.

Vergnes, L., Phan, J., Strauss, M., Tafuri, S., & Reue, K. (2003). Cholesterol and cholate components of an atherogenic diet induce distinct stages of hepatic inflammatory gene expression. J Biol Chem, 278(44), 42774–42784. doi: 10.1074/jbc.M306022200

Wang, Y. X., Martin-McNulty, B., Huw, L. Y., da Cunha, V., Post, J., Hinchman, J., . . . Kauser, K. (2002). Anti-atherosclerotic effect of simvastatin depends on the presence of apolipoprotein E. Atherosclerosis, 162(1), 23–31.

Weber, C., & Noels, H. (2011). Atherosclerosis: current pathogenesis and therapeutic options. Nat Med, 17(11), 1410–1422. doi: 10.1038/nm.2538

Wouters, K., van Gorp, P. J., Bieghs, V., Gijbels, M. J., Duimel, H., Lutjohann, D., . . . Hofker, M. H. (2008). Dietary cholesterol, rather than liver steatosis, leads to hepatic inflammation in hyperlipidemic mouse models of nonalcoholic steatohepatitis. Hepatology, 48(2), 474–486.

Wu, B. J., Yan, L., Charlton, F., Witting, P., Barter, P. J., & Rye, K. A. (2010). Evidence that niacin inhibits acute vascular inflammation and improves endothelial dysfunction independent of changes in plasma lipids. Arterioscler Thromb Vasc Biol, 30(5), 968–975.

Yancey, P. G., & Jerome, W. G. (2001). Lysosomal cholesterol derived from mildly oxidized low density lipoprotein is resistant to efflux. Journal of lipid research, 42(3), 317–327.

Yancey, P. G., Miles, S., Schwegel, J., & Jerome, W. G. (2002). Uptake and trafficking of mildly oxidized LDL and acetylated LDL in THP-1 cells does not explain the differences in lysosomal metabolism of these two lipoproteins. Microscopy and microanalysis : the official journal of Microscopy Society of America, Microbeam Analysis Society, Microscopical Society of Canada, 8(2), 81–93. doi: 10.1017.S1431927601020013

Yasutake, K., Nakamuta, M., Shima, Y., Ohyama, A., Masuda, K., Haruta, N., . . . Enjoji, M. (2009). Nutritional investigation of non-obese patients with non-alcoholic fatty liver disease: the significance of dietary cholesterol. Scand J Gastroenterol, 44(4), 471–477. doi: 10.1080/00365520802588133

Yimin, Furumaki, H., Matsuoka, S., Sakurai, T., Kohanawa, M., Zhao, S., . . . Chiba, H. (2011).

A novel murine model for non-alcoholic steatohepatitis developed by combination of a high-fat diet and oxidized low-density lipoprotein. Lab Invest, 92(2), 265–281.

Yla-Herttuala, S., Palinski, W., Rosenfeld, M. E., Parthasarathy, S., Carew, T. E., Butler, S., . . . Steinberg, D. (1989). Evidence for the presence of oxidatively modified low density lipoprotein in atherosclerotic lesions of rabbit and man. The Journal of clinical investigation, 84(4), 1086–1095. doi: 10.1172/JCI114271

Yoshida, H., Quehenberger, O., Kondratenko, N., Green, S., & Steinberg, D. (1998). Minimally oxidized low-density lipoprotein increases expression of scavenger receptor A, CD36, and macrosialin in resident mouse peritoneal macrophages. Arterioscler Thromb Vasc Biol, 18(5), 794–802.

Zambon, A., & Cusi, K. (2007). The role of fenofibrate in clinical practice. Diabetes and Vascular Disease Research, 4 Suppl 3, S15–20.

Zhang, J. R., Coleman, T., Langmade, S. J., Scherrer, D. E., Lane, L., Lanier, M. H., . . . Ory, D. S. (2008). Niemann-Pick C1 protects against atherosclerosis in mice via regulation of macrophage intracellular cholesterol trafficking. The Journal of clinical investigation, 118(6), 2281–2290. doi: 10.1172/JCI32561

Zwijsen, R. M., Oudenhoven, I. M., & de Haan, L. H. (1992). Effects of cholesterol and oxysterols on gap junctional communication between human smooth muscle cells. Eur J Pharmacol, 228(2–3), 115–120.

Chapter 8

Trends in Bone Tissue Engineering: Proteins for Osteogenic Differentiation and the Respective Scaffolding

Vera Grotheer[1], Margit Schulze[2] and Edda Tobiasch[2]

1 Introduction

Bone tissue engineering is one of the most promising areas in stem cell research, giving rise to possible clinical application curing bone defects. There is a requirement for bone replacement due to bone defects caused by trauma, degenerative disorders, or infections, and because of the demographic development of the industrial nations this interest will further increase in the future. The current gold standard for bone defect repair is a tissue autograft from the patient (Khan *et al.*, 2008). However this is not always possible and it requires an additional surgery for the patient. Thus another method would be favorable. Different mesenchymal stem cell sources including bone marrow-derived stem cells (BMSCs), adipose-derived stem cells (ASCs), dental pulp stem cells (DPSCs), umbilical cord blood cells (UCBs) but also induced pluripotent stem cells (iPSs) got into focus of bone regeneration due to their ability to differentiate into the osteogenic lineage. Understanding the differentiation process in detail is necessary to achieve a tight control needed for safe clinical applications in the future. In addition selecting an appropriate source for cells for bone tissue engineering and the design of a suitable scaffolding material in which cells will reside needs careful consideration (Amini *et al.*, 2012). This overview will summarize major cell sources, important proteins, transcription factors and signaling cascades, which govern mesenchymal stromal cell (MSC) fate

[1] Department of Trauma and Hand Surgery, Medical Faculty, University Hospital Düsseldorf, Germany

[2] Department of Natural Sciences, University of Applied Sciences Bonn-Rhine-Sieg, Germany

towards the osteogenic lineage as well as new trends in the development of scaffold materials with osteo-conductive and osteoinductive properties.

2 Mesenchymal Stromal Cell Sources for Osteogenic Differentiation

MSCs are multipotent cells capable of self-renewal and multilineage differentiation and meanwhile transdifferentiation potential is assumed by some authors (Barzilay *et al.*, 2009; Jackson *et al.*, 2012). For bone tissue engineering MSCs are a very attractive cell source, because they have substantial advantages in comparison to embryonic stem cells (Murry & Keller, 2008). They are ethical unproblematic (Monti & Redi, 2011) and an autologous stem cell graft is possible. In addition MSCs exert potent immunosuppressive and anti-inflammatory effects through interactions with both, the innate and adaptive immune system (De Miguel *et al.*, 2012). In brief they are capable of regulating immune cells, such as T-cells, B-cells, dendritic cells and natural killer cells (Ren *et al.*, 2008; Yamaza *et al.*, 2010; Zhao *et al.*, 2010).

A huge variety of markers are published to describe mesenchymal stem cells. To facilitate their comparability the International Society for Cellular Therapy has published a position statement defining minimal criteria for MSC characterization (Dominici *et al.*, 2006). Following their suggestion MSCs are depicted by their ability to be plastic adherent and differentiate into osteoblasts, adipocytes and chondroblasts *in vitro*. Next to this MSCs have to express specific cell surface markers namely CD105, CD73, CD90 and lack the expression of CD45, CD34, CD14 or CD11B, CD79 α or Cd19 and HLA-DR surface molecules. But nowadays it is known that the expression of surface antigens is dependent on culture senescence and can vary according to the source of tissue (Keating, 2012; Mitchell *et al.*, 2006). Adult stem cells and particular MSCs can be isolated from a wide variety of tissues (Pansky *et al.*, 2007). In the following a short overview about the most promising MSC sources (see Table 1) and isolation techniques for future bone tissue engineering is given.

BMSC are the oldest and still most commonly used stem cell source for tissue engineering (Baksh *et al.*, 2007; Seong *et al.*, 2010). BMSCs express a variety of cell surface markers, such as STRO-1, CD105, SH3, CD29, CD44, CD71, CD90, CD106, CD120a, and CD124 (Pittenger *et al.*, 1999; Seong *et al.*, 2010). Isolating BMSCs from bone marrow has been mainly based on following methods: cultivating only adherent cells on tissue culture plates after isolation, collecting STRO-1 or CD105 positive cell populations or cultivating CD45 or Gly-A negativ populations (Seong *et al.*, 2010). But the availability of BMSCs for autologous use is limited and combined with donor side morbidity.

The preparation of UCBCs is completely noninvasive, because the umbilical cord is considered as medical waste. UCBCs have been reported to be positive for various markers such as CD9, CD13, CD29, CD44, CD54, CD73, CD90, and CD105, which is a very similar expression pattern as observed in BMSCs (Rebelatto *et al.*, 2008; Seong *et al.*, 2010). To obtain UBCs from umbilical cord, the tissue can be either minced into small fragments and seeded in culture dishes (Marmotti *et al.*, 2012) or the cells can be ob-

	BMSC	ASC	UCB	DPSC	iPS
Cell features	painful, invasive procedure	less invasive	not invasive, medical waste	less invasive	minimal invasive
Osteogenic differentiation	not restricted	not restricted	restricted	not restricted	not restricted
Apoptosis tolerance	not high	high	not high	not high	sensitive
Proliferation	low	high	dependent of origin	very high	low; connected with genetic instability
Immunosuppressiv	+	+	+	+	-
Immunomodulatory	+	+	+	+	- (+ MSC)
Immunogenetic	-	-	-	-	+
Autologous graft possible	+	+	restricted	restricted	+

Table 1: Comparison of MSCs derived from different sources.

tained by enzymatic digestion. Therefore Wharton's jelly or pieces of it will be exposed to collagenase (He *et al.*, 2014; Kikuchi-Taura *et al.*, 2012) (and hyaluronidase) with or without trypsin, or to a combination of collagenase, hyaluronidase and dispase II (Salehinejad *et al.*, 2012; Tsagias *et al.*, 2011). Next to this, stem cells from the umbilical cord can be collected from patients using heparinized tubes and proper salt-based solutions. Then mononuclear cells can be isolated by Ficoll density centrifugation (Markov *et al.*, 2007). But UCBCs yield is relatively low and the cells show delayed and insufficient differentiation into osteocytes (Hsieh *et al.*, 2013; Nagamura-Inoue & He, 2014).

Another interesting source for adult stem cell are teeth (Haddouti *et al.*, 2009). Due to their ecto-mesenchymal origin they are pre-committed toward hard tissues. Different stem cells can be isolated either from the dental follicle or from various tissue layer of the adult tooth. The most commonly used DPSCs originate form the dental pulp of the adult tooth. DPSCs are prepared by first cleaning the teeth with ethanol. Each tooth is cut into two pieces, the pulp tissue will remove, minced, and digested with a collagenase solution (Alkaisi *et al.*, 2013). Dental pulp stem cell are reported to be positive for STRO-1, CD146 and pericyte antigen 3G5 (Petrovic & Stefanovic, 2009). They are highly proliferative and display the typical immunoreactivity profile of MSCs (Gronthos *et al.*, 2000). During adolescence molares will sometimes be extracted, often because of cosmetic reasons. Nevertheless, the availability of autologous DPSCs extracted from pulpa tissue is limited.

A new and very interesting stem cells source has been created by Takahasi and Yamanaka. These induced pluripotent stem cells (iPSs) (Takahashi & Yamanaka, 2006) are generated by reprogramming differentiated somatic cells of adult tissue with specific transcription factors namely Oct4, Sox2, Klf4 and c-myc (Takahashi *et al.*, 2007). Or Oct4, Sox2, Lin28 and Nanog (Yu *et al.*, 2007). More recently, this reprogramming could be managed by less and less factors, up to one factor only, dependent on the tissue (Kim *et al.*, 2009). The iPS-technology used for reprogramming transcription factor overexpression via retroviral vectors, thus integrating into unknown positions in the genome could not be avoided. This can lead to an overexpression of proto-oncogenes or destruction of tumor-suppressor genes and therefore tumor formation. Due to this a current goal in iPS research is to avoid the use of integrating vectors to achieve safer cell reprogramming (de Lazaro *et al.*, 2014). Nevertheless an application *in vivo* is still problematic because iPS, having the same potency as ESC, also display the same problems: They can easily form teratomas (Knoepfler, 2009). Next to this derivatives of iPSs stimulate a T-cell–dependent immune response (Zhao *et al.*, 2011).

Adipose-derived stem cells can be isolated from either from adipose tissue or from liposuction aspirates. Fat tissue can be minced and then digested with collagenase or liposuction aspirates can directly digested with enzymes. In the following ASCs can be isolated through several centrifugation steps and a filtration process with cell strainer (Bunnell *et al.*, 2008). ASC express the following cell surface marker, which vary according to the passage number and isolation techniques: CD13, CD29, CD34, CD44, CD54, CD73, CD90, CD105, CD144, CD166 and others. ASCs are a promising autologous cell source in tissue engineering and regenerative medicine, because of it's availability in huge cell numbers and easy accessibility (Zhang *et al*, 2012).

3   Osteogenic Differentiation Factors

The major culture supplements for osteogenic differentiation are β–glycerophosphate, ascorbic acid and dexamethasone (Bosnakovski *et al.*, 2005). The concentration of these supplements vary from research group to research group, but it's undoubtable that these factors are the main inducers of osteogenic differentiation. In addition to these common supplements, further factors such as recombinant human BMP-2 (Yamagiwa *et al.*, 2001) or parathyroid hormone-related peptide have been reported to facilitate osteogenic proliferation and differentiation in both, in *in vitro* and in *in vivo* studies (Miao *et al.*, 2001).

In line with the topic of the book, this review will focus on cytokine signaling that governs osteogenic differentiation. But it should be mentioned that this differentiation pathway, as others, can be directed by multiple microenvironmental factors (Zhang *et al.*, 2012) such as hyperbaric oxygen (Lin *et al.*, 2014a, 2014b), pH, stiffness of the surface, mechanical forces (Adamo & Garcia-Cardena, 2011; Boccafoschi *et al.*, 2013; Kanno *et al.*, 2007; Nakamura *et al.*, 2013; Tsai *et al.*, 2009), or electrical currents (Fickert *et al.*, 2011), electromagnetic radiation (Alexandrov *et al.*, 2013) and magnetic fields (Yan *et al.*, 2010). For more information on these factors the given publications are recommended.

4   The Signaling Cascades of Osteogenic Differentiation

The osteogenic differentiation is tightly regulated by several pathways promoting osteoblastic development, albeit with notable mechanistical differences. In the following a short overview about these interwining pathways contributing to osteogenesis is given.

4.1   The Smad-Dependent Bone Morphogenic Protein Pathway in Osteogenesis

The bone morphogenic protein (BMP) pathway induces the lineage commitment of MSCs to multipotent osteochondroprogenitors (Abzhanov et al., 2007). First BMP ligands (e.g. BMP-2) bind to two specific heterogenic serine/threonin transmembrane receptors of the transforming growth factor (TGF)-β-receptor superfamily: BMPR-1 and BMPR-2. For each of them three receptors types have been identified so far: for BMPR-1: Alk2, Alk3, Alk6, and for BMPR-2: BR2, ActR2 and ActrR2B (Nohe et al., 2004). BMPR-2 phosphorylates BMPR-1, which then leads to phosphorylation of the receptor regulated Smad proteins (Gilboa et al., 2000; Marcellini et al., 2012) (see Figure 1). Phosphorylated Receptor-regulated Smad-1, -5, or -8 form heteromeric complexes with the common key mediator Smad 4 and localize into the nucleus regulating the transcription of specific target genes, especially the master regulator of osteogenic differentiation: the Runt-related transcription factor 2 (RUNX2) (Javed et al., 2008; Miyazono et al., 2005).

4.2   The Canonical Wnt Pathway in Osteogenesis

Dependent on the local concentration, Wnt (combined name: *wingless*-gen and *Int*-gen) has different functions. An elevated level of Wnt stimulates proliferation instead of differentiation and the presence of inhibitors can initiate osteogenesis by reducing Wnt signaling and inhibits both, the adipogenic and chondrogenic potential in pre-osteoblasts. Thus the Wnt pathway acts to drive the osteochondro-progenitors towards an osteoblastic fate (Mak et al., 2006). To activate the Wnt pathway, Wnt ligands bind to the cognate seven-pass transmembrane G-protein-coupled frizzled receptor linking it to its co-receptor, the low-density related protein LRP-5/6 (Mao et al., 2001). This activation leads to an assembly of glycogen synthase kinase-3β (GSK3β) and adenomatous polyposis coli (APC) protein with the membrane (see Figure 2). In consequence GSK3β cannot induce the subsequent degradation of β-catenin leading to its accumulation in the cytoplasm and within the nucleus. In the nucleus, β-catenin interacts with a repressor of transcription, the lymphoid enhancer-binding factor/T-cell-specific transcription factor (LEF/TCF). This interaction permits recruitment of the histone acetylase CBP/p300 (CREB) binding protein which activates gene transcription (Deschaseaux et al., 2009). The expression of alkaline phosphatase (ALP) is one of the major marker genes for osteogenesis regulated via this pathway (Rawadi et al., 2003).

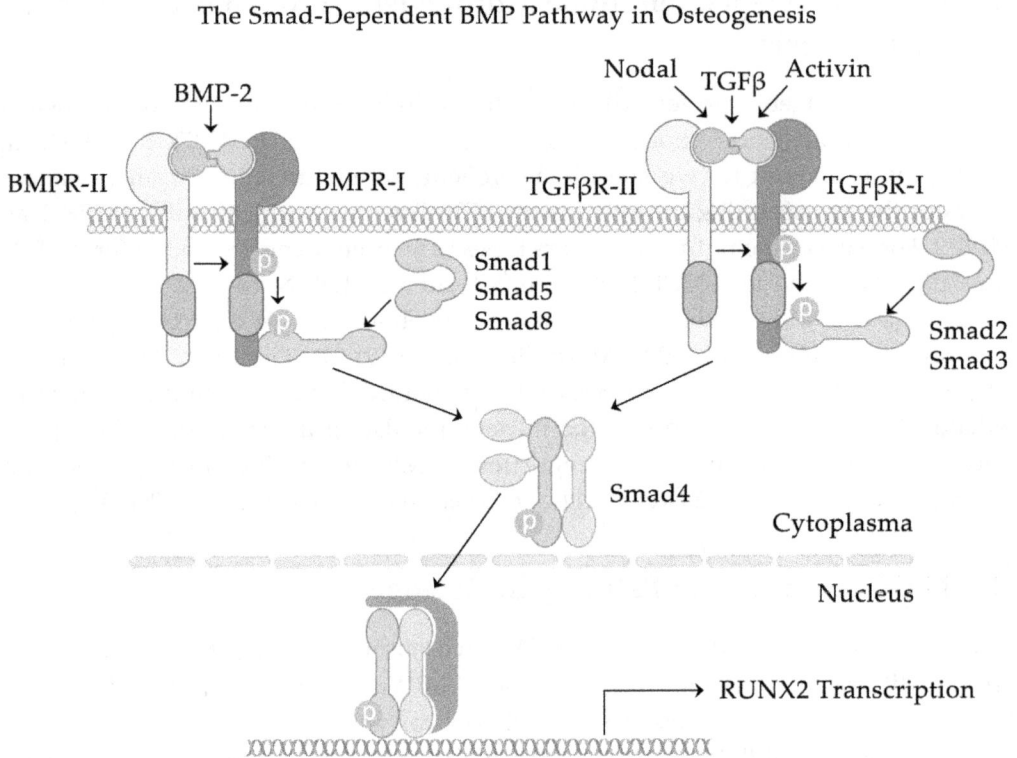

Figure 1: BMP-signaling induces by involving SMAD-proteins important osteo-genic transcription factors: BMPR-2 phosphorylates BMPR-1, which then phos-phorylates Smad proteins. Phosphorylated R-Smad-1, -5, or -8 form heteromeric complexes with the common key mediator Smad 4 and localize to the nucleus regulating the transcription of RUNX2. Furthermore Nodal, TGF-β and Activin can induce the same receptor familiy (TGFβR-I and TGFβR-II) Smad-2 and Smad-3 which form a heteromeric complex with Smad 4 and regulates RUNX2 expres-sion, too.

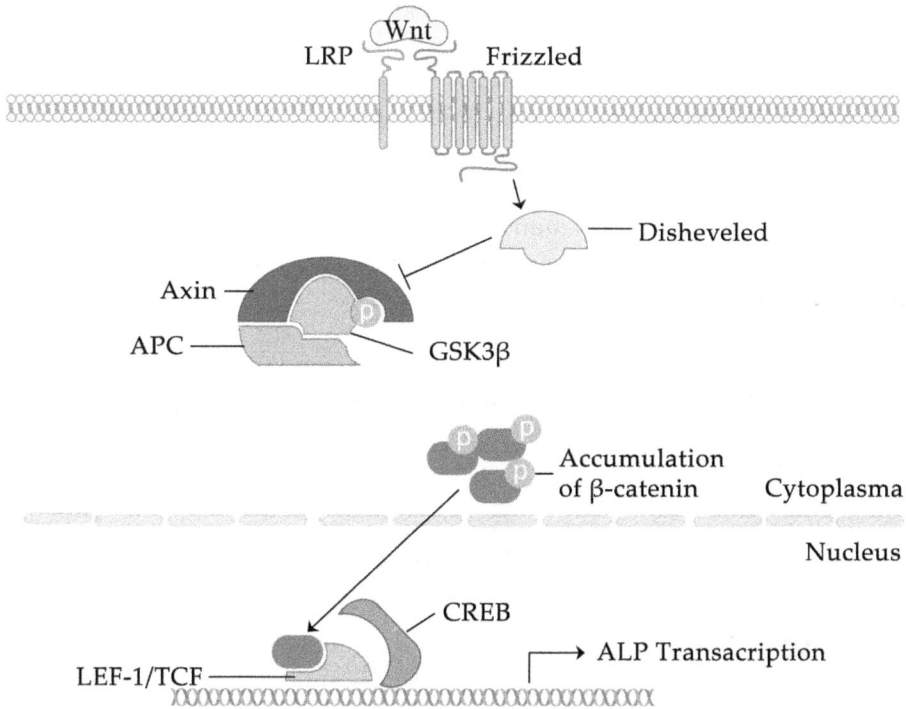

Figure 2: Activated WNT signaling leads to an accumulation of β-catenin, that in consequence activates the transcription of osteogenic genes: Wnt ligands bind to the receptor linking it to its co-receptor, LRP-5/6. This activation leads to an assembly of GSK3β and APC protein with the membrane. In consequence GSK3β is phosphorylated by disheveled and so it´s inactivated. So subsequent degradation of β-catenin is abolished leading to its accumulation in the cytoplasm and within the nucleus. In the nucleus, β-catenin interacts with a repressor of transcription LEF/TCF. This interaction permits recruitment of CREB binding protein, which activates gene transcription of ALP.

4.3   The Mitogen Activated Protein Kinase Pathway in Osteogenesis

The Mitogen-Activated-Protein-Kinase (MAPK) pathway plays a crucial role in bone formation, because it interferes with other major osteogenic pathways (e.g. Ihh, BMP, Wnt-signaling). The MAPK pathway transduces signals from several growth factors or adhesion molecules (e.g. Fibroblast Growth Factor (FGF), Insulin-like growth factor (IGF) to the MAP-Kinase. In consequence of the activation of MAPK GSK3β is inactivated thereby accumulating β-catenin (Thornton *et al.*, 2008) (see Figure 3). Furthermore ERK can stimulate the phosphorylation and thus activation of RUNX2 and distal less homebox5 (Dlx5). This is in line with BMP signaling which can also activate RUNX2 and Dlx5. After phosphorylating RUNX2 or Dlx5 the expression of Osterix, a key marker of osteogenesis, can further mediate independently osteoblastic cell maturation. RUNX2 can also be activated by p38. In contrast to this, the activation of MAPK signaling can also antagonize bone formation by inhibition of BMP-induced Smad phosphorylation and therefore inhibit translocation of the Smad complex into the nucleus (Schindeler & Little, 2006).

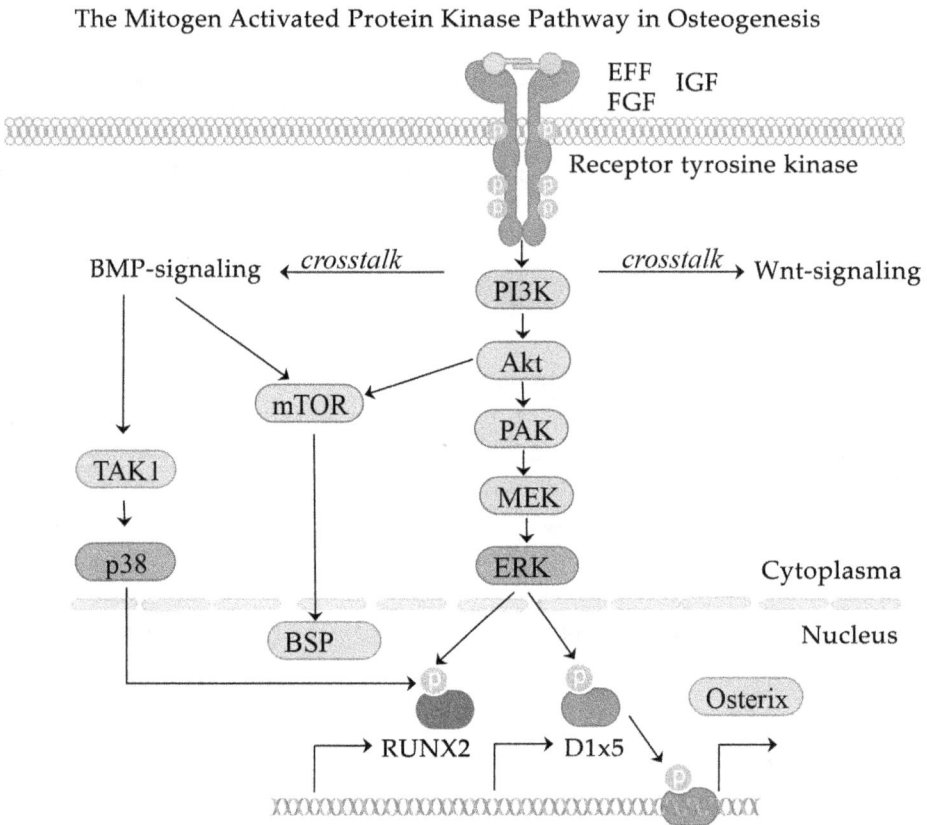

Figure 3: MAPK-signaling can induce phosphorylation of RUNX2 and Dlx5 and furthermore Osterix expression. And MAPK-signaling can inhibit BMP- and Wnt-signaling (see Figure 2 and 3).

4.4   The Hedgehog Pathway in Osteogenesis

The Hedgehog pathway regulates both chondrocyte and osteoblast differentiation during endochondral bone formation. This pathway is triggered by binding of Hedgehog to its receptor Patched (Ptch) causing the removal of the inhibition of Smoothened (Smo), which in turn inactivates GSK-3β (see Figure 4). In consequence intra-cytoplasmatic Glioma-associated oncogene homolog (Gli) proteins will not be cleaved, thus GliA an activator of transcription can localize into the nucleus. GSK-3β is required for the inhibition of Hedghog-signaling but also crucial for regulating the Wnt-/β-catenin pathway (see Figure 2).

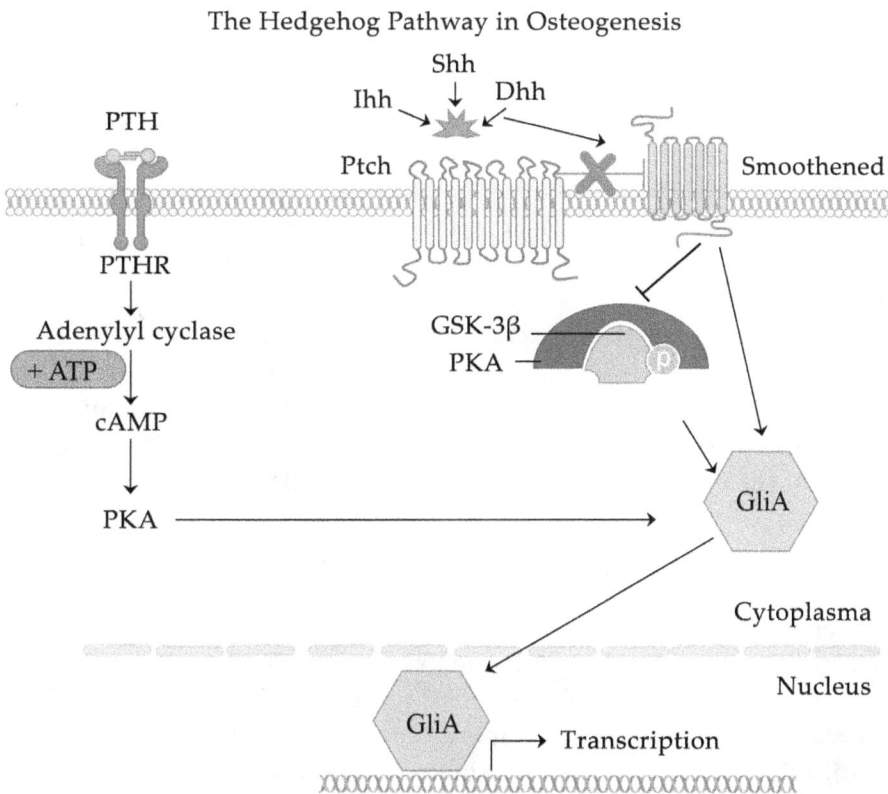

Figure 4: Indian- Sonic-, Desert-Hedgehog binds to its receptor Patched (Ptch) causing the removal of the inhibition of Smo, which in turn inactivates GSK-3β. So Gli proteins will not be cleaved, thus GliA an activator of transcription can localize into the nucleus. Parathyroid hormon (PTH) binding to the parathyroid receptor (PTHR) activates several downstream effectors, such as Proteinkinase A (PKA), which can activate GliA, too.

4.5   The Notch and the Cadherin Pathway in Osteogenesis

Highly conserved Notch Signaling plays a crucial role in osteogenic differentiation. Upon binding of Delta or Jagged to the Notch receptor a series of cleavages mediated by γ-secretase occurs resulting in a release of the Notch intracellular domain (NCID). NCID translocates into the nucleus and activates the transcription of Notch target genes. Notch maintains MSCs in an undifferentiated state by repressing RUNX2 (Engin & Lee, 2010). Furthermore it is known that Notch-pathway regulates BMP-2-signaling (Viale-Bouroncle *et al.*, 2014).

Differentiation causes changes in cells shape. MSCs need in general cell adhesion to an extracellular matrix (ECM) via integrins for differentiation (Schwartz & Ginsberg, 2002). When MSC are exposed to an osteogenic differentiation culture medium, the cells spread physically and flattened during cell adhesion to support the differentiation. For this integrin ligation is required. Integrins can activate Rho-associated protein kinase (ROCK) mediated by Ras homolog gene family member A (RhoA). Furthermore RhoA can be activated by the noncanonical Wnt-pathway. RhoA effector proteins regulate actomyosin contractility via a direct phosphorylation of myosin light chain and phosphorylation and inactivation of the myosin binding subunit of myosin phosphatase which in fact leads to an reorganization of the cytoskeleton (McBeath *et al.*, 2004.)

5   Purinergic Receptors and Osteogenic Differentiation

Although is has been proposed already in the early 1990s that extracellular ATP could modulate events crucial to maintain normal bone homeostasis and it was suggested already then that the effect might be via purinoceptors (Schöfl *et al.*, 1992), it was only acknowledged recently that extracellular nucleotides (eNTPs) and their metabolites which exist transiently in the extracellular environment are active as ligands on both, ionotropic and metabotropic purinoreceptors, having significant regulatory effects in osteoblasts and osteoclasts.

The metabolism of eNTPs is regulated via nucleotide processing ectoenzymes on the plasma membrane of bone cells and their precursor. Thus, from their niche, MSCs have a substantial influence on the complex signaling network of eNTPs and its derivatives (Scarfi, 2013). So is ATP metabolized into adenosine by human primary osteoblast or mesenchymal stem cells via CD73 a GPI-anchored cell surface protein with ecto-5'-nucleotidase activity which is in addition a major marker of MSCs character (Dominici *et al.*, 2006).

There are three classes of puringeric receptors. Depending on their ligand they are divided into four G protein-coupled P1 receptors (A1, A2A, A2B and A3) preferentially activated by adenosine, and P2 receptors where nucleotides such as ATP serve as preferred ligands. The P2 receptors are divided into seven P2X receptors (P2X1 to P2X7) that are ligand-gated ion channels and twelve G protein-coupled P2Y receptors (P2Y1, P2Y2, P2Y4 to P2Y6, P2Y8 to P2Y14) (see Table 2).

P1 Receptor	Present in	References
A1	(h) DPSCs	D'Alimonte *et al.*, 2013
	(h) BM-derived mononuclear cells	He *et al.*, 2013
	Osteoclast	He & Cronstein., 2011
A2A	(m) BMSCs	Ode *et al.*, 2013
A2B	(m) BMSCs	Carroll *et al.*, 2012, Gharibi *et al.*, 2011
	(h) BMSCs	Ciciarello *et al.*, 2013; He *et al.*, 2013; Shih *et al.*, 2014
	(h) BM-derived mononuclear cells	He *et al.*, 2013
	(h) Osteoblasts	Costa *et al.*, 2011
	Mouse organism	Takedachi *et al.*, 2012
P2X1	Osteoblasts	Orriss *et al.*, 2012
P2X5	(h) ASCs, DFCs	Zippel *et al.*, 2012
P2X6	(h) ASCs	Zippel *et al.*, 2012
P2X7	(h) ASCs, DFCs	Zippel *et al.*, 2012
	Mouse organism	Ke *et al.*, 2003, Li *et al.*, 2005
	Osteoblasts	Orriss *et al.*, 2012
	MC3T3-E1 osteoblast-like cells	Grol *et al.*, 2012
P2Y1	(h) ASCs, DFCs	Zippel *et al.*, 2012
P2Y2	(h) ASCs, DFCs	Zippel *et al.*, 2012
	Osteoblasts	Orriss *et al.*, 2006
P2Y4	(h) ASCs	Zippel *et al.*, 2012
	Osteoblasts	Orriss *et al.*, 2012''0)
P2Y6	Osteoblasts	Orriss *et al.*, 2012''06
P2Y13	(m) BM-MSCs	Biver *et al.*, 2013
	(m) Osteoblasts	Wang *et al.*, 2013
P2Y14	(h) ASCs	Zippel *et al.*, 2012

Abbreviations: Adipose tissue-derived stem cells (ASCs); bone marrow-derived mesenchymal stem cells (BMSCs); dental follicle-derived cells (DFCs); human (h); mouse (m); rat (r)

Table 2: Involvement of purinergic receptors during osteogenic differentiation.

The secretion of adenosine and the presence of its four receptors in bone cells have been well documented (He & Cronstein, 2011). Osteogenic differentiation is stimulated by the nucleoside adenosine, resulting from ATP degradation induced by CD39 and CD73 ectonucleotidases expressed on the MSC membrane (Ciciarello *et al.*, 2013). Moreover adenosine receptors also regulate chondrocyte and cartilage homeostasis (Mediero & Cronstein, 2013). In this process CD73 seem to be involved too, because treatment with an CD73 inhibitor increases chondrogenic matrix deposition while reducing mineral matrix deposition as well as osteogenic markers expression (Ode *et al.*, 2013).

Osteoblasts are also known to express multiple P2 receptor subtypes. But both, P1 and P2 receptors do not only play a role in the mature cell types, they are also crucial in their precursor cells and respective lineage commitment and lineage-specific differentiation (Gharibi *et al.*, 2011; Zippel *et al.*, 2012).

The abundant A2B receptor seems to play a role in MSC differentiation, which may be also influenced via the A1 or A2A receptor, defining whether osteoblasts are driven into proliferation or differentiation (Costa *et al.*, 2011). A1 receptor activation enhances RUNX-2 and alkaline phosphatase expression via activation of dishevelled protein and glycogen synthase kinase-3β of the canonical Wnt signaling pathway (see Figure 2). This effect can be abolished by siRNA treatment of Dickkopf-1 in osteogenic differentiation of dental pulp stem cells (D'Alimonte *et al.*, 2013). A2B expression positively regulated by CD73, and its activity is transiently upregulated at early stages of osteoblastic differentiation inducing the expression of osteoblast-related genes such as Runx2, ALP, osteocalcin (OC) and bone sialoprotein (see Chapter 6 for details) (Takedachi *et al.*, 2012). This mechanism at least partially involves cAMP signaling (see Figure 4) (Carroll *et al.*, 2012). On the other hand, MSCs differentiation towards adipocytes shows an increase in A1 and A2A receptor expression (Gharibi *et al.*, 2011).

A similar receptor type specificity was shown for the P2X ion channels where P2X1 and P2X7 receptors where reported to negatively regulate bone mineralization (Orriss *et al.*, 2012). This is in contrast to the finding of another group which stated that the activation of P2X7 stimulates osteoblast differentiation and matrix mineralization in vitro via a Ca^{2+}-dependent stimulation of metabolic acid production that is dependent on glucose and phosphatidylinositol 3-kinase activity (see Figure 3) (Grol *et al.*, 2012). During osteoblast maturation there is a decrease of the cell proliferation associated P2X5 and a shift from P2X to P2Y expression.

Mature osteoblasts preferentially express the G protein-coupled P2Y2 receptor but also P2Y4 and P2Y6, which might function as 'off-switches' for mineralized bone formation (Orriss *et al.*, 2006). Osteoblasts release ATP and act on ATP via P2 receptors blocking bone mineralisation of the collagenous matrix by inhibiting alkaline phosphatase expression and activity. But the blocking also works via a receptor-independent mechanism: the ATP hydrolysis product pyrophosphate (Orriss *et al.*, 2013; Burnstock *et al.*, 2013). The P2Y2 receptor stimulation sensitizes mechanical stress activated calcium channels, leading to calcium influx and activation of the MAPK pathways ERK 1/2 and p38 (see Figure 3) via the upstream mediators PI-PLC, PKC and Src (Katz *et al.* 2006). This mechanism has been suggested to be one of the key transduction pathways activated by mechanical stimulation of bone. Another P2 receptor involved in this process is P2Y13. ADP stimulation of this receptor leads to the expression of osterix, alkaline phosphatase, and collagen type I, which are involved in the maturation of osteoblasts (Biver *et al.*, 2013). Deletion of this receptor leads to an enhanced osteogenic response to mechanical loading in vivo, possibly because of the reduced extracellular ATP degradation by ALP (Wang *et al.*, 2013). This is in line with findings in osteoblasts of KO mice of this receptor where a down-regulation of RhoA/ROCK I signaling (see Figure 5) and a

The Notch and Cadherin Pathway in Osteogenesis

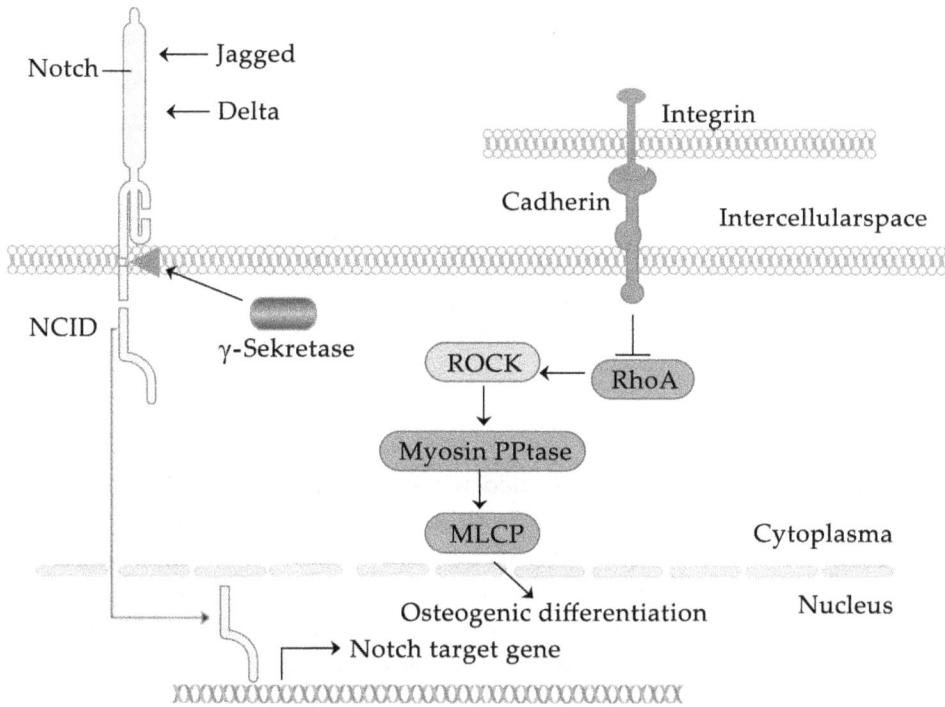

Figure 5: The Notch-Signaling induced by Jagged or Delta regulates Notch targets genes (e.g. NF-κB and BMP-signaling. RhoA/Rock activation is necessary for osteogenic differentiation by mediating reorganization of cytoskeleton.

reduced ratio of receptor activator of nuclear factor κB ligand/osteoprotegerin leads to reduced bone turnover rates (Wang *et al.*, 2012). CD73 and adenosine receptors are also involved in MSCs reaction to mechanical stimulation leading to a down-regulation of Adora2a (Ode *et al.*, 2013).

Several signaling pathways seem to be combined in the concerted action of P1 and P2 receptors in osteogenic precursor cells. P2Y2 receptors enhance osteoblast differentiation through the PI3K/AKT signaling pathway activation (see Figure 3) and consecutive induction of ALP and BSP but also BMP-2, BMP-4, BMP-5 (see Figure 1) gene expression (Ayala-Peña *et al.*, 2013). Nucleotide stimulation can also potentiate signals via parathyroid hormone (PTH), a principal regulator of bone resorption and formation (Buckley *et al.*, 2001) and influence MSCs differentiation via parathyroid hormone-related protein (Longo *et al.*, 2013). A synergistic effect of ATP and PTH on c-fos induction is observed through intracellular cAMP levels via a non-mitogen-activated protein kinase/ternary complex factor pathway (Bowler *et al.*, 1999).

Taken together bone is a dynamic organ that undergoes continuous remodeling via osteoclast resorption and osteoblast synthesis leading to mineralization of new bone. Recent data suggests that purinergic signaling is important not only in this process but also in joint disorders such as osteoporosis, rheumatoid arthritis and cancers (Burnstock *et al.*, 2013) and last not least the maturation of the key cell types involved in these processes (Zippel *et al.*, 2012).

6   Essential Transcription Factors for Osteogenic Differentiation

The differentiation from mesenchymal stem cells to osteoblasts and further bone formation requires coordinated activities of multiple signaling pathways and the activation of essential transcription factors. In the following a short overview about crucial transcription factors, which regulate the differentiation from MSCs to mature osteoblasts is given.

RUNX2 is the master transcription factor regulating early osteogenesis (Liu & Lee, 2013). RUNX2 KO-mice embryos died without bone formation. This transcription factor enhances the expression of collagen type 1, osteocalcin and bone sialoprotein three well established marker genes for osteogenesis. On the other hand RUNX2 over-expression in osteoblasts severely reduces osteocalcin expression and osteoblast maturation. Taken together RUNX2 is required committing undifferentiated cells towards the osteogenic lineage, but appears to maintain these cells in an immature stage (Komori, 2006). Other transcription factors and co-regulators include CCAAT/Enhancer-Binding-Protein (C/EBP), Distal-less homebox 3 (Dlx3), Muscle segment homeobox 2 (Msx2), PPARγ, Twist-related protein 1 (Twist), Signal transducer and activator of transcription (Stat1), Smad3, Yamaguchi sarcoma viral oncogene homolog (Yes) and Transducin-like enhancer of Split (TLE) decrease the transcriptional activity of RUNX2. RUNX2 directs mesenchymal progenitor cells towards osteoblasts while inhibiting their differentiation towards adipocytes.

Osterix (Osx) is the master regulator of late osteogenesis, inhibiting chondrogenesis required for bone formation. It is a downstream gene of RUNX2 and inhibits osteoblast proliferation while inducing osteoblast terminal differentiation (Sinha & Zhou, 2013; Tang *et al.*, 2011).

This inhibition is partial connected by acting as a feedback control mechanism involved in bone formation, by inhibiting Wnt-signaling by at least three different ways (Zhang *et al.*, 2008): So Osx inhibits the binding of T-cell-factor (Tcf) to the DNA where Tcf forms a functional DNA binding complex with β-catenin and initiates transcription. Furthermore Osx is needed for the expression of two antagonists of Wnt-signaling, the major player Dickkopf (Dkk1) and Sclerostin (Sost). Other targets controlled by Osx are the special AT-rich sequence binding protein 2 (Satb2), the nuclear steroid vitamin D receptor (VDR) and the vascular endothelial growth factor (VEGF). The first and second are involved directly in bone development and metabolism respectively, while the last has an indirect effect being involved in angiogenesis.

SatB2 directly interacts with and augments the activity of both, RUNX2 and ATF4. It regulates the craniofacial and osteoblast differentiation and function. It is shown to be a downstream target of Osterix and it can upregulate Osteocalcin and Osx promoter activity. Taken together Osx and Satb2 can influence each others promoter activity (Zhang, 2012).

Peroxysome proliferator-activated receptor γ (PPARγ) expression is connected with adipogenesis. Doing so it inhibits the transcription of RUNX2 and facilitates the proteasomal degradation of β-catenin (Lee *et al.*, 2013). The pro-adipocyte function relies on the inhibition of β-catenin, but the anti-osteoblastic activity is independent of this interaction. On the other hand it was shown that PPARγ2 could enhance osteogenic differentiation if co-incubated with BMP-2 in C3H10T1/2 (Yu *et al.*, 2012).

Activating transcription factor 4 (ATF4) regulates the terminal differentiation and function of osteoblasts, including the synthesis of collagen. ATF4 directly binds to the promoter of osteocalcin activating gene transcription (Nakamura *et al.*, 2013).

Dlx5 The osteogenic homebox protein induces osteoblast maturation and inhibits osteocyte formation. Dlx5 is immediately activated by the BMP-signaling pathway and triggers the expression of RUNX2, osteopontin and alkaline phosphatase thus supports osteogenesis.

Nuclear factor "kappa-light-chain-enhancer" of activated B-cells (NF-κB) is an important regulator of the immune system. It was found that proinflammatory cytokines (especially TNF-α) inhibit osteogenic differentiation by increasing the expression of NF-κB. NF-κB inhibits the differentiation of MSCs and commits them towards osteoblastic cells. This effect is mediated by promoting the degradation of β-catenin.

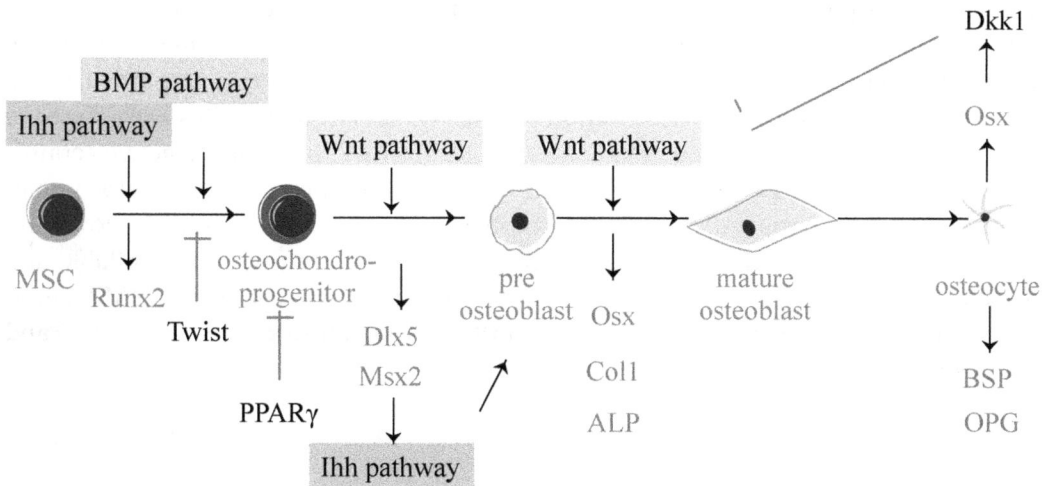

Figure 6: Distribution and effects of signaling pathways and transcription factors. Twist proteins interact with RUNX2 und inhibit RUNX2 function. Msx2 promotes osteoblast formation. Dlx5 leads to maturation of osteoblast cells. Osteoprotegerin (OPG) is preferentially expressed by mature osteoblasts. Osx inhibits in a feedback loop Wnt-pathway.

7   Osteogenic Differentiation and Respective Scaffolding

Scaffolds for tissue engineering are defined as porous 3D substrate materials guiding cell adhesion, differentiation, proliferation, and growth. A potential scaffold should be osteoconductive, osteoinductive, and osteogenic for enhanced bone formation (Kolk *et al.*, 2012; Scaglione *et al.*, 2012). Autografts, still the gold standard today, include the risk of immune rejections, blood coagulation or tissue hypertrophy, thus artificial materials are a very attractive alternative. Today, a broad variety of artificial materials has been developed and tested that can mainly be classified according to their chemical nature into metals, inorganic ceramics, and organic polymers and corresponding composites, i.e. ceramic-polymer and metal-polymer composites (Ricciardi and Bostrom, *et al.*, 2013, Polo-Corrales *et al.* 2014). In the following a short overview will be given focusing recently published studies on most promising scaffold material candidates for osteogenic differentiations, their chemical composition, 3D fabrication and bioactivation.

7.1   Scaffold Materials

Ceramics and Glasses

Ceramics and Glasses are widely used for bone regeneration and based on hydroxy apatite (HA), calcium phosphates, in particular tricalcium phosphate (TCP) (Kaur *et al.*, 2014). Additionally, they are often combined with metals and/or natural or synthetic polymers since pure ceramic materials are brittle and lack interconnected pores required for cell proliferation, and angiogenesis, limiting the use of ceramic scaffolds to rather small defects (Jones, 2013). **Bioglasses**, their biological response, in particular cell attachment influenced by ionic dissolution products from HA spherulites were tested *in vivo* for large bone tissue engineering (Zhi *et al.*, 2013). Novel triphasic bioactive ceramic scaffolds were synthesized and tested in vitro and in vivo concerning their cytocompatibility and osteogenesis influenced by fibroblast growth factor-2 release (Roohani-Esfahani *et al.*, 2014). Cements of varying composition are commercially available and tested *in vitro* and *in vivo* regarding their osteogenic properties, e.g. PMMA-based Gentafix®, calcium phosphates Calcibon®, Graftys®, calcium sulphates MIIG-115® and nanocrystalline HA Ostim® (Drosos *et al.*, 2012).

Metals

Current research on metals used for bone grafts include sintered metallic foams as part of biodegradable bone replacement materials (Orinak *et al.*, 2014), porous titanium with entangled wire structure for load-bearing biomedical applications (Jiang and He, 2014), low elastic modulus titanium-nickel scaffolds (Li *et al.*, 2014b) and novel layered HA/TCP-zirconia scaffold composites with high bending strength for load-bearing bone implant applications (Yang *et al.*, 2014).

Natural Polymers

Beside metals and inorganic ceramic materials, there are a huge number of organic polymers synthesized to be used as artificial bone grafts. They are classified into natural and artificial polymers, degradable and non-degradable materials.

Natural polypeptides and polysaccharides for bone regeneration include various types of collagens, gelatin, fibrin, fibronectin, chitosan, silk, alginates, hyaluronic acid, and corresponding derivatives (Polo-Corrales et al., 2014). Natural chitosan is used in different combinations to prepare bionic bone structures: e.g. chitosan/hydroxyapatite composites (Zhang et al., 2014, Jiang T. et al., 2014. Osteogenic differentiation of bone marrow-derived stem cells could be demonstrated using mixed gelatin and chitosan-oligosaccharide scaffolds (Sandeep et al., 2014). Silk proteins, and silk/forsterite composites are recently tested in vitro (Kundu et al. 2014, Teimouri et al., 2014).

Synthetic Polymers

Synthetic polymers provide the opportunity to tailor physical properties such as molecular weight, molecular weight distribution and correlated mechanical properties. Major challenges are the design of tailored 3D architectures with defined porosity and appropriate surface for cell adhesion. In general, the polymers themselves are biocompatible, many of them are bioresorbable. Further requirements can include injectability and biodegradability. For bone regeneration, scaffolds have to possess appropriate mechanical stability. Via variation of molecular weight (MW) and MW distribution, biodegradation rate and mechanical properties can be influenced. Depending on the polymer synthesis methods, linear and branched structures and three dimensional networks can be prepared. One of the remaining problems is the formation and accumulation of certain amounts of degradation products in a short time period due to bulk degradation. Although some of the degradation products (e.g. lactic and glycolic acids) are also present in normal metabolic pathways, these amounts may result in local inflammation. Synthetic polymers used as scaffolds for bone grafts include *polyesters,* mainly poly-lactic acid (PLA) and poly-glycolic acid (PGA) (Clark et al 2014, Tahriri et al. 2014), poly(caprolactone) (PCL) (Mkhabela et al. 2014), PLGA doped PCL microspheres with a layered architecture and an island-sea topography (Cheng et al., 2014), *polyurethane* and corresponding composites (Mi et al., 2014, Buschmann et al., 2011) and corresponding copolymers. PCL scaffolds engineered for sustained drug release and evaluated in vitro using human bone marrow-derived mesenchymal stem cells. Alkaline phosphatase activity showed a significant increase in activity and increased mineralization in PCL matrices (Mkhabela and Ray, 2014). *Polyether–ester* co-polymers tested as bone filling materials for clinical applications (PolyActive™, IsoTis Orthopaedics) are studied regarding the influence of porosity, molecular network mesh size and swelling on dynamic mechanical properties (Moroni et al. 2008).

Composite Materials

Composites are designed to gain synergetic effects by combining required mechanical properties with osteoconductive characteristics. Within the last two decades, a broad variety of composites was tested for their osteogenic potential, e.g.: synthetic PLA mineralized with calcium phosphate (Kim *et al.* 2011a), biomimetic collagen-apatite composites with a multi-level lamellar structure (Xia *et al.* 2014), silane-modified chitosan-silica hybrid scaffolds (Connell *et al.* 2014), biopolymer/calcium phosphate composites (Li *et al.* 2014a) and pre-vascularized constructs using pre-differentiated rADSCs, arteriovenous vascular bundle and porous nano-HA/polyamide-66 scaffolds (Yang *et al.*, 2013).

Nanomaterials

Nanomaterials, e.g. carbon nanotubes (Martins-Junior *et al.* 2013) and nano-HA-based bioglasses (Erol-Taygun *et al.* 2013) were developed within the last two decades and tested in tissue regeneration, i.e. cardiac, skin, bone, cartilage and nerve) (Peran *et al.* 2013, Li *et al.* 2013). Again, the most promising approaches are represented by nano-based composites. Applications are mainly focused on utilization of nanomaterials to improve mechanical properties of scaffold materials. Thus, nanofibers are prepared via electrospinning, phase separation or self-assembling techniques mimicking the nanofibrillar structure of ECM. Nanostructured mesoporous silicon can be used for discriminating *in vitro* calcification of electrospun scaffold composites (Fan *et al.* 2014). Enhancement of cell-based therapeutic angiogenesis was reported using a novel type of injectable scaffolds based on HA/polymer nanocomposite microspheres and nanofibers (Mima *et al.*, 2012). Direct-write assembly of 3D silk/HA scaffolds for bone co-cultures were tested *in vitro* (Sun *et al.*, 2012).). Composites of HA-silica nanoparticles reinforcing PLA scaffolds were synthesized and tested regarding their influence on scaffold bioactivity (Guerzoni *et al.* 2014 The influence of HA nanoparticle content and initial cell seeding density on early osteogenic signal expression of rat bone marrow stromal cells was studied by (Kim *et al.* 2011b).

7.2   Scaffold fabrication techniques

A special focus in scaffold fabrication is given to vary the ***porosity*** and investigate resulting mechanical and morphological properties (Hoseini *et al.* 2014, Loh *et al.* 2013). Porous scaffolds were prepared based on a hydroxyl functionalized polymer, poly(hydroxymethyl glycolide-co-ε-caprolactone) (PHMGCL) produced via 3D plotting resulting in a high porosity and an interconnected pore structure. Human mesenchymal stem cells were seeded onto the scaffolds filled the pores of the PHMGCL scaffold within one week, displayed increased metabolic activity and supported osteogenic differentiation (Seyednejad *et al.* 2011). Porous nanocomposites based on poly(vinylalcohol) and colloidal HA nanoparticles were prepared via controlled synthesis methods; *in vitro* experiments with osteoblast cells indicated an appropriate penetration of the cells into the scaffold's pores and cell growth support (Poursamar *et al.* 2011). Pore expanded mesoporous HA via auxiliary solubilizing template method were developed by Zeng (Zeng *et al.* 2014). Current research of material scientists is focused on strategies for directing the structure and function of 3D interconnected polymer sponges and foams. Some recently published examples should be given: differently organized collagen fibers within newly formed bone under unloading conditions could be generated depending on differently architectured scaffolds (Walters and Stegemann 2014); novel ß-TCP/PLA composite scaffolds with high strength and enhanced permeability were prepared by a modified salt leaching method (Rakovsky *et al.* 2014); a bottom-up approach to construct microfabricated multilayer scaffolds for bone tissue engineering (Lima *et al.*, 2014), cell viability enhancement in 3D hydrogel scaffolds fabricated via cell-dispersing technique supplemented by preosteoblast-laden microbeads (Lee *et al.*, 2014). Effects of fabrication approaches on HA particle size were studied in addition to mechanical properties and mineralization of rigid thermoplastic polyurethane/HA composites (Mi *et al.*, 2014). Hafezi and colleagues investigated the influence of sintering temperature and cooling rate on the morphology, mechanical behavior and apatite-forming ability of a novel nanostructured Mg/Ca silicate scaffold prepared by a freeze casting method (Hafezi *et al.* 2014). Porous 3D shape memory polymers (SMP) were synthesized as foams and meshes and tested regarding the influence of fabrication parameters on pore size and macrostructural porosity (Hearon *et al.*, 2013). In addition to experimental fabrication, computational studies are performed for scaffold design optimization (Dias *et al.*, 2014, Giannitelli *et al.*, 2014).

Polymeric Gels and Hydrogels

Concerning fabrication of 3D polymer structures, polymeric gels and hydrogels are the most widely used forms providing the possibility to encapsulate drugs and/or cells (Fang *et al.*, 2014). Due to limited mechanical and viscoelastic properties, gels and hydrogels are mainly used for controlled drug release. Regarding their chemical nature, gels and hydrogels are prepared from natural polysaccharides, e.g. hyaluronic acid derivatives, synthetic polymers, e.g. poly(hydroxyethyl methacrylate) or semi-synthetic derivatives, e.g. collagen-PLA composites. Three dimensional network formation is performed via radical or photopolymerization induced by ultraviolet irradiation. Self-assembling peptide hydrogel structures can support the differentiation and transdifferentiation of cells. Stem or progenitor cells are encapsulated within these self-assembling peptide hydrogel structures. The peptide hydrogel nanoscale environment renders the cells permissive for instruction by differentiation factors such as growth factors or ECM components enabling the cells to differentiate or transdifferentiate within the structures (Dreifke *et al.*, 2013). Recently published hydrogels include the following: multifunctional hydrogels based on ß-cyclodextrins with effects on biomineralization (Liu *et al.* 2014), degradable, injectable, porous, and cell-responsive gelatin cryogels capable of controlled release of proteins (Sandeep *et al.* 2014), and sol-gel derived bioactive glass scaffolds prepared by freeze casting method (Mozafari and Moztarzadeh, 2014). Injectability is one of the significant advances of gels and hydrogels, leading to a broad variety of investigated polymers. Examples include injectable composite microspheres of HA/PLGA (Hu *et al.*, 2014), or injectable thermosensitive calcium phosphate-based hydrogels (Fan *et al.*, 2014).

Foams

Besides gels and hydrogels, foams are developed as scaffolds and drug delivery matrices. One of the few synthetic polymers approved for human clinical use are porous foams made of a racemic poly(lactide-co-glycolide) copolymer (Ma *et al.* 2008). Microcellular foams are made from biodegradable or non-biodegradable polymers with pores throughout the material having a diameter of about 1 to 200 microns. In addition, polymer surfaces may be textured as a result of foaming. This is of vital interest, since surface morphology and roughness have been demonstrated to influence the physiological response to an implant, including cell attachment, morphology and differentiation.

Injectable foams have attracted considerable attention in recent years. Many injectable biomaterials, such as hydrogels and calcium phosphate cements (CPCs), have nanoscale pores that limit the rate of cellular migration and proliferation. While introduction of macroporosity has been suggested to increase cellular infiltration and tissue healing, many conventional methods for generating macropores often require harsh processing conditions that preclude their use in injectable foams. In recent years, processes such as porogen leaching, gas foaming, and emulsion-templating have been adapted to generate macroporosity in injectable CPCs, hydrogels, and hydrophobic polymers. While some of the more mature injectable foam technologies have been evaluated in clinical trials, there are challenges remaining to be addressed, such as the biocompatibility and ultimate fate of the sacrificial phase used to generate pores within the foam after it sets *in situ*. Furthermore, while implantable scaffolds can be washed extensively to remove undesirable impurities, all of the components required to synthesize injectable foams must be injected into the defect. Thus, every compound in the foam must be biocompatible and noncytotoxic at the concentrations utilized. As future research addresses these critical challenges, injectable macroporous foams are anticipated to have an increasingly significant impact on improving patient outcomes for a number of clinical procedures (Prieto *et al.* 2014).

Nanobased Fabrication Techniques

Various nanobased fabrication techniques have been developed in the past decade that open new opportunities for 3D scaffold design. In particular, electrospinning and different rapid prototyping technique including three dimensional printing, fused deposition modeling (FDM), stereolithography, selective laser ablation (SLA) and selective laser sintering (SLS) are considered to be the most promising techniques for smart scaffold fabrication resulting in new materials, nanostructured surfaces, and novel 3D architectures (L. Zhang & Webster, 2009). Various material classes were tested including 3D printed synthetic polymers (An *et al.* 2013, Hribar *et al.* 2014), porous electrospun 3D PCL/ß-TCP composites (Kim and Kim, 2014) *in vitro* and *in vivo* evaluation of bone formation using solid freeform fabrication-based bone morphogenic protein-2 releasing PCL/PLGA scaffolds (Kim, T. *et al.* 2014), direct 3D powder printing of biphasic calcium phosphate scaffolds for substitution of complex bone defects (Castilho *et al.*, 2014), apatite formation and osteogenic activity of electrospun composites for bone TE (Patlolla *et al.* 2014), HA nanofibers fabricated through electrospinning and sol-gel process (Lee and

Kim, 2014). Computational modeling studies were performed for predicting the elastic properties of selective laser sintered (SLS) PCL/beta-TCP bone scaffolds (Doyle *et al.* 2014).

7.3   Scaffold bioactivation

Biomimetic Surfaces

First approaches to develop biomimetic surfaces include conventional surface coating performed via chemical and physical vapor deposition methods, well-known techniques used in microelectronic industry to modify surfaces in a controlled manner (Ma *et al.*, 2008). A platform of thin polymer coatings was introduced for the functional modulation of immobilized bioactive molecules at solid/liquid interfaces. Heparinization was one of the first approaches for biomimetic surface modification. Koenig and colleagues compared the integration of heparin during matrix synthesis versus adsorptive post surface modification to gain biomimetic bone grafts (Koenig *et al.*, 2014). Another well-known system for surface functionalization are hyaluronic acid and corresponding derivatives, e.g. fibrin-hyaluronic acid hydrogel on solid-free form-based scaffolds followed by BMP-2 loading to enhance bone regeneration (Kong *et al.* 2011). Another approach is based on covalently attached alternating maleic acid anhydride (MAA) copolymers with a variety of co-monomers and extended through conversion of the anhydride moieties by hydrolysis or reaction with functional amines. Within the last two decades, extensive research has been performed on the incorporation of adhesion promoting oligopeptides into biomaterial surfaces and/or bulk. For individual control of the release kinetics of bioactive agents, the appropriate combination of bioactive factors needed at different time points during tissue regeneration has still to be studied in more detail. Furthermore, the therapeutic application of growth factors can be accompanied by undesirable side effects due to the difficulty to control the release in an appropriate dose-depending manner. Bioactive factors are extensively investigated for their effects on angiogenesis, cell growth or stem cell differentiation. Both, native and artificial receptor ligands, i.e. extracellular nucleotides are known to induce stem cell differentiation or growth, e.g. bone morphogenic proteins and transforming growth factor-ß used in bone and cartilage regeneration. BMPs have been shown to influence cell adhesion and migration (Crouzier *et al.* 2011, Su *et al.*, 2014) and to recruit mesenchymal stem cells from bone marrow and periosteum to the site of repair and to support proliferation and differentiation of these cells, inducing vascularization, bone formation, remodeling, and marrow differentiation (Carroll and Ravid 2013, Schober *et al.* 2013), reviewed with specific focus on dental pulp (Carreira *et al.* 2014). Studies demonstrated significant influence of scaffold composition on growth and differentiation of bone marrow-derived mesenchymal stem cells. *In vitro* mineralization and *in vivo* bone regeneration studies were performed in a rat calvarial defect model using an acrylic acid-functionalized porous resveratrol-conjugated PCL composite material showing increased osteogenesis (Kamath *et al*, 2014). Dishowitz and colleagues studied Jagged1 immobilization to an osteoconductive polymer and found an activating effect on the Notch signaling pathway and induction effect on osteogenesis (Dishowitz *et al.* 2014). Bioerodible systems for sequential release of multiple drugs (growth or transcription factors, receptors and corresponding ligands) were recently tested for bone applications (Sundararaj *et al.* 2014).

Nanoscaled Drug Release Systems

Nanoscaled drug release systems include hyaluronic acid, acrylic acid, dextran methacrylic acid, polyethylene glycol acrylate/methacrylate, polyethylene glycol diacrylates and dimethacrylates. Dendron-like nanoparticles have been synthesized and tested including *in vivo* studies of stem cell differentiation into osteoblasts (Oliveira *et al.*, 2011). Biodegradable dexamethasone-loaded dendron-like nanoparticles of carboxymethylchitosan/poly (amido amine) dendrimer have been synthesized and used as intracellular drug delivery systems. Results proved a non-cytotoxic *in vitro* behavior, supporting cell attachment and incorporation. *In vivo* experiments using rats could demonstrate a good performance of dendron-like nanoparticles for intracellular delivery of dexamethasone. Modeling vascularized bone regeneration within a porous biodegradable CaP scaffold loaded with growth factors (Sun *et al.*, 2013). Angiogenic/osteogenic response of bmMSCs on bone-derived scaffold including effect of hypoxia and role of PI3K/Akt-mediated VEGF-VEGFR pathway (Zhou *et al.*, 2014) controlled multiple growth factor delivery via designed affinity (Suarez-Gonzalez *et al.*, 2013) intrafibrillar silicification of collagen scaffolds for sustained release of stem cell homing chemokine in hard tissue regeneration (Niu *et al.*, 2012). Engineered microenvironments have been designed for controlled stem cell differentiation including biomimetics and controlled release, e.g. fibrin/hyaluronic acid hydrogels on solid freeform-based scaffolds loaded with BMP-2 (Kong *et al.* 2011), dual release of stromal cell-derived factor-1 and BMP-2 from hydrogels (Ratanavaraporn *et al.* 2011), glycosaminoglycans as regulators for stem cell differentiation (Smith *et al.* 2011). So called 'integrated biomimetic systems' combine conventional materials and fabrication methods, respectively with nanomaterials and nanotechnologies: e.g. chitosan/hyaluronic acid composites (Huang *et al.* 2011).

Surface Patterning

Surface topography and roughness in micro- and even nanoscale is known to influence biocompatibility of synthetic materials used for tissue engineering applications. Furthermore, adhesion and alignment strongly depends on micro- and nanotopographical features (Scharnagl *et al.* 2010). Symmetry and regularity of surface patterns (isotropic versus anisotropic grinding) causes differences in cell responses. Conventional surface modification strategies can be divided into two groups: methods that are changing surface chemistry and topography e.g. chemical adsorption, plasma treatment methods and chemical etching and secondly methods altering the surface topography: mechanical roughening, the so-called substrate templating methods (e.g. lithography), electro and vapor deposition methods, and novel moulding processes. In the last decade, material surfaces used for tissue engineering applications are micro- and nanostructured during scaffold fabrication via solid freeform techniques, e.g. 3D printing, 3D plotting. Rapid prototyping processes do show differences in resolution and all are characterized by advantages and certain limitations (Peltola *et al.* 2008). So, the highest resolutions can be realized via SLA (70-250 µm). However SLA requires appropriate liquid photopolymers that are still limited in availability whereas 3D print is a rather fast process but characterized by weak bonding between powder particles. Surface patterning of novel polyesters to be used in bone tissue engineering is realized via 3D print process (Seydnejad *et al.* 2011). Whitesides and co-worker first described the patterning of proteins and cells using the so-called soft lithography (Whitesides, 2001). Patterning via electrospinning was used to study the role of nanostructured mesoporous silicon in discriminating *in vitro* calcification for electrospun scaffold composites (Fan *et al.* 2011). Electrospun scaffold composites consisting of PCL/gelatine nanofiber were produced and micropatterned by femtosecond laser ablation for tissue engineering applications (Lim *et al.* 2011). Geometry and size of ECM structures do have significant effects on various cell properties including attachment/adhesion, migration, and proliferation. Differences in height of nanotopographic features influence cell behavior through secondary effects, such as alterations in the effective substrate stiffness. Gerecht and co-workers could demonstrate that nanotopographic structured ECM alters the morphology and proliferation of human embryonic stem cells through cytoskeletal-mediated mechanisms (Gerecht *et al.* 2007). Poly(dimethylsiloxane) gratings with 600 nm features and spacing are designed that are able to induce embryonic stem cells alignment and elongation. In addition, they could also show that nanotopographic features altered the organization of various cytoskeletal components, such as F-actin, vimentin, and tubulin. Changes in proliferation and morphology were abolished by the effect of actin-disrupting agents. Furthermore, the influence of nanotopographic features may be mediated through secondary effects as alterations in the effective stiffness perceived by the cell or differences in protein adsorption caused by ECM nanotopographics.

Self-Assembled Composites

Surface patterning via self-assembled composites enables surface chemistry and topography variation in a very controlled manner. Thus, the influence of PCL-based hybrid scaffold on hMSC seeding efficiency, proliferation, distribution and differentiation was investigated. Porous PCL meshes were prepared by fused deposition modeling embedded in a matrix of hyaluronic acid, methylated collagen and terpolymer via polyelectrolyte complex co-acervation. Embedded scaffolds provided a higher cell seeding efficiency, a more homogeneous cell distribution and more osteogenically differentiated cells, verified by a more pronounced gene expression of the bone markers alkaline phosphatase, osteocalcin, bone sialoprotein I and bone sialoprotein II (Chen *et al.* 2010). Organic/inorganic colloidal composite gels were fabricated from self-assembling gelatin nanospheres and calcium phosphate nanocrystals (Wang *et al.* 2014). Novel 2D and 3D biointerfaces using self-organization to control cell behavior, direct patterning of protein- and cell-resistant polymeric monolayers and microstructures and concave pit-containing scaffold surfaces that improve stem cell-derived osteoblast performance and lead to significant bone tissue formation (Tanaka 2011).

The layer-by-layer technique using polyelectrolytes was used for positioning an anchoring of biomolecules (e.g. BMP-2) onto scaffold surfaces using multiple functional-ities of polyelectrolyte multilayer films. Assembling polyelectrolyte multilayers and their effects on self-assembly of particles in a so-called bottom-up approach is reported for polymers, particles, nanoparticles, and carbon nanotubes. Depositing methods in-clude dip coating, spin coating, spraying and a new dewetting method, which appears to be efficient, economical, and fast and could be used to create unique adsorption to-pographies, including fractal networks and aligned fibers. Min and colleagues reported tunable staged release of therapeutics from layer-by-layer coatings with clay interlayer barrier (Min *et al.*, 2014).

Recent In Vivo Studies

Recent in vivo studies on scaffold-based biomimetic approaches including commercially produced bone grafts are performed (Ghasemi-Mobarakeh *et al.* 2013, Rao and Stegemann 2013, Ricciardi and Bostrom, 2013, Polo-Corrales *et al.* 2014). However, there are still many detailed problems to be solved in future development of artificial bone replacement materials, e.g. combining osteoinductive proteins with an osteoconductive scaffold to perform timed-released delivery of proteins like growth and transcription factors in a tightly controlled manner. Tailoring chemical and mechanical properties by different manufacturing techniques offers the ability to adjust specific material specifi-cations to the application site, e.g. via variation of pore size, mechanical strength, bio-degradation and bioresorption rate. In addition, scaffold topography has to be adjusted to optimize cellular adhesion and proliferation. Osteoinductive growth factors support regeneration of defects, however, due to associated insufficient vascularization, scaffold materials have to be designed that support both, osteogenesis and angiogenesis. Recent-ly reported approaches include 3D scaffolds co-seeded with human endothelial progen-itor and mesenchymal stem cells (Duttenhoefer *et al.*, 2013), porous bioceramics scaffold by accumulating HA spherulites for large bone tissue engineering (Zhi *et al.* 2013) and 2-N,6-O-sulfated chitosan nanoparticles incorporating BMP-2 for vascularization and bone regeneration in critical sized defects (Cao *et al.*, 2014).

8   Proteins used for Clinical Application of Mesenchymal Stem Cells for Bone Healing

The ideal graft for bone healing would possess three main characteristics: it would be osteogenic, osteoinductive, and osteoconductive. Although the perfect artificial graft has been created yet scientist try to meet these criteria. To do so todays engineered bone tissue normally consists of three components: scaffold, stem cells, and proteins (growth factors). In this section a short overview about major proteins used for osteo-genic induction will be given.

Fibronectin

Fibronectin (FN) is an adhesive glycoprotein involved in early stages of osteogen-esis (Ribeiro *et al.*, 2010). FN increases cell adhesion (Pierschbacher & Ruoslahti, 1984) and migration (Humphries *et al.*, 1989) and furthermore promotes osteoblastic differentiation (Ding *et al.*, 2006). It has been shown that *in vitro* attachment and proliferation of bone forming cells on hydroxyapatite scaffolds is significantly increased with FN and fetal calf serum. For *in vivo* studies hydroxyapatite disks coated with FN and fetal calf serum were seeded with green fluorescent protein-expressing cells and implanted in mice. Schonmeyr and colleagues (Schonmeyr *et al.*, 2008) stated that this difference less profound and not significant *in vivo*. In a mouse model plasma FN could elevate direct bone formation faster. This is to some extent in line with the *in vitro* results indicating that plasma FN significantly promoted BMSC chemotaxis, but has no effect on differentiation and proliferation. Another group, while using anodized titanium implants coated with a fibroblast growth factor (FGF)-FN fusion protein, could demonstrate that the implants enhance osseointegration *in vivo* (Park *et al.*, 2006). So it can be concluded that plasma FN regulates chemotaxis of osteogenic cells and coating implant with pFN enhances early osseointegration (Jimbo *et al.*, 2007).

BMP-2

BMP-2 induces osteoblast differentiation of mesenchymal precursor cells and enhances bone matrix production by osteoblastic cells (Susperregui *et al.*, 2008). It stimulates RUNX2-deficient cells to express makers related to osteoblasts differentiation using a RUNX-independent pathway. But it failed to induce these cells to differentiate into bone-forming osteoblasts and mature chondrocytes (Liu *et al.*, 2007). BMP-2 elevates the expression of one of the master regulators of osteogenic differentiation: Osterix. This induction is mediated by Dlx5 (Lee *et al.*, 2003). BMSC transfected with BMP-2 have the potential to enhance bone repair and bone regeneration *in vivo* (Ding *et al.*, 2007). Keibl and co-worker (Keibl *et al.*, 2011) showed in a rodent model that the transplantation of ASCs modulates the callus induction by BMP-2 to a normal volume. In a canine *in vivo* model, ASCs transduced with a vector expressing the BMP-2 gene enhanced the repair of critical-sized bone defect, too. Furthermore it was shown that BMP-2 gene therapy together with beta-tricalciumphosphate scaffold could be used to promote mandibular repair and bone regeneration in a rat model (Zhao *et al.*, 2010).

Osteopontin

Osteopontin (OPN) is a non-collagenous bone matrix protein which promotes osteoblast and osteoclast adhesion, differentiation, and function (Giachelli *et al.*, 2002). It was demonstrated that OPN found in mineralized tissues, modulates osteoclast functions (Li *et al.*, 2009). On the one hand Grimm and colleagues found that the early human response to systemic endotoxemia boosts OPN levels and modifies bone markers, indicating a decrease in the lytic activity of osteoclasts, accompanied by an induction of osteoblasts activity (Grimm *et al.*, 2010). And on the other hand OPN inhibits mineral crystallization both, *in vivo* and *in vitro*. In addition *in vitro* experiments with OPN show conflicting activities. The specific binding of OPN to collagen I influences osteoblast adhesion (Liu *et al.*, 2007). A study found that OPN is more important for osteoblast adhesion to the collagen matrix than bone Sialoprotein (BSP) (Bernards *et al.*, 2008). Furthermore another study comparing the cell binding activity of absorbed BSP and OPN bound to hydroxyapatite concluded that there is a preference for cellular binding to hydroxyapatite with absorbed BSP compared to OPN (Bernards *et al.*, 2008)

Bone Sialoprotein

Bone Sialoprotein (BSP) is a major non-collagenous glycosylated phosphoprotein of the extracellular bone matrix (Wang *et al.*, 2006). It is expressed in differentiated osteoblasts and seems to function in the initial mineralization of bone (Wang *et al.*, 2011). It can induce osteoblast differentiation through Arginyl-glycyl-aspartic(RGD)-mediated cell interactions to promote mineralization. Also by serving as a matrix-associated signal that promotes increasing production of mineralized matrix (Gordon *et al.*, 2007). Therefore BSP deficiency is accompanied with impaired bone growth and mineralization (Malaval *et al.*, 2008). In addition BSP plays a role in primary bone formation and mineralization of newly formed bone during the process of cortical bone healing *in vivo* (Monfoulet *et al.*, 2010). But unfortunately coating a variety of scaffolds with BSP was not directly associated with an enhancement of osteoprogenitor cell differentiation neither *in vitro* nor *in vivo*. Thus presentation of BSP on substrates is not sufficient to prime BMSC in functional osteoblastic differentiation (Schaeren *et al.*, 2010).

In conclusion pretreatment of biomaterials with FN in the initial phase of osteogenic differentiation, improved results for all types of surfaces providing an ideal microenvironment that enhances the adhesion and proliferation of pluripotent cells. In the second stage of differentiation surface coating with BMP-2 increases better adhesion and reduced proliferation of MSCs (Chatakun *et al.*, 2014).

9   Conclusions

There is a high interest for biomedical research on developing optimal cell therapeutics for bone healing due to an increasing need for bone regeneration and replacement. Engineering bone tissue is a complex process not only based on cellular and molecular developmental biology approaches, but also guided by bioengineering and biomechanical projections. For an *in vivo* application every simple component (MSC source, scaffold, and growth factor) must fulfill distinct requirements and the interaction of these components must be optimized needing to act in concert to perfectly match for a safe application in humans. These challenges are guiding and will certainly also drive future research in this fast developing scientific field.

Acknowledgement

Supported by the Bundesministerium für Bildung und Forschung (BMBF)-FHprofUnt,

[FKZ: 03FH012PB2 to E.T]; NRW FH-Extra, [FKZ: z1112fh012 to E.T]; DAAD PPP Vigoni, [FKZ: 314-vigoni-dr and FKZ: 54669218 to E.T]; BMBF-AIF, [FKZ: 1720X06 to E.T]. The figures are made with motifolio.com©.

References

Abzhanov, A., Rodda, S. J., McMahon, A. P., & Tabin, C. J. (2007). Regulation of skeletogenic differentiation in cranial dermal bone. Development, 134, 3133–3144.

Adamo, L., & Garcia-Cardena, G. (2011). Directed stem cell differentiation by fluid mechanical forces. Antioxidants & Redox Signaling, 15, 1463–1473.

Alkaisi, A., Ismail, A. R., Mutum, S. S., Ahmad, Z. A., Masudi, S., & Abd Razak, N. H. (2013). Transplantation of human dental pulp stem cells: enhance bone consolidation in mandibular distraction osteogenesis. Journal of Oral Maxillofacial Surgery, 71, 1758.e1751–1713.

Amini, A. R., Laurencin, C. T., & Nukavarapu, S. P. (2012). Bone tissue engineering: recent advances and challenges. Critical Reviws in Biomedical Engineering, 40, 363–408.

An, J., Chua, C. K., Yu, T. et al. (2013) Advanced nanobiomaterial strategies for the development of organized tissue engineering constructs. Nanomedicine, 8, 591–602

Audoly L. P., Gabel C. A., Jee W. S., Dixon S. J., Sims S. M., & Thompson D. D. (2003). Deletion of the P2X7 nucleotide receptor reveals its regulatory roles in bone formation and resorption. Molecular Endocrinology, 17, 1356–1367.

Ayala-Peña, V. B., Scolaro, L. A., & Santillán, G. E. (2013). ATP and UTP stimulate bone morphogenetic protein-2,-4 and -5 gene expression and mineralization by rat primary osteoblasts involving PI3K/AKT pathway. Experimental Cell Research, 319, 2028–2036.

Baksh, D., Yao, R., & Tuan, R. S. (2007). Comparison of proliferative and multilineage differentiation potential of human mesenchymal stem cells derived from umbilical cord and bone marrow. Stem Cells, 25, 1384–1392.

Barzilay, R., Melamed, E., & Offen, D. (2009). Introducing transcription factors to multipotent mesenchymal stem cells: making transdifferentiation possible. Stem Cells, 27, 2509–2515.

Bernards, M. T., Qin, C., & Jiang, S. (2008). MC3T3-E1 cell adhesion to hydroxyapatite with adsorbed bone sialoprotein, bone osteopontin, and bovine serum albumin. Colloids and Surfaces B: Biointerfaces, 64, 236–247.

Bernards, M. T., Qin, C., Ratner, B. D., & Jiang, S. (2008). Adhesion of MC3T3-E1 cells to bone sialoprotein and bone osteopontin specifically bound to collagen I. Journal of Biomedical Materials Research Part A, 86, 779–787.

Biver, G., Wang, N., Gartland, A., Orriss, I., Arnett, T. R, Boeynaems, J. M., Robaye, B. (2013). Role of the P2Y13 receptor in the differentiation of bone marrow stromal cells into osteoblasts and adipocytes. Stem Cells, 12, 2747–2758.

Boccafoschi, F., Mosca, C., Ramella, M., Valente, G., & Cannas, M. (2013). The effect of mechanical strain on soft (cardiovascular) and hard (bone) tissues: common pathways for different biological outcomes. Cell Adhesion & Migration, 7, 165–173.

Bosnakovski, D., Mizuno, M., Kim, G., Takagi, S., Okumura, M., & Fujinaga, T. (2005). Isolation and multilineage differentiation of bovine bone marrow mesenchymal stem cells. Cell and Tissue Research, 319, 243–253.

Bowler, W. B., Dixon, C. J., Halleux, C., Maier, R., Bilbe, G., Fraser, W. D., Gallagher, J. A., & Hipskind, R. A. (1999). Signaling in human osteoblasts by extracellular nucleotides. Their weak induction of the c-fos proto-oncogene via Ca2+ mobilization is strongly potentiated by a parathyroid hormone/cAMP-dependent protein kinase pathway independently of mitogen-activated protein kinase. Journal of Biological Chemistry, 274, 14315–14324.

Buckley, K. A., Wagstaff, S. C., McKay, G., Gaw, A., Hipskind, R. A., Bilbe, G., Gallagher, J. A., & Bowler, W. B. (2001). Parathyroid hormone potentiates nucleotide-induced [Ca2+]i release in rat osteoblasts independently of Gq activation or cyclic monophosphate accumulation. A mechanism for localizing systemic responses in bone. Journal of Biological Chemistry, 276, 9565–9571.

Bunnell, B. A., Flaat, M., Gagliardi, C., Patel, B., & Ripoll, C. (2008). Adipose-derived stem cells: isolation, expansion and differentiation. Methods, 45, 115–120.

Burnstock, G., Arnett, T. R., & Orriss, I. R. (2013). Purinergic signalling in the musculoskeletal system. Purinergic Signalling, 9, 541–572.

Buschmann, J., Welti, M., Hemmi, S., Neuenschwander, P., Baltes, C., & Giovanoli, P. (2011) Three-dimensional co-cultures of osteoblasts and endothelial cells in DegraPol foam: histological and high-field magnetic resonance imaging analyses of pre-engineered capillary networks in bone grafts. Tissue Engineering Part A, 17, 291–299.

Cao, L., Wang, J., Hou, J., Xing, W., & Liu, C. (2014) Vascularization and bone regeneration in a critical sized defect using 2-N,6-O-sulfated chitosan nanoparticles incorporating BMP-2. Biomaterials 35, 684–98.

Carreira, A.C., Lojudice, E., Halcsik, E., Navarro, R.D., Sogayar, M.C., & Granjeiro, J.M. (2014) Bone Morphogenic Proteins: Facts, Challenges, and Future Perspectives. Journal of Dental Research, 93, 335–345.

Carroll, S.H. & Ravid, K. (2013) Differentiation of mesenchymal stem cells to osteoblasts and chondrocytes: a focus on adenosine receptors. Expert Rev Molecular Medicine, 15, 1–12.

Carroll, S. H., Wigner, N. A., Kulkarni, N., Johnston-Cox, H., Gerstenfeld, L. C., & Ravid, K. (2012). A2B adenosine receptor promotes mesenchymal stem cell differentiation to osteoblasts and bone formation in vivo. Journal of Biological Chemistry, 287, 15718–15727.

Castilho, M., Moseke, C., Ewald, A., Gbureck, U., Groll, J., Pires, I., Tessmar, J., & Vorndran, E. (2014) Biofabrication, 6, Article Number 015006.

Chen, M., Le, D.Q., Baatrup, A., Nygaard, J. V., Hein, S., Bjerre, L., Kassem, M., Zou, X., & Bünger, C. (2011) Self-assembled composite matrix in a hierarchical 3-D scaffold for bone tissue engineering. Acta Biomaterialia, 7,2244–2255.

Cheng, D., Cao, X., & Gao, H. (2014) Engineering PLGA doped PCL microspheres with a layered architecture and an island-sea topography. RSC Advances, 4, 9031–9038.

Ciciarello, M., Zini, R., Ross,i L., Salvestrini, V., Ferrari, D., Manfredini, R., & Lemoli, R. M. (2013). *Extracellular purines promote the differentiation of human bone marrow-derived mesenchymal stem cells to the osteogenic and adipogenic lineages. Stem Cells and Development, 22, 1097–1111.*

Clark, A., Milbrandt, T.A., & Hilt, J.Z. (2014) *Tailoring properties of microsphere-based poly(lactic-co-glycolic acid) scaffolds. Journal of Biomedical Materials Research Part A, 102, 348–357.*

Connell, L.S., Romer, F., & Suarez, M. (2014) *Chemical characterisation and fabrication of chitosan-silica hybrid scaffolds with 3-glycidoxypropyl trimethoxysilane. Journal of Materials Chemistry Part B, 2, 668–680.*

Costa, M. A., Barbosa, A., Neto, E., Sá-e-Sousa, A., Freitas, R., Neves, J. M,, Magalhães-Cardoso, T., Ferreirinha, F., & Correia-de-Sá, P. (2011). *On the role of subtype selective adenosine receptor agonists during proliferation and osteogenic differentiation of human primary bone marrow stromal cells. Journal of Cellular Physiology, 226, 1353–1366.*

Crouzier, T., Fourel, L., Boudou, T., Albigès-Rizo, C., & Picart, C. (2011) *Presentation of BMP-2 from a Soft Biopolymeric Film Unveils its Activity on Cell Adhesion and Migration. Advanced Materials, 23, 111–118.*

D'Alimonte, I., Nargi, E., Lannutti, A., Marchisio, M., Pierdomenico, L., Costanzo, G., Iorio, P. D., Ballerini, P., Giuliani, P., Caciagli, F., & Ciccarelli, R. (2013). *Adenosine A1 receptor stimulation enhances osteogenic differentiation of human dental pulp-derived mesenchymal stem cells via WNT signaling. Stem Cell Research, 11, 611–624.*

de Lazaro, I., Yilmazer, A., & Kostarelos, K. (2014). *Induced pluripotent stem (iPS) cells: A new source for cell–based therapeutics? Journal of Controlled Release, 185C, 37–44.*

De Miguel, M. P., Fuentes-Julian, S., Blazquez-Martinez, A., Pascual, C. Y., Aller, M. A., Arias, J., & Arnalich-Montiel, F. (2012). *Immunosuppressive properties of mesenchymal stem cells: advances and applications. Current Molecular Medicine, 12, 574–591.*

Deschaseaux, F., Sensebe, L., & Heymann, D. (2009). *Mechanisms of bone repair and regeneration. Trends in Molecular Medicine, 15, 417–429.*

Dias, M.R., Guedes, J.M., & Flanagan, C.L. (2014) *Optimization of scaffold design for bone tissue engineering: A computational and experimental study. Medical Engineering and Physics, 36, 448–457.*

Ding, H. F., Liu, R., Li, B. G., Lou, J. R., Dai, K. R., & Tang, T. T. (2007). *Biologic effect and immunoisolating behavior of BMP-2 gene-transfected bone marrow-derived mesenchymal stem cells in APA microcapsules. Biochemical and Biophysical Research Communications, 362, 923–927.*

Ding, H. T., Wang, C. G., Zhang, T. L., & Wang, K. (2006). *Fibronectin enhances in vitro vascular calcification by promoting osteoblastic differentiation of vascular smooth muscle cells via ERK pathway. Journal of Cellular Biochemistry, 99, 1343–1352.*

Dishowitz, M.I., Zhu, F., & Sundararaghavan, H.G. (2014) Jagged1 immobilization to an osteoconductive polymer activates the Notch signaling pathway and induces osteogenesis. Journal of Biomedecial Materials Research Part A, 102, 1558–1567.

Doyle, H., Lohfeld, S., & McHugh, P. (2014) Predicting the Elastic Properties of Selective Laser Sintered PCL/beta-TCP Bone Scaffold Materials Using Computational Modelling. Annals in Biomedical Engineering, 42, 661–677.

Dreifke, M.l B., Ebraheim, N.A., & Jayasuriya, A.C. (2013) Investigation of potential injectable polymeric biomaterials for bone regeneration. Journal of Biomedical Materials Research Part A, 101A, 2436–2447.

Drosos, G.I., Babourda, E., Magnissalis, E.A., Giatromanolaki, A., Kazakos, K., & Verettas, D.A. (2012) Mechanical characterization of bone graft substitute ceramic cements. Injury, International Journal of Care Injured, 43, 266–271.

Duttenhoefer, F., Lara de Freitas, R., Meury, T., Loibl, M., Benneker, L.M., Richards, R.G., Alini, M., & Verrier, S. (2013) 3D scaffolds co-seeded with human endothelial progenitor and mesenchymal stem cells: evidence of prevascularisation within 7 days. European Cell Materials, 26, 49–64.

Engin, F., Lee, B. (2010) NOTCHing the bone: insights into multi-functionality. Bone, 46, 274–280

Erol-Taygun, M., Zheng, K., & Boccaccini, A.R. (2013) Nanoscale Bioactive Glasses in Medical Applications. International Journal of Applied Glass Science, 4, 136–148.

Fang, J., Yang, Z., & Tan, S. (2014) Injectable gel graft for bone defect repair. Regenerative Medicine, 9, 41–51.

Fan, D.M., Akkaraju, G.R., & Couch, E.F. (2011) The role of nanostructured mesoporous silicon in discriminating in vitro calcification for electrospun composite tissue engineering scaffolds. Nanoscale, 3, 354–361.

Fan, R., Deng, X., & Zhou, L. (2014) Injectable thermosensitive hydrogel composite with surface-functionalized calcium phosphate as raw materials. International Journal of Nanomedicine, 9, 615–626.

Fickert, S., Schroter-Bobsin, U., Gross, A. F., Hempel, U., Wojciechowski, C., Rentsch, C., Corbeil, D., Gunther, K. P. (2011). Human mesenchymal stem cell proliferation and osteogenic differentiation during long-term ex vivo cultivation is not age dependent. Journal of Bone and Mineral Metabolism, 29, 224–235.

Gharibi, B., Abraham, A. A., Ham, J., & Evans, B. A. (2011). Adenosine receptor subtype expression and activation influence the differentiation of mesenchymal stem cells to osteoblasts and adipocytes. Journal of Bone and Mineral Research, 26, 2112–2124.

Ghasemi-Mobarakeh, L., Prabhakaran, M.P., & Balasubramanian, P. (2013) Advances in Electrospun Nanofibers for Bone and Cartilage Regeneration. Journal of Nanoscience and Nanotechnology 13(7), 4656–4671.

Giachelli, C. M., & Steitz, S. (2000). Osteopontin: a versatile regulator of inflammation and *biomineralization. Matrix Biology, 19, 615–622.*

Giannitelli, S.M., Accoto, D., Trombetta, M., & Rainer, A. (2014) Current trends in the design of scaffolds for computer-aided tissue engineering. Acta Biomaterialia, 10, 580–594.

Gilboa, L., Nohe, A., Geissendorfer, T., Sebald, W., Henis, Y. I., & Knaus, P. (2000). Bone morphogenetic protein receptor complexes on the surface of live cells: a new oligomerization mode for serine/threonine kinase receptors. Molecular Biology of the Cell, 11, 1023–1035.

Gordon, J. A., Tye, C. E., Sampaio, A. V., Underhill, T. M., Hunter, G. K., & Goldberg, H. A. (2007). Bone sialoprotein expression enhances osteoblast differentiation and matrix mineralization in vitro. Bone, 41, 462–473.

Grimm, G., Vila, G., Bieglmayer, C., Riedl, M., Luger, A., & Clodi, M. (2010). Changes in osteopontin and in biomarkers of bone turnover during human endotoxemia. Bone, 47, 388–391.

Grol, M. W., Zelner, I., & Dixon, S. J. (2012). $P2X_7$-mediated calcium influx triggers a sustained, PI3K-dependent increase in metabolic acid production by osteoblast-like cells. American Journal of Physiology - Endocrinology and Metabolism 302, E561–E575.

Gronthos, S., Mankani, M., Brahim, J., Robey, P. G., & Shi, S. (2000). Postnatal human dental pulp stem cells (DPSCs) in vitro and in vivo. Proceedings of the National Academy of Science of the United States of America, 97, 13625–13630.

Guerzoni, S., Deplaine, H., & El Haskouri, J. (2014) Combination of silica nanoparticles with hydroxyapatite reinforces poly (L-lactide acid) scaffolds without loss of bioactivity. Journal of Bioactive Compatible Polymers, 29, 15–31.

Haddouti, E.-M., Skroch, M., Zippel, N., Müller, C., Birova, B., Pansky, A., Kleinfeld, C., Winter, M., & Tobiasch, E. (2009). Human Dental Follicle Precursor Cells of Wisdom Teeth: Isolation and Differentiation towards Osteoblasts for Implants with and without Scaffolds. Material Science Engineering and Technology, 40, 732–737.

Hafezi, M., Nezafati, N., & Nadernezhad, A. (2014) Effect of sintering temperature and cooling rate on the morphology, mechanical behavior and apatite-forming ability of a novel nanostructured magnesium calcium silicate scaffold prepared by a freeze casting method. Journal of Material Science, 49, 1297–1305.

He, H., Nagamura-Inoue, T., Tsunoda, H., Yuzawa, M., Yamamoto, Y., Yorozu, P., Agata, H., Tojo, A. (2014). Stage-Specific Embryonic Antigen 4 in Wharton's Jelly-Derived Mesenchymal Stem Cells Is Not a Marker for Proliferation and Multipotency. Tissue Engineering Part A, 20, 1314–1324.

He, W., & Cronstein, B. (2011). The roles of adenosine and adenosine receptors in bone remodeling. Frontiers in Bioscience, (Elite Ed). 3, 888–895.

He W., Mazumder A., Wilder T., & Cronstein B. N. (2013). Adenosine regulates bone metabolism via A1, A2A, and A2B receptors in bone marrow cells from normal humans and patients with multiple myeloma. FASEB Journal, 27, 3446–3454.

Hearon, K., Singhal, P., & Horn, J. (2013) Porous Shape-Memory Polymers. Polymer Revision,

53, 41–75.

Hoseini, J., Kaka, G., & Sadraie, S.H. (2014) Fabrication of Variable Porous Hydroxyapatite Scaffolds to Investigate Appropriate Mechanical and Morphological Properties for Bone Tissue Engineering. Journal of Biomaterials Tissue Engineering, 4, 138–142.

Hribar, K.C., Soman, P., & Warner, J. (2014) Light-assisted direct-write of 3D functional biomaterials. Lab On A Chip, 14, 268–275.

Hsieh, J. Y., Wang, H. W., Chang, S. J., Liao, K. H., Lee, I. H., Lin, W. S., Wu, C., Lin, W., Cheng, S. M. (2013). Mesenchymal stem cells from human umbilical cord express preferentially secreted factors related to neuroprotection, neurogenesis, and angiogenesis. PLoS One, 8, e72604.

Hu, X., Shen, H., & Yang, F. (2014) Modified composite microspheres of hydroxyapatite and poly(lactide-co-glycolide) as an injectable scaffold. Applied Surface Science, 292, 764–772.

Huang, Z., Feng, Q., Yu, B., & Li, S. (2011) Biomimetic properties of an injectable chitosan/nano-hydroxyapatite/collagen composite. Material Science and Engineering: C, 31, 683–687.

Humphries, M. J., Obara, M., Olden, K., & Yamada, K. M. (1989). Role of fibronectin in adhesion, migration, and metastasis. Cancer Investigations, 7, 373–393.

Islam, A., Yasin, T., & Rehman, I. (2014) Synthesis of hybrid polymer networks of irradiated chitosan/poly(vinyl alcohol) for biomedical applications. Radiation Physics and Chemistry, 96, 115–119.

Jackson, W. M., Nesti, L. J., & Tuan, R. S. (2012). Concise review: clinical translation of wound healing therapies based on mesenchymal stem cells. Stem Cells Translational Medicine, 1, 44–50.

Javed, A., Bae, J. S., Afzal, F., Gutierrez, S., Pratap, J., Zaidi, S. K., Lou, Y., van Wijnen, A., Stein, J., Stein, G., Lian, J. B. (2008). Structural coupling of Smad and RUNX2 for execution of the BMP2 osteogenic signal. Journal of Biological Chemistry, 283, 8412–8422.

Jiang, G. & He, G. (2014) Enhancement of the porous titanium with entangled wire structure for load-bearing biomedical applications. Material Design 56, 241–244.

Jiang, T., Deng, M., & James, R. (2014) Micro- and nanofabrication of chitosan structures for regenerative engineering. Acta Biomaterialia 10(4), 1632–1645.

Jimbo, R., Sawase, T., Shibata, Y., Hirata, K., Hishikawa, Y., Tanaka, Y., Bessho, K., Ikeda, T., Atsuta, M. (2007). Enhanced osseointegration by the chemotactic activity of plasma fibronectin for cellular fibronectin positive cells. Biomaterials, 28, 3469–3477.

Jones, J.R. (2013) Review of bioactive glass: From Hench to hybrids. Acta Biomaterialia 9(1), 4457–4486.

Kamath, M.S., Ahmed, S.S.S.J., Dhanasekaran, M., & Santosh, S.W. (2014) Polycaprolactone scaffold engineered for sustained release of resveratrol: therapeutic enhancement in bone tissue engineering. International Journal of Nanomedicine, 9, 183–195.

Kanno, T., Takahashi, T., Tsujisawa, T., Ariyoshi, W., & Nishihara, T. (2007). Mechanical stress-mediated RUNX2 activation is dependent on Ras/ERK1/2 MAPK signaling in osteoblasts. Journal of Biological Chemistry, 101, 1266–1277.

Katz, S., Boland, R., & Santillán, G. (2006). *Modulation of ERK 1/2 and p38 MAPK signaling pathways by ATP in osteoblasts: involvement of mechanical stress-activated calcium influx, PKC and Src activation. International Journal of Biochemistry and Cell Biology, 38, 2082–2091.*

Kaur, G., Pandey, O.P., & Singh, K. (2014) *A review of bioactive glasses: Their structure, properties, fabrication, and apatite formation. Journal of Biomedical Material Research Part A, 102, 254–274.*

Ke H. Z., Qi H., Weidema A. F., Zhang Q., Panupinthu N., Crawford D. T., Grasser W. A., Paralkar V. M., Li M.,

Keating, A. (2012). *Mesenchymal stromal cells: new directions. Cell Stem Cell, 10, 709–716.*

Keibl, C., Fugl, A., Zanoni, G., Tangl, S., Wolbank, S., Redl, H., & van Griensven, M. (2011). *Human adipose derived stem cells reduce callus volume upon BMP-2 administration in bone regeneration. Injury, 42, 814–820.*

Khan, Y., Yaszemski, M. J., Mikos, A. G., & Laurencin, C. T. (2008). *Tissue engineering of bone: material and matrix considerations. The Journal of Bone & Joint Surgery Am, 90, 36–42.*

Kikuchi-Taura, A., Taguchi, A., Kanda, T., Inoue, T., Kasahara, Y., Hirose, H., Sato, I., Matsuyama, T., Nakagomi, T., Yamahara, K., Stern, D., Ogawa, H., Soma, T. (2012). *Human umbilical cord provides a significant source of unexpanded mesenchymal stromal cells. Cytotherapy, 14, 441–450.*

Kim, J. B., Greber, B., Arauzo-Bravo, M. J., Meyer, J., Park, K. I., Zaehres, H., Scholer, H. R. (2009). *Direct reprogramming of human neural stem cells by OCT4. Nature, 461, 649–643.*

Kim, K., Dean, D., & Lu, A.Q. (2011b) *Early osteogenic signal expression of rat bone marrow stromal cells is influenced by both hydroxyapatite nanoparticles content and initial cell seeding density in biodegradable nanocomposites scaffolds. Acta Biomaterialia, 7, 1249–1264.*

Kim, M.S. & Kim, G.H. (2014) *Highly porous electrospun 3D polycaprolactone/beta-TCP biocomposites for tissue regeneration. Material Letters, 120, 246–250.*

Kim, S.H., Oh, S.A., & Lee, W.K. (2011a) *Poly(lactic acid) porous scaffold with calcium phosphate mineralized surface and bone marrow mesenchymal stem cell growth and differentiation. Material Science and Engineering: C, 31, 612–619.*

Kim, T.-H., Yun, Y.-P., & Park, Y.-E. (2014) *In vitro and in vivo evaluation of bone formation using solid freeform fabrication-based bone morphogenic protein-2 releasing PCL/PLGA scaffolds. Biomedical Materials, 9, Article Number: 025008.*

Knoepfler, P. S. (2009). *Deconstructing stem cell tumorigenicity: a roadmap to safe regenerative medicine. Stem Cells, 27, 1050–1056.*

Koenig, U., Lode, A., & Welzel, P.B. (2014) *Heparinization of a biomimetic bone matrix: integration of heparin during matrix synthesis versus adsorptive post surface modification.*

Journal of Material Sciences - Materials in Medicine, 25, 607–621.

Kolk, A., Handschel, J., Drescher, W., Rothamel, D., Kloss, F., Blessmann, M., Heiland, M., Wolff, K.-D., & Smeets, R. (2012) Current trends and future perspectives of bone substitute materials: From space holders to innovative biomaterials. Journal in Cranio-Maxillo facial Surgery, 40, 706–718.

Komori, T. (2006). Regulation of osteoblast differentiation by transcription factors. Journal of Cellular Biochemistry, 99, 1233–1239.

Kong, S.W., Kim, J.S., & Park, K.S. (2011) Surface modification with fibrin hyaluronic acid hydrogel on solid-free form-based scaffolds followed by BMP-2 loading to enhance bone regeneration. Bone, 48, 298–306.

Kundu, B., Kurland, N.E., & Bano, S. (2014) Silk proteins for biomedical applications: Bioengineering perspectives. Progress in Polymer Science, 39, 251–267.

Lee, H., Jin., Ahn, S.H., & Chun, W. (2014) Enhancement of cell viability by fabrication of macroscopic 3D hydrogel scaffolds using an innovative cell-dispensing technique supplemented by preosteoblast-laden micro-beads. Carbohydrate Polymers, 104, 191–198.

Lee, J.H. & Kim, Y.J. (2014) Hydroxyapatite nanofibers fabricated through electrospinning and sol-gel process. Ceramics International, 40, 3361–3369.

Lee, M. H., Kwon, T. G., Park, H. S., Wozney, J. M., & Ryoo, H. M. (2003). BMP-2-induced Osterix expression is mediated by Dlx5 but is independent of RUNX2. Biochemical and Biophysical Research Communications, 309, 689–694.

Lee, M. J., Chen, H. T., Ho, M. L., Chen, C. H., Chuang, S. C., Huang, S. C., Tu,Y., Wang, G., Kang, L., Chang, J. K. (2013). PPARgamma silencing enhances osteogenic differentiation of human adipose-derived mesenchymal stem cells. Journal of Cellular and Molecular Medicine, 17, 1188–1193.

Li, H., Liu, Y., Zhang, Q., Jing, Y., Chen, S., Song, Z., Yan, J., Li, Y., Wu, X., Zhang, X., Zhang, Y., Case, J., Yu, M., Ingram, D., Yang, F. C. (2009). Ras dependent paracrine secretion of osteopontin by Nf1+/− osteoblasts promote osteoclast activation in a neurofibromatosis type I murine model. Pediatric Research, 65, 613–618.

Li, J., Baker, B.A., & Mou, X. (2014a) Biopolymer/Calcium Phosphate Scaffolds for Bone Tissue Engineering. Advances in Health Care Materials, 3, 469–484.

Li J., Liu D., Ke H. Z., Duncan R. L., & Turner C. H. (2005). The P2X7 nucleotide receptor mediates skeletal

mechanotransduction. Journal of Biological Chemistry, 280, 42952–42959.

Li, J., Yang, H., & Wang, H. (2014b) Low elastic modulus titanium-nickel scaffolds for bone implants. Materials Sciences and Engineering: C, 34, 110–114.

Li, X., Wang, Lu., & Fan, Y. (2013) Nanostructured scaffolds for bone tissue engineering. Journal of Biomedical Materials Research Part A, 101A, 2424–2435.

Lima, M.J., Pirraco, R.P., & Sousa, R.A. (2014) Bottom-up approach to construct microfabricated multi-layer scaffolds for bone tissue engineering. Biomedical Microdevices,

16, 69–78.

Lin, S. S., Ueng, S. W., Niu, C. C., Yuan, L. J., Yang, C. Y., Chen, W. J., Chen, J. K. (2014a). *Effects of hyperbaric oxygen on the osteogenic differentiation of mesenchymal stem cells. BMC Musculoskeletal Disorders, 15, 56.*

Lin, S. S., Ueng, S. W., Niu, C. C., Yuan, L. J., Yang, C. Y., Chen, W. J., Lee, M., Chen, J. K. (2014b). *Hyperbaric oxygen promotes osteogenic differentiation of bone marrow stromal cells by regulating Wnt3a/beta-catenin signaling - an in vitro and in vivo study. Stem Cell Research, 12, 260–274.*

Liu, L., Qin, C., Butler, W. T., Ratner, B. D., & Jiang, S. (2007). *Controlling the orientation of bone osteopontin via its specific binding with collagen I to modulate osteoblast adhesion. Journal of Biomedical Materials Research Part A, 80, 102–110.*

Liu, S., Chen, X., & Zhang, Q. (2014) *Multifunctional hydrogels based on beta-cyclodextrin with both biomineralization and anti-inflammatory properties. Carbohydrate Polymers, 102, 869–876.*

Liu, T., Gao, Y., Sakamoto, K., Minamizato, T., Furukawa, K., Tsukazaki, T., Shibata, Y., Bessho, K., Komori, T., Yamaguchi, A. (2007). *BMP-2 promotes differentiation of osteoblasts and chondroblasts in RUNX2-deficient cell lines. Journal of Cellular Physiology, 211, 728–735.*

Liu, T. M., & Lee, E. H. (2013). *Transcriptional regulatory cascades in RUNX2-dependent bone development. Tissue Engineering Part B Review, 19, 254–263.*

Loh, Q.L., & Choong, C. (2013) *Three-Dimensional Scaffolds for Tissue Engineering Applications: Role of Porosity and Pore Size. Tissue Engineering B - Reviews, 19, 485–502.*

Longo, A., Librizzi, M., Naselli, F., Caradonna, F., Tobiasch, E., & Luparello, C. (2013). *PTHrP in differentiating human mesenchymal stem cells: transcript isoform expression, promoter methylation, and protein accumulation. Biochemie, 95, 1888–1896.*

Ma, P.X. (2008) *Biomimetic materials for tissue engineering. Advances in Drug Delivery Revision, 60, 184–98.*

Mak, K. K., Chen, M. H., Day, T. F., Chuang, P. T., & Yang, Y. (2006). *Wnt/beta-catenin signaling interacts differentially with Ihh signaling in controlling endochondral bone and synovial joint formation. Development, 133, 3695–3707.*

Malaval, L., Wade-Gueye, N. M., Boudiffa, M., Fei, J., Zirngibl, R., Chen, F., Laroche, N., Roux, J., Burt-Pichat, B., Duboeuf, F., Boivin, G., Jurdic, P., Lafage-Proust, M., Amedee, J., Vico, L., Tossant, J., Aubin, J. E. (2008). *Bone sialoprotein plays a functional role in bone formation and osteoclastogenesis. The Journal of Experimental Medicine, 205, 1145–1153.*

Mao, J., Wang, J., Liu, B., Pan, W., Farr, G. H., 3rd, Flynn, C., Yuan, H., Takada, S., Kimlemann, D., Li, L., Wu, D. (2001). *Low-density lipoprotein receptor-related protein-5 binds to Axin and regulates the canonical Wnt signaling pathway. Molecular Cell, 7, 801–809.*

Marcellini, S., Henriquez, J. P., & Bertin, A. (2012). *Control of osteogenesis by the canonical Wnt and BMP pathways in vivo. Bioessays, 34, 953–962.*

Markov, V., Kusumi, K., Tadesse, M. G., William, D. A., Hall, D. M., Lounev, V., Carlton, A., Leonard, J., Cohen, R.I., Rappaport, E.F., Saitta, B. (2007). Identification of cord blood-derived mesenchymal stem/stromal cell populations with distinct growth kinetics, differentiation potentials, and gene expression profiles. Stem Cells and Development, 16, 53–73.

Marmotti, A., Mattia, S., Bruzzone, M., Buttiglieri, S., Risso, A., Bonasia, D. E., Blonna, D., Castoldi, F., Rossi, R., Zanini, C., Ercole, E., Defabiani, E., Tarella, C., Peretti, G. M. (2012). Minced umbilical cord fragments as a source of cells for orthopaedic tissue engineering: an in vitro study. Stem Cells International, 2012, 326813.

Martins-Junior, P.A., Alcantara, C.E., & Resende, R.R. (2013) Carbon Nanotubes: Directions and Perspectives in Oral Regenerative Medicine. Journal in Dental Research, 92, 575–583.

McBeath, R., Pirone, D.M., Nelson, C.M., Bhadriraju, K., Chen, C.S. (2004) Cell shape, cytoskeletal tension, and RhoA regulate stem cell lineage commitment. Developmental Cell 6: 483–495

Mediero, A., & Cronstein, B. N. (2013). Adenosine and bone metabolism. Trends in Endocrinology and Metabolism, 24, 290–300.

Mi, H.-Y., Jing, X., & Salick, M.R. (2014) Morphology, mechanical properties, and mineralization of rigid thermoplastic polyurethane/hydroxyapatite scaffolds for bone tissue applications: effects of fabrication approaches and hydroxyapatite size. Journal of Material Sciences, 49, 2324–2337.

Miao, D., Tong, X. K., Chan, G. K., Panda, D., McPherson, P. S., & Goltzman, D. (2001). Parathyroid hormone-related peptide stimulates osteogenic cell proliferation through protein kinase C activation of the Ras/mitogen-activated protein kinase signaling pathway. The Journal of Biological Chemistry, 276, 32204–32213.

Mima, Y., Fukumolo, S., Koyama, H., Okada, M., Tanaka, S., Shoi, T., Emoto, M., Furuzono, T., Nishizawa, Y., & Inaba, M. (2012) Enhancement of cell-based therapeutic angiogenesis using a novel type of injectable scaffolds of hydroxyapatite-polymer nanocomposite microspheres. PLoS One, 7, e35199.

Min, J., Braatz, R.D., & Hammond, P.T. (2014) Tunable staged release of therapeutics from layer-by-layer coatings with clay interlayer barrier. Biomaterials, 35, 2507–2517.

Mitchell, J. B., McIntosh, K., Zvonic, S., Garrett, S., Floyd, Z. E., Kloster, A., Di Halvorsen, Y., Storms, R., Goh, B., Kilroy, G. Wu, X., Gimble, J. M. (2006). Immunophenotype of human adipose-derived cells: temporal changes in stromal-associated and stem cell-associated markers. Stem Cells, 24, 376–385.

Miyazono, K., Maeda, S., & Imamura, T. (2005). BMP receptor signaling: transcriptional targets, regulation of signals, and signaling cross-talk. Cytokine & Growth Factor Reviews, 16, 251–263.

Mkhabela, V.J. & Ray, S.S. (2014) Poly(epsilon-caprolactone) Nanocomposite Scaffolds for Tissue Engineering: A Brief Overview. Journal of Nanoscience and Nanotechnology, 14, 535–545.

Monfoulet, L., Malaval, L., Aubin, J. E., Rittling, S. R., Gadeau, A. P., Fricain, J. C., & Chassande, O. (2010). Bone sialoprotein, but not osteopontin, deficiency impairs the mineralization of regenerating bone during cortical defect healing. Bone, 46, 447–452.

Monti, M., & Redi, C. A. (2011). The biopolitics of frozen embryos. The International Journal of Developmental Biology, 55, 243–247.

Moroni, L., Wijn, J., & Van Blitterswijkc, A. (2008) Integrating novel technologies to fabricate smart scaffolds. Journal of Biomaterial Science Polymer Edition, 19, 543–572.

Murry, C. E., & Keller, G. (2008). Differentiation of embryonic stem cells to clinically relevant populations: lessons from embryonic development. Cell, 132, 661–680.

Nagamura-Inoue, T., & He, H. (2014). Umbilical cord-derived mesenchymal stem cells: Their advantages and potential clinical utility. World Journal of Stem Cells, 6, 195–202.

Nakamura, S., Miki, H., Kido, S., Nakano, A., Hiasa, M., Oda, A., Amou, H., Watanabe, K., Harada, T., Fuji, S., Takeuchi, K., Kagawa, K., Ozaki, S., Matsumoto, T., Abe, M. (2013). Activating transcription factor 4, an ER stress mediator, is required for, but excessive ER stress suppresses osteoblastogenesis by bortezomib. International Journal of Hematology, 98, 66–73.

Niu, L.N., Jiao, K., & Qi, Y.P. (2012) Intrafibrillar silicification of collagen scaffolds for sustained release of stem cell homing chemokine in hard tissue regeneration. FASEB J 11, 4517–29.

Nohe, A., Keating, E., Knaus, P., & Petersen, N. O. (2004). Signal transduction of bone morphogenetic protein receptors. Cell Signal, 16, 291–299.

Ode, A., Schoon, J., Kurtz, A., Gaetjen, M., Ode, J. E., Geissler, S., & Duda, G. N. (2013). CD73/5'-ecto-nucleotidase acts as a regulatory factor in osteo-/chondrogenic differentiation of mechanically stimulated mesenchymal stromal cells. European Cells and Materials, 25, 37–47.

Oliveira, J. M., Sousa, R. A., Malafaya, P. B., Silva, S. S., Kotobuki, N., Hirose, M., Ohgushi, H., Mang, J. F., & Reis, R. L. (2011) In vivo study of dendron-like nanoparticles for stem cells "tune-up": From nano to tissues. Nanomedicine, 7, 914–924.

Orinak, A., Orinakova, R., & Kralova, Z.O. (2014) Sintered metallic foams for biodegradable bone replacement materials. Journal of Porous Materials, 21, 131–140.

Orriss, I. R., Key, M. L., Brandao-Burch, A., Patel, J. J., Burnstock, G., & Arnett, T. R. (2012). The regulation of osteoblast function and bone mineralisation by extracellular nucleotides: The role of p2x receptors. Bone, 51, 389–400.

Orriss, I. R., Key, M. L., Hajjawi, M. O., & Arnett, T. R. (2013). Extracellular ATP released by osteoblasts is a key local inhibitor of bone mineralization. Public Library of Science One, 8, e69057.

Orriss, I. R., Knight, G. E., Ranasinghe, S., Burnstock, G., & Arnett, T. R. (2006). Osteoblast responses to nucleotides increase during differentiation. Bone, 39, 300–309.

Pansky, A., Roitzheim, B., & Tobiasch, E. (2007). Differentiation potential of adult of human *mesenchymal stem cells. Clinical Laboratory, 53, 81–84.*

Park, J. M., Koak, J. Y., Jang, J. H., Han, C. H., Kim, S. K., & Heo, S. J. (2006). *Osseointegration of anodized titanium implants coated with fibroblast growth factor-fibronectin (FGF–FN) fusion protein. The International Journal of Oral & Maxillofacial Implants, 21, 859–866.*

Patlolla, A., & Arinzeh, T.L. (2014) *Evaluating Apatite Formation and Osteogenic Activity of Electrospun Composites for Bone Tissue Engineering. Biotechnology and Bioengineering, 111, 1000–1017.*

Peran, M., Angel-Garcia, M., & Lopez-Ruiz, E. (2013) *How can nanotechnology help to repair the body? Advances in cardiac, skin, bone, cartilage and nerve. Tissue Regeneration Materials, 6, 1333–1359.*

Petrovic, V., & Stefanovic, V. (2009). *Dental Tissue — New Source for Stem Cells. TheScientificWorldJOURNAL, 9, 1167–1177.*

Pierschbacher, M. D., & Ruoslahti, E. (1984). *Variants of the cell recognition site of fibronectin that retain attachment-promoting activity. Proceedings of th National Adacemy of Science of the United States of America, 81, 5985–5988.*

Pittenger, M. F., Mackay, A. M., Beck, S. C., Jaiswal, R. K., Douglas, R., Mosca, J. D., Moorman, M. A., Simonetti, D. W., Craig, S., Marshak, D. R. (1999). *Multilineage potential of adult human mesenchymal stem cells. Science, 284, 143–147.*

Polo-Corrales, L., Latorre-Esteves, M., & Ramirez-Vick, J.E. (2014) *Scaffold Design for Bone Regeneration. Journal of Nanoscience and Nanotechnology, 14, 15–56.*

Poursamar, S.A., Azami, M., & Mozafari, M. (2011) *Controllable synthesis and characterization of porous polyvinyl alcohol/hydroxyapatite nanocomposite scaffolds via an in situ colloidal technique. Colloids Surfaces Part B Biointerfaces, 84, 310–316.*

Prieto, E. M., Page, J. M., Harmata, A. J., & Guelcher, S. A. (2014) *Injectable foams for regenerative medicine. WIREs Nanomedicine Nanobiotechnology, 6, 136–154.*

Rao, R.R. & Stegemann, J.P. (2013) *Cell-based approaches to the engineering of vascularized bone tissue. Cytotherapy, 15, 1309–1322.*

Rakovsky, A., Gotman, I., & Rabkin, E. (2014) *beta-TCP-polylactide composite scaffolds with high strength and enhanced permeability prepared by a modified salt leaching method. Journal of Mechanical Behavior and Biomedical Materials, 32, 89–98.*

Ratanavaraporn, J., Furuya, H., & Kohara, H. (2011) *Synergistic effects of the dual release of stromal cell-derived factor-1 and bone morphogenic protein-2 from hydrogels on bone regeneration. Biomaterials, 32, 2797–2811.*

Rawadi, G., Vayssiere, B., Dunn, F., Baron, R., & Roman-Roman, S. (2003). *BMP-2 controls alkaline phosphatase expression and osteoblast mineralization by a Wnt autocrine loop. Journal of Bone and Mineral Research, 18, 1842–1853.*

Rebelatto, C. K., Aguiar, A. M., Moretao, M. P., Senegaglia, A. C., Hansen, P., Barchiki, F., Oliveira, J., Martins, J., Kuligovski, C., Mansur, F., Christofis, A., Amaral, V.G., Brofman,

P. S., Goldenberg, S., Nakao, L.S., Correa, A. (2008). Dissimilar differentiation of mesenchymal stem cells from bone marrow, umbilical cord blood, and adipose tissue. Experimental Biology and Medicine (Maywood), 233, 901–913.

Ribeiro, N., Sousa, S. R., & Monteiro, F. J. (2010). Influence of crystallite size of nanophased hydroxyapatite on fibronectin and osteonectin adsorption and on MC3T3-E1 osteoblast adhesion and morphology. Journal of Colloid Interface Science, 351, 398–406.

Ricciardi, B.F. & Bostrom, M.P. (2013) Bone graft substitutes: Claims and credibility. Seminars in Arthroplasty, 24, 119–123.

Roohani-Esfahani, S., Wong, K,Y., & Lu, Z. (2014) Fabrication of a novel triphasic and bioactive ceramic and evaluation of its in vitro and in vivo cytocompatibility and osteogenesis. Journal of Material Chemistry Part B, 2, 1866–1878.

Salehinejad, P., Alitheen, N. B., Ali, A. M., Omar, A. R., Mohit, M., Janzamin, E., Samani, F. S., Torshizi, Z., Nematollahi-Mahani, S. N. (2012). Comparison of different methods for the isolation of mesenchymal stem cells from human umbilical cord Wharton's jelly. In Vitro Cellular & Development Biology - Animal, 48, 75–83.

Sandeep, T., Koshy, T.C., Ferrante, S.A., Lewin, D., & Mooney, J. (2014) Injectable, porous, and cell-responsive gelatin cryogels. Biomaterials, 35, 2477–2487.

Scaglione, S., Giannoni, P., Bianchini, P., Sandri, M., Marotta, R., Firpo, G., Valbusa, U., Tampieri, A., Diaspro, A., Bioanco, P., & Quarto, R. (2012) Order versus Disorder: in vivo bone formation within osteoconductive scaffolds. Scientific Reports, 2, 274.

Scarfi, S. (2014). Purinergic receptors and nucleotide processing ectoenzymes: Their roles in regulating mesenchymal stem cell functions. World Journal of Stem Cells, 6, 153–162.

Schaeren, S., Jaquiery, C., Wolf, F., Papadimitropoulos, A., Barbero, A., Schultz-Thater, E., Heberer, M., Martin, I. (2010). Effect of bone sialoprotein coating of ceramic and synthetic polymer materials on in vitro osteogenic cell differentiation and in vivo bone formation. Journal of Biomedical Material Research Part A, 92, 1461–1467.

Scharnagl, N., Lee, S., & Hiebl, B. (2010) Design principles for polymers as substratum for adherent cells. Journal of Material Chemistry, 20, 8789–8802.

Schindeler, A., & Little, D. G. (2006). Ras-MAPK signaling in osteogenic differentiation: friend or foe? Journal of Bone Mineral Research, 21, 1331–1338.

Schober, A., Fernekorn, U., & Singh, S. (2013) Mimicking the biological world: Methods for the 3D structuring of artificial cellular environments. Engineering Life Science, 13, 352–367.Schöfl, C., Cuthbertson, K. S., Walsh, C. A., Mayne, C., Cobbold, P., von zur Mühlen, A., Hesch, R. D., & Gallagher J. A. (1992). Evidence for P2-purinoceptors on human osteoblast-like cells. Journal of Bone and Mineral Research, 7, 485–491.

Schonmeyr, B. H., Wong, A. K., Li, S., Gewalli, F., Cordiero, P. G., & Mehrara, B. J. (2008). Treatment of hydroxyapatite scaffolds with fibronectin and fetal calf serum increases osteoblast adhesion and proliferation in vitro. Plastic and Reconstructive Surgery, 121, 751–762.

Schwartz, M. A. & Ginsberg, M. H. (2002) Networks and Crosstalks: integrin signaling spreads. Nature Cell Biology 4: E65–68

Seong, J. M., Kim, B. C., Park, J. H., Kwon, I. K., Mantalaris, A., & Hwang, Y. S. (2010). Stem cells in bone tissue engineering. Biomedical Material, 5, 062001.

Seyednejad, H., Gawlitta, D., Dhert, W. J. A., van Nostrum, C. F., Vermonden, T., & Hennink, W. (2011) Preparation and characterization of a three-dimensional printed scaffold based on a functionalized polyester for bone tissue engineering applications. Acta Biomaterialia, 7, 1999–2006.

Shih Y. R. , Hwang Y., Phadke A., Kang H., Hwang N.S., Caro E. J., Nguyen S., Siu M., Theodorakis E. A., Gianneschi

N. C., Vecchio K. S., Chien S., Lee O. K., & Varghese S. (2014). Calcium phosphate-bearing matrices induce osteogenic differentiation of stem cells through adenosine signaling. Proceedings of the National Academy Science U S A, 111, 990–995.

Sinha, K. M., & Zhou, X. (2013). Genetic and molecular control of osterix in skeletal formation. Journal of Cellular Biochemistry, 114, 975–984.

Smith, R. A., Meade, K., Pickford, C. E., Holley, R. J., & Merry, C. L. (2011) Glycosaminoglycans as regulators of stem cell differentiation. Biochemical Society Transactions, 39, 383–387.

Su, C.C., Kao, C.T., & Hung, C.J. (2014) Regulation of physicochemical properties, osteogenesis activity, and fibroblast growth factor-2 release ability of beta-tricalcium phosphate for bone cement by calcium silicate. Materials Science and Engineering: C - Materials in Biology Applications, 37, 156–163.

Suarez-Gonzalez, D., Lee, J. S., Diggs, A., Nemke, B., Markel, M., Hollister, S. J., & Murphy, W. L. (2013) Controlled Multiple Growth Factor Delivery from Bone Tissue Engineering Scaffolds Via Designed Affinity. Tissue Engineering Part A, 2013 Dec 18 [Epub ahead of print].

Sun, L., Parker, S.T., Syoji, D. Wang, X., Lewis, J.A., & Kaplan, D.L. (2012) Direct-write assembly of 3D silk/hydroxyapatite scaffolds for bone co-cultures. Advances in Health Care Materials, 1, 729–35.

Sundararaj, S.C., Thomas, M.V., & Dziubla, T.D. (2014) Bioerodible system for sequential release of multiple drugs. Acta Biomaterialia, 10, 115–125.

Susperregui, A. R., Vinals, F., Ho, P. W., Gillespie, M. T., Martin, T. J., & Ventura, F. (2008). BMP-2 regulation of PTHrP and osteoclastogenic factors during osteoblast differentiation of C2C12 cells. Journal of Cellular Physiology, 216, 144–152.

Suzuki, K., Zhu, B., Rittling, S. R., Denhardt, D. T., Goldberg, H. A., McCulloch, C. A., & Sodek, J. (2002). Colocalization of intracellular osteopontin with CD44 is associated with migration, cell fusion, and resorption in osteoclasts. Journal of Bone and Mineral Research, 17, 1486–1497.

Tahriri, M. & Moztarzadeh, F. (2014) Preparation, Characterization, and In Vitro Biological

Evaluation of PLGA/Nano-Fluorohydroxyapatite (FHA) Microsphere-Sintered Scaffolds for Biomedical Applications. Applied Biochemistry and Biotechnology, 172, 2465–2479.

Takahashi, K., Tanabe, K., Ohnuki, M., Narita, M., Ichisaka, T., Tomoda, K., Yamanaka, S. (2007). *Induction of pluripotent stem cells from adult human fibroblasts by defined factors. Cell, 131, 861–872.*

Takahashi, K., & Yamanaka, S. (2006). *Induction of pluripotent stem cells from mouse embryonic and adult fibroblast cultures by defined factors. Cell, 126, 663–676.*

Takedachi, M., Oohara, H., Smith, B. J., Iyama, M., Kobashi, M., Maeda, K., Long, C. L., Humphrey, M. B., Stoecker, B. J., Toyosawa, S., Thompson, L. F., & Murakami, S. (2012). *CD73-generated adenosine promotes osteoblast differentiation. Journal of Cellular Physiology, 227, 2622–2631.*

Tang, W., Li, Y., Osimiri, L., & Zhang, C. (2011). *Osteoblast-specific transcription factor Osterix (Osx) is an upstream regulator of Satb2 during bone formation. The Journal of Biological Chemistry, 286, 32995–33002.*

Teimouri, A., Ghorbanian, L., & Chermahini, A.N. (2014) *Fabrication and characterization of silk/forsterite composites for tissue engineering applications. Ceramics International, 40, 6405–6411.*

Thornton, T. M., Pedraza-Alva, G., Deng, B., Wood, C. D., Aronshtam, A., Clements, J. L., Sabio, G. Davis, R. J., Matthews, D. E., Doble, B., Rincon, M. (2008). *Phosphorylation by p38 MAPK as an alternative pathway for GSK3beta inactivation. Science, 320, 667–670.*

Tsagias, N., Koliakos, I., Karagiannis, V., Eleftheriadou, M., & Koliakos, G. G. (2011). *Isolation of mesenchymal stem cells using the total length of umbilical cord for transplantation purposes. Transfusion Medicine, 21, 253–261.*

Tsai, M. T., Li, W. J., Tuan, R. S., & Chang, W. H. (2009). *Modulation of osteogenesis in human mesenchymal stem cells by specific pulsed electromagnetic field stimulation. Journal Orthopedic Research, 27, 1169–1174.*

Viale-Bouroncle, S., Gosau, M., Morsczeck, C. (2014) *NOTCH1 signaling regulates the BMP2/DLX3 directed osteogenic differentiation of dental follicle cells. Biochemical and Biophysical Research Communications 443: 500–504*

Walters, B.D. & Stegemann, J.P. (2014) *Strategies for directing the structure and function of three–dimensional collagen biomaterials across length scales. Acta Biomaterialia, 10, 1488–1501.*

Wang, H., Bongio, M., & Farbod, K. (2014) *Development of injectable organic/inorganic colloidal composite gels made of self-assembling gelatin nanospheres and calcium phosphate nanocrystals. Acata Biomaterialia, 10, 508–519.*

Wang, J., Zhou, H. Y., Salih, E., Xu, L., Wunderlich, L., Gu, X., HOfstaetter, J.G., Torres, M., Glimcher, M. J. (2006). *Site-specific in vivo calcification and osteogenesis stimulated by bone sialoprotein. Calcified Tissue International, 79, 179–189.*

Wang, N., Robaye, B., Agrawal, A., Skerry, T. M., Boeynaems, J. M., & Gartland, A. (2012).

Reduced bone turnover in mice lacking the P2Y(13) receptor of ADP. Molecular Endocrinology, 26, 142–152.

Wang, N., Rumney, R. M., Yang, L., Robaye, B., Boeynaems, J. M., Skerry, T.M., Gartland, A. (2013). The P2Y(13) receptor regulates extracellular ATP metabolism and the osteogenic response to mechanical loading. Journal Bone and Mineral Research, 28, 1446–1456.

Wang, S., Sasaki, Y., Zhou, L., Matsumura, H., Araki, S., Mezawa, M., Takai, H., Chen, Z., Ogata, Y. (2011). Transcriptional regulation of bone sialoprotein gene by interleukin-11. Gene, 476, 46–55.

Whitesides, G.M., Ostuni, E., & Takayama, S. (2001) Soft lithography in biology and biochemistry. Annual Review of Biomedical Engineering, 3, 335–373.

Xia, Z., Villa, M.M., & Wei, M. (2014) A biomimetic collagen-apatite scaffold with a multi-level lamellar structure for bone tissue engineering. Journal of Materials Chemistry Part B, 2, 1998–2007.

Yamagiwa, H., Endo, N., Tokunaga, K., Hayami, T., Hatano, H., & Takahashi, H. E. (2001). In vivo bone-forming capacity of human bone marrow-derived stromal cells is stimulated by recombinant human bone morphogenetic protein-2. Journal of Bone and Mineral Metabolism, 19, 20–28.

Yan, J., Dong, L., Zhang, B., & Qi, N. (2010). Effects of extremely low-frequency magnetic field on growth and differentiation of human mesenchymal stem cells. Electromagnetic Biology and Medicine, 29, 165–176.

Yang, J.Z., Sultana, R., & Hu, X.Z. (2014) Novel Layered Hydroxyapatite/Tri-Calcium Phosphate-Zirconia Scaffold Composite with High Bending Strength for Load-Bearing Bone Implant Application. International Journal of Applied Ceramic Technology, 11, 22–30.

Yang, P, Huang, X., Shen, J., Wang, C., Dang, X., Mankin, H., Duan, Z., & Wang, K. (2013) Development of a new pre-vascularized tissue-engineered construct using pre-differentiated rADSCs, arteriovenous vascularbundle and porous nano-hydroxyapatide-polyamide 66 scaffold. BMC Musculoskeletal Disorder, 14, 318.

Yu, J., Vodyanik, M. A., Smuga-Otto, K., Antosiewicz-Bourget, J., Frane, J. L., Tian, S., Thomson, J. A. (2007). Induced pluripotent stem cell lines derived from human somatic cells. Science, 318, 1917–1920.

Yu, W. H., Li, F. G., Chen, X. Y., Li, J. T., Wu, Y. H., Huang, L. H., Wang, Z., Li, P., Wang, T., Lahn, B.T., Xiang, A. P. (2012). PPARgamma suppression inhibits adipogenesis but does not promote osteogenesis of human mesenchymal stem cells. The International Journal of Biochemistry & Cell Biology, 44, 377–384.

Zeng, F., Wang, J., & Wu, Y. (2014) Preparation of pore expanded mesoporous hydroxyapatite via auxiliary solubilizing template method. Colloids at Surfaces Part A — Physiochemical Engineering Aspects 441, 737–743.

Zhang, C. (2012). Molecular mechanisms of osteoblast-specific transcription factor Osterix effect on bone formation. Beijing Da Xue Xue Bao, 44, 659–665.

Zhang, C., Cho, K., Huang, Y., Lyons, J. P., Zhou, X., Sinha, K., McCrea, P. D., de Crombrugghe, B. (2008). Inhibition of Wnt signaling by the osteoblast-specific transcription factor Osterix. Proceedings of the National Academy of Science of the United States of America, 105, 6936–6941.

Zhang, J., Nie, J., & Zhang, Q. (2014) Preparation and characterization of bionic bone structure chitosan/hydroxyapatite scaffold for bone tissue engineering. Journal of Biomaterials Science - Polymer Edition, 25, 61–74.

Zhang, L., & Webster, T. (2009). Nanotechnology and nanomaterials: Promises for improved tissue regeneration. Nano Today, 4, 66–80.

Zhang, Y., Khan, D., Delling, J., & Tobiasch, E. (2012). Mechanisms underlying the osteo- and adipo-differentiation of human mesenchymal stem cells. The Scientific World Journal, 2012, 793823.

Zhao, J., Hu, J., Wang, S., Sun, X., Xia, L., Zhang, X., Zhang, Z., Jiang, X. (2010). Combination of beta-TCP and BMP-2 gene-modified bMSCs to heal critical size mandibular defects in rats. Oral Diseases, 16, 46–54.

Zhao, T., Zhang, Z. N., Rong, Z., & Xu, Y. (2011). Immunogenicity of induced pluripotent stem cells. Nature, 474, 212–215.

Zhi, W., Zhang, C., Duan, K., Li, X., Qu, S., Wang, J., Zhu, Z., Huang, P., Xia, T., Liao, G., & Weng, J. (2013) A novel porous bioceramics scaffold by accumulating hydroxyapatite spherulites for large bone tissue engineering in vivo. II. Construct large volume of bone grafts. Journal of biomedical materials research. Part A., 2013, Aug 14, [Epub ahead of print].

Zhou, Y., Guan, X., Yu, M., Wang, X., Zhu, W., Wang, C., Yu, M., & Wang, H. Angiogenic/osteogenic response of BMMSCs on bone-derived scaffold: Effect of hypoxia and role of PI3K/Akt-mediated VEGF-VEGFR pathway. Biotechnology Journal. 2014 Jan 14. doi: 10.1002/biot.201300310

Zippel, N., Limbach, C. A., Ratajski, N., Urban, C., Luparello, C., Pansky, A., Kassack, M. U., and Tobiasch, E. (2012). Purinergic receptors influence the differentiation of human mesenchymal stem cells. Stem Cells and Development, 12, 884–900.

Zippel, N., Schulze, M., & Tobiasch, E. (2010). Biomaterials and Mesenchymal Stem Cells for Regenerative Medicine. Recent Patents in Biotechnology, 4, 1–22.

Chapter 9

Intracellular Tau Modifications and Cell-based Sensors for Monitoring Tau Aggregation

Mamunul Haque[1,2], Sungsu Lim[2], Dohee Kim[3,2], Dong Jin Kim[2] and Yun Kyung Kim[2,1]

1 Introduction

Tau is a neuron-specific microtubule-binding protein that stabilizes microtubules (Kolarova *et al.*, 2012). When pathologically modified, tau dissociates from microtubules and becomes insoluble aggregates called neurofibrillary tangles (NFTs). NFTs are accumulated in neuronal perikarya or dystrophic neurites in axons and dendrites, causing degeneration of tangle-bearing neurons. The NFT formation is one of the most significant pathological signatures in Alzheimer's Disease (AD) and multiple neurodegenerative disorders classified as tauopathies. Accordingly, great efforts have been made to investigate the mechanism of tau aggregation and to identify the pathogenic tau species. Accumulating evidences suggest that soluble tau oligomers, rather than large insoluble aggregates, are the pathogenic forms responsible for neuronal degeneration and cognitive impairment. Formation of the fibrillary inclusions might serve as a neuronal defense mechanism to quarantine the toxic oligomers. In addition, tau oligomers propagate in neurons acting as a seed for native tau aggregation. Due to the pathological implication, tau oligomers become an important therapeutic target to cure tauopathies. However, progress has been slow due to the lack of understating tau aggregation mechanism. Tau is an intrinsically soluble protein. To become a neurotoxic aggregate, tau undergoes a number of harmful modifications. In this book chapter, we will look for

[1] Biological Chemistry, University of Science and Technology, Korea
[2] Center for Neuro-medicine, Korea Institute of Science and Technology, Korea
[3] Department of Biotechnology, Translational Research Center for Protein Function Control, College of Life Science and Biotechnology, Yonsei University, Seoul, Korea

various tau modifications associated with aggregation and also introduce cell models for monitoring tau aggregation in cells.

2   Tau and Neuro-degeneration

Tau protein is highly expressed in neurons, but also expressed in low levels in non-neuronal cells such as astrocytes and oligodendrocytes (Shin *et al.*, 1991). Tau stabilizes microtubule and promotes microtubule assembly that is critical for neuronal outgrowth (Cleveland *et al.*, 1977; Kolarova *et al.*, 2012; Mazanetz & Fischer, 2007; Obulesu *et al.*, 2011). Tau also has a role in anchoring microtubules to other cytoskeletal filaments and cytoplasmic organelles such as mitochondria for the structural supports (Jung *et al.*, 1993; Miyata *et al.*, 1986). Full-length human tau contains four tandem repeat seqeunces (R1–R4) containing a number of lysine residues (Figure 1). The postively charged lysine residues are critical for binding to microtubules, which are highly negatively charged (20 to 30 electrons per αβ-tubulin dimer) (Kolarova *et al.*, 2012). Thus, the repeat sequences are called as a microtubule-binding domain.

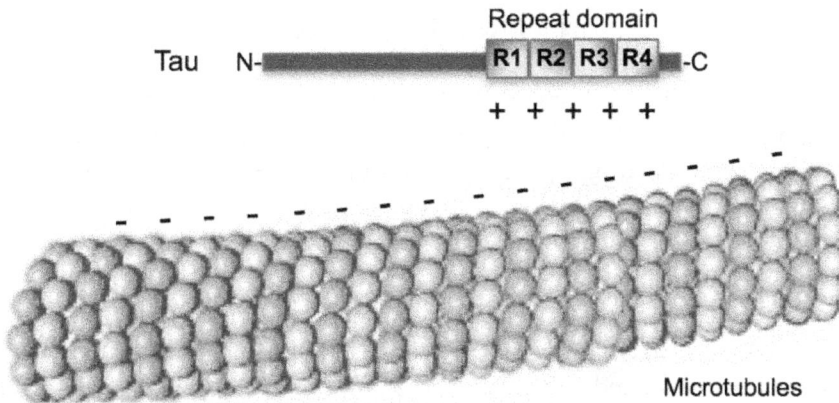

Figure 1: The schematic representation of tau and its repeat domain (R1–R4). The positively charged repeat domain binds to hightly negatively charged microtubules.

Microtubules are highly dynamic structures that continuously assemble and dissemble in cells. To maintain microtubule dynamics, tau's binding affinity to microtubules is tightly controlled by a number of kinases and phosphatases. By introducing one or two phosphates, tau controls its binding affinity to a microtubule (Brandt *et al.*, 2005; Kenessey & Yen, 1993) (Figure 2). However, when tau is abnormally hyper-phosphorylated, tau loses its binding affinity to a microtubule and become aggregated into NFTs (LaPointe *et al.*, 2009; Mandelkow *et al.*, 2003).

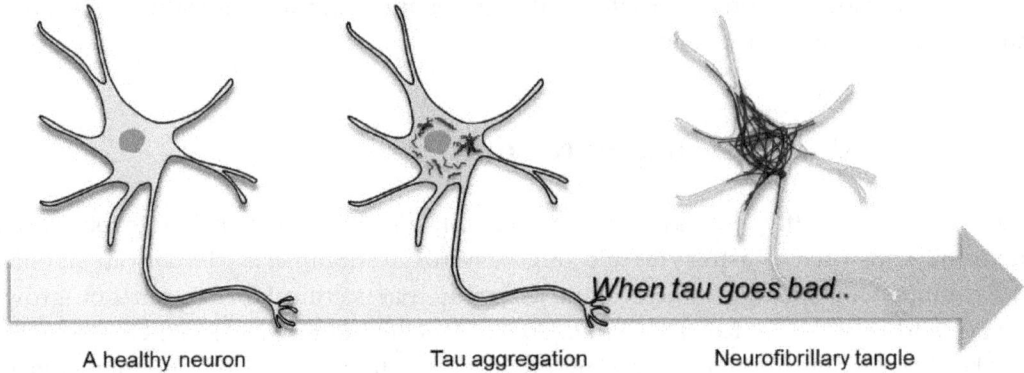

Figure 2: Tau physiological conditions. In healthy neuron, tau is associated with microtubules, promotes axonal outgrowth and synaptic vesicle transportation. In diseased neuron, tau becomes dissociated from microtubules, loses its function and form neurotoxic oligomers to aggregates.

Accumulation of tau aggregates is one of the most significant pathological events in tauopathies including AD. Hence, there has been great effort to identify the pathogenic tau aggregates that cause neurodegeneration. Tau induces neuro-degeneration in various mechanisms. Firstly, neuronal degeneration is initiated with the hyper-phosphorylated tau. The hyper-phosphorylated tau destabilizes microtubules and the disruption of microtubule directly induces neuronal dysfunctions (Reddy, 2011). Second, neuro-degeneration is mediated by diverse tau aggregates. Accumulation of NFTs in neuron might be toxic by acting as physical barriers in the cytoplasm. However, it is become apparent that soluble tau oligomers, rather than the large filamentous aggregates, are the pathogenic forms that initiate and also propagate tau pathogenesis in a brain (Kopeikina *et al.*, 2012; Lasagna-Reeves *et al.*, 2012). In addition, intracellular accumulation of phosphorylated tau might be a burden to the endoplasmic reticulum (ER), leading to induce ER-stress or unfolded protein response (Grune *et al.*, 2004).

3   Post-translational Modifications of Tau

Contradictory to the pathological aggregation, tau is a naturally "unfolded" protein, which is highly soluble in physiological conditions. To become a susceptible substrate for paired helical filaments (PHFs), tau protein undergoes a series of abnormal modifications and conformational changes (Garcia-Sierra *et al.*, 2008). Phosphorylation is the most studied tau modifications as numerous studies have suggested that tau aggregation is initiated by tau phosphorylation (Kim *et al.*, 2012). Tau hyper-phosphorylation might be important for initiating tau pathology by detaching tau from microtubules, however, hyper-phosphorylated tau does not aggregate spontaneously in cells. Diverse post-translational modifications are required to facilitate tau aggregation (Liu *et al.*,

2002; Reynolds *et al.*, 2007; Walker *et al.*, 2012). Recent evidences show that intermolecular disulfide cross-linking is critical in generating tau oligomers that serve as a building block for higher-order aggregates (Haque *et al.*, 2014). Also, a proteolytic cleavage is known to facilitate filamentous tau aggregation by removing the fluctuating N-and C-terminal ends (von Bergen *et al.*, 2006).

Cells also activate diverse defense mechanisms to prevent or reduce tau aggregates. In healthy neurons, tau phosphorylation residues are pre-sealed with glycosylation, thus the phosphorylation sites are protected from kinase attack. Also, hyperphosphorylated tau and its aggregates are degraded by ubiquitin-proteasome pathway or autophagosis (Sergeant *et al.*, 2008; Wang *et al.*, 2009). Here we will review diverse tau modification that promote or prevent tau aggregation (Figure 3).

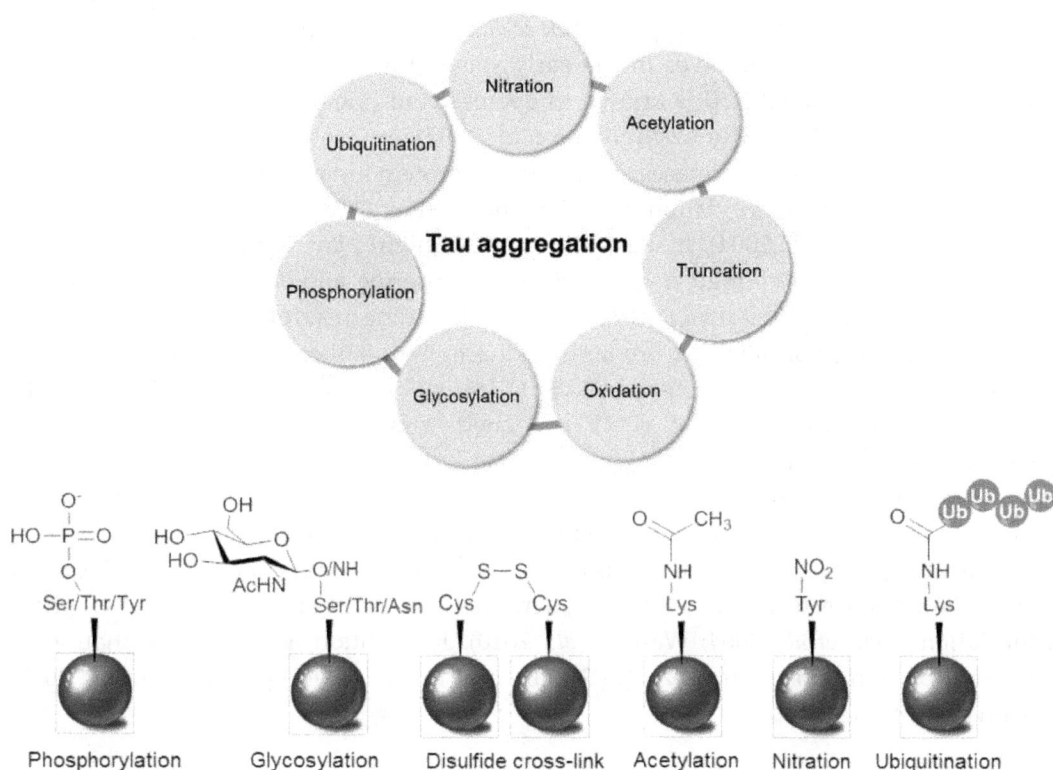

Figure 3: Schematic diagram of tau post-translational modifications.

3.1 Phosphorylation

Full-length human tau contains total 85 putative phosphorylation sites; 45 serine (ser), 35 threonine (thr), and 5 tyrosine (tyr) residues. Among the 85 residues, so far 67 residues were experimentally identified as phosphorylation sites of tau; 38 ser, 26 thr, and 3 tyr (Table 1). In neurons, tau phosphorylation is tightly regulated by multiple protein kinases and phosphatases. When the regulation is imbalanced, tau becomes hyper-phosphorylated. Evidences have showed that tau protein isolated from a healthy brain is also partially phosphorylated with an average of about 2 moles of phosphate per a mole of protein (Drechsel *et al.*, 1992; Mazanetz & Fischer, 2007). In contrast, tau isolated from the AD patient's brain contains 6 to 8 moles of phosphate per mole of protein (Mazanetz & Fischer, 2007). Hyper-phosphorylated tau dissociates from microtubules and initiates tau pathology.

Tau phosphorylation is mediated by kinases or phosphatases (Buee *et al.*, 2000; Trojanowski & Lee, 1995). Among many kinases, proline-directed kinases such as GSK-3β (glycogen synthase kinase 3), CDK5 (cyclin-dependent kinase 5) have received the most attention due to the selectivity to tau (Dhavan & Tsai, 2001; Perry *et al.*, 1999; Shelton & Johnson, 2004; Spittaels *et al.*, 2000). GSK-3β is highly expressed in brains associated with tauopathies (Bhat *et al.*, 2004) and also the elevated activity of CDK5 was observed in AD brain tissues (Augustinack *et al.*, 2002; Tseng *et al.*, 2002). This suggests that GSK-3β and CDK5 involves in the early stage of NFT formation during AD progression. Inhibition of GSK3β is known to decrease tau phosphorylation and NFT formation (Hong *et al.*, 1997; Munoz-Montano *et al.*, 1997).

Non-proline directed kinases such as PKA (protein kinase A), CK1 (casein kinase) also regulates tau phosphorylation. It is also known that CK1 is highly expressed in AD patient's brain (Li *et al.*, 2004). It suggests that CK1 might play an important role in tau phosphorylation in AD (Singh *et al.*, 1995). Besides serine and threonine residues, tau contains five tyrosine residues. Among the five-tyrosine residues, three residues are known to be phosphorylated. A Src-family kinase, Fyn, is the mostly studied tyrosine kinase that phosphorylates tyrosine-18 (Y18) of tau (Lee *et al.*, 2004). Y18-phosphorylation was also found in NFTs isolated from AD brains and also AD transgenic mice (Bhaskar *et al.*, 2010).

Among many phosphatases, protein phosphatase 2A (PP2A) is the major tau phosphatase in the AD pathology. Inhibition of PP2A induces tau hyper-phosphorylation and disrupts neuronal cytoskeleton and neuritic outgrowth (Chen *et al.*, 2008; Saito *et al.*, 1995). The decrease of PP2A also increases GSK3β level that induces tau phosphorylation (Tian *et al.*, 2004; Wang *et al.*, 2010). In addition, protein phosphatases 1 (PP1) and protein phosphatases 2B (PP2B) are also related in AD process (Chung, 2009; Martin *et al.*, 2013).

3.2   Glycosylation

Glycosylation is a key post-translational modification and mediates covalent attachment of oligosaccharides to the protein backbone. There are two types of glycosylation involved in tau pathology. N-glycosylation adds sugars to asparagine (Asn) residues and O-glycosylation adds sugars to serine or threonine residues (Arnold *et al.*, 1996; Wang *et al.*, 1996) (Figure 4).

Recent evidences have suggested the role of O-glycosylation in preventing tau aggregation. O-glycosylation prevents tau phosphorylation by the pre-acquisition of serine and threonine residues. Actually in AD, a negative correlation between O-

Domain	Amino acid position	Glycosylation	Non-proline directed					Proline directed				Tyrosine			Phosphorylation kinase — Phosphatase		
			CK1δ	CK2	PKA	PKC	CaMPK II	GSK-3β	CDK2	CDK5	MAPK	Fyn	Syk	c-Abl	PP1	PP2A	PP2B
	T17		•														
	Y18											•	•				
	T39		•	•													
	S46		•					•	•		•					•	•
	T50		•					•			•						
	T52			•													
Acidic domain	S56		•	•													
	T69																
	T95		•					•			•						
	T101		•					•			•						
	T102		•														
	S113		•														
	T123					•		•			•						
	S129							•									•
	S131		•				•	•									
	T149		•					•									
	T153							•		•	•						
	T169		•					•									•
	T175							•		•	•						
	T181	•	•					•	•	•	•						
	S184		•					•		•	•						
	S195							•	•	•	•						
	Y197			•									•				
	S198		•		•			•	•	•	•				•	•	•
Proline-rich domain	S199	•			•			•	•	•	•				•	•	•
	S202	•	•		•			•	•	•	•					•	
	T205				•			•									
	S208		•		•												
	S210		•		•												
	T212	•	•		•		•	•	•	•	•						•
	S214	•	•		•			•		•							•
	T217	•	•		•			•	•								
	T220				•			•									
	T231							•	•	•	•				•		•
	S235							•	•	•	•						•
	S237		•					•									
	S238		•					•									

Continued on next page…

... continued from previous page

Domain	Amino acid position	Glycosylation	CK1δ	CK2	PKA	PKC	CaMPK II	GSK-3β	CDK2	CDK5	MAPK	Fyn	Syk	c-Abl	PP1	PP2A	PP2B
Microtubule-binding domain	S241		●														
	T245				●												
	S258		●		●	●		●									
	S262	●	●		●	●	●	●									
	T263		●				●	●			●						
	S285		●					●									
	S289		●					●									
	S293				●	●											
	S305				●	●		●									
	S320				●	●											
	S324		●		●	●		●									
	S341		●		●			●									
	S352		●		●		●	●			●						
	S356	●	●		●			●									
	T361		●														
	T373		●							●							
	T386		●	●													
	Y394													●			
C-terminal domain	S396		●	●		●		●	●	●	●						●
	S400			●				●								●	●
	T403			●				●									
	S404	●	●	●		●		●	●	●	●				●	●	●
	S409			●	●		●	●									
	S412		●	●	●			●									
	S413		●	●	●			●									
	T414		●		●		●	●									
	S416		●		●		●	●									
	S422	●									●						
	S433		●		●												
	S435		●														

Table 1: Single letter amino acid abbreviations indicate the sites of important phosphorylation kinase, phosphatase and glycosylation residues in tau (S, serine; T, threonine; Y, tyrosine). Numbering is based on the sequence of the largest isoform of human central nervous system tau (441 amino acids long). (Avila, 2006; Gong *et al.*, 2005; Hanger *et al.*, 2009; Morishima-Kawashima *et al.*, 1995; Sergeant *et al.*, 2008).

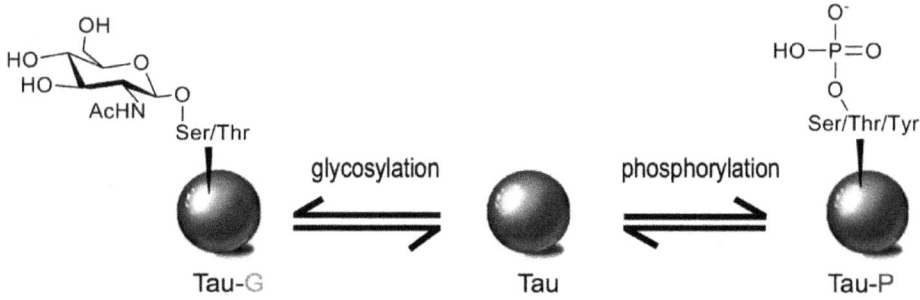

Figure 4: O-glycosylation prevents tau phosphorylation.

Glycosylation and tau phosphorylation has been reported (Lefebvre *et al.*, 2003; Liu *et al.*, 2009; Robertson *et al.*, 2004). It is worth mentioning that impaired glucose metabolism in AD brain results in the reduction of O-Glycosylation, leading to tau hyper-phosphorylation (Deng *et al.*, 2009; Gong *et al.*, 2006; Liu *et al.*, 2009). Therefore, O-glycosylation may protect tau from hyperphosphorylation and consequently is expected to prevent NFT formation. Compared to O-glycosylation, the role of N-glycosylation is not clear in tau pathology. However, N-glycosylation was found in PHFs isolated AD brain (Liu *et al.*, 2002), and this suggests that N-glycosylation might be associated with tau pathology (Selkoe, 2004; Suzuki *et al.*, 2006).

3.3   Disulfide Bond Cross-linking

Full-length human tau (441 a.a.) contains two cysteine residues that can form both intra- and inter-molecular disulfide bonds. When tau is exposed to oxidizing conditions such as H_2O_2, a series of inter- and intramolecular disulfide bonds are formed (Zambrano *et al.*, 2004). Intramolecular disulfide bonds lead to the formation of compact monomers that cannot form extended structure. However, intermolecular disulfide-bonds lead to form higher-order oligomers. The intermolecular cross-linked oligomers serve as "nuclei" for further tau aggregation (Walker *et al.*, 2012) (Figure 5).

Oxidative stress is one of the key factors contributing to neuro-degeneration (Uttara *et al.*, 2009). It is highly possible that the disruption of cellular redox potential induces tau oxidetion to form intermolecular disulfide cross-links. Although the precise role that disulfide cross-linked tau play in vivo is not clear, the cross-linked tau oligomers promote tau aggregation in vitro (Zhao & Zhao, 2013). Recent studies reported that the soluble tau oligomers are presumed to be neuro-toxic than large insoluble aggregates and propagate into other brain regions and induce aggregation of normal tau proteins. Therefore, the generation of disulfide cross-linked tau oligomer might be the most critical event in the initiation and progression of neuro-degeneration (Walker *et al.*, 2012).

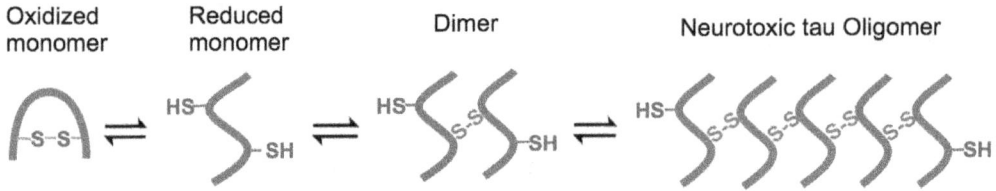

Figure 5: Tau disulfide cross-links generates tau oligomers (Haque *et al.*, 2014).

3.4   Proteolytic Cleavage (Truncation)

A number of studies have shown that tau is a substrate for various proteases and prote-olysis affects tau toxicity and aggregation. Evidence exists that tau proteins isolated from AD patient's brain contain the mixture of C-truncated and N-truncated tau species (Novak *et al.*, 1993). The N-terminal of tau is highly sensitive to proteolysis that quickly digested to small peptides. In contrast, the C-terminal cleavage sites are near the micro-tubule-binding domain, thus the cleavage is semi-protected when tau is binding to a microtubule. When tau protein detaches from a microtubule, C-terminus is exposed and digested by proteases. Evidence also suggest that the proteolytic cleavages facilitate tau polymerization (Garcia-Sierra *et al.*, 2008). N- and C- terminal ends of tau might be too soluble to form compact aggregates (von Bergen *et al.*, 2006). By removing the flickering N- and C-terminal ends, tau could be aggregated into compact filaments.

Abnormal proteolytic cleavages occur as part of the aging process and cell death in many neurodegenerative disorders. A major participant is a family of serine-aspartyl proteases called caspases, which are activated during apoptosis (Dickson, 2004). It is known that caspases are activated and also over expressed in AD brains (Chung *et al.*, 2001; Horowitz *et al.*, 2004). Researchers have found tau truncation in AD patients' brains, especially at aspartic acids (D13 and D421), and glutamic acid (E391).

This truncation contributes to neuronal apoptosis and tau polymerization (Fasulo *et al.*, 2000; Garcia-Sierra *et al.*, 2008; Horowitz *et al.*, 2004; Martin *et al.*, 2011). In addition, tau truncation might recruit other modifications such as glycation (Ledesma *et al.*, 1994), ubiquitination (Morishimakawashima *et al.*, 1993), accumulation of hyperphosphory-lated tau in tangles (de Calignon *et al.*, 2010), alterations in the organizations and functions of some membrane organelles like mitochondria (Quintanilla *et al.*, 2009) and endoplasmic reticulum (Matthews-Roberson *et al.*, 2008).

3.5   Acetylation

Acetylation is the introduction of an acetyl group to a lysine residue of a protein. Recently, acetylation has been highlighted as a potentially harmful modification of tau facilitating aggregation. The microtubule-binding domain of tau contains 45 lysine residues, of which positive charges are critical for microtubule binding. Acetylation removes the positive charge on tau, and accordingly acetylated tau lose its binding affinity to microtubule (Cohen *et al.*, 2011; Irwin *et al.*, 2012). Mass spectrometry analysis identified that lysine residues (Lys280, Lys281, Lys369) in the microtubule-binding motif as the major sites for acetylation (Cohen *et al.*, 2011). Researchers also showed that the increase acetylation on Lys280 in AD patient's brain, and the acetylation on Lys280 is known to facilitate tau tangle formation (Irwin *et al.*, 2012). Acetylation impairs tau's binding affinity to microtubules, prevents tau degradation by blocking ubiquitinylation, and promotes tau aggregation (Cohen *et al.*, 2011; Min *et al.*, 2010; Wang *et al.*, 2013). Therefore, acetylation is critical for leading to tau pathology (Kolarova *et al.*, 2012; Min *et al.*, 2010).

3.6   Nitration

Oxidative/nitrative injury has been implicated in the pathogenesis of tauopathies (Horiguchi *et al.*, 2003). Reactive oxygen and nitrogen species produce nitrating agents that nitrates tyrosine residues of tau (Figure 3). Actually, nitration on tyrosine-29 was found in tau isolated from AD patient brain (Reynolds *et al.*, 2007; Reynolds *et al.*, 2006). Nitration could promote a conformation change in tau that may promote fibril assembly. In addition, nitration might induce o-o' dityrosine cross-linking that stabilizes tau polymers at several stages of filament maturation. Although the exact mechanism is still in debate, tau nitration is known to promote tau aggregation, and tau nitration might provide a links between the oxidative/nitrative damages and tau pathology.

3.7   Ubiquitination

Ubiquitin-proteasome system (UPS) has implicated in removal of mis-folded proteins in a number of neurodegenerative diseases (Korhonen & Lindholm, 2004). Recent studies also suggested that UPS is responsible for degrading abnormally modified tau protein in neurons. Several lysine residues (K254, K311, and K353) located in the microtubule-binding region have been identified as ubiquitinylation sites of tau (Cripps *et al.*, 2006; de Vrij *et al.*, 2004; Morishimakawashima *et al.*, 1993). The ubiquitinylation sites imply that when tau is binding to a microtubule, tau ubiquitinylation is prohibited. When tau is released from a microtubule via hyper-phosphorylation, the lysine residues are exposed and become ubiquitinylated. Ubiquitinylated tau protein is degraded by proteasome complex. Recent evidences have shown that the proteasome activity is actually down-regulated or inhibited in AD patients (de Vrij *et al.*, 2004; Keck *et al.*, 2003). The down-regulation of UPS system results in the accumulation of mis-folded tau in neurons.

In addition to UPS, autophagosis has been highlighted as an important pathway that participate in the degradation of tau aggregates. Autophagy is a catabolism-based mechanism that degrades unnecessary and dysfunctional components in cells. Recent evidence has shown that mutant tau and tau aggregates are degraded by autophagosis in N2a cell model (Wang *et al.*, 2009). It seems that large tau aggregates are degraded by autophagosis rather than proteasome complex (Feuillette *et al.*, 2005; Kruger *et al.*, 2012).

4   Cell-based Models to Investigate Intracellular Tau Interactions & Aggregation

To investigate tau aggregation processes in cells, diverse cell-models expressing tau have been developed. For the live cell observation, various fluorescence proteins (GFP, CFP and YFP) conjugated to tau were expressed in cells (Lu & Kosik, 2001; Nonaka *et al.*, 2010). The exogenously expressed tau showed aggregated phenotypes upon the diverse stimulation inducing tauopathies. However, in the fluorescence protein conjugated systems, majority of tau molecules exist as monomers presenting strong fluorescence signals in cytosol. Thus it was difficult to distinguish oligomeric tau aggregates from monomeric tau in the early stage of aggregation. It is becoming apparent that oligomeric tau species play a critical role in the initiation and progression of tau pathology. Therefore, a cell-based sensor, which is able to discriminate pathological tau aggregates in cells, would be beneficial to investigate tau pathogenesis. Here we will introduce advanced cell-based sensors that could monitor and quantify tau assembly in living cells by using fluorescence resonance energy transfer (FRET) or fluorescence complementation techniques (split-GFP and BiFC) (Figure 6).

4.1   FRET-based Sensor to Investigate Tau-tau Interaction

Fluorescence resonance energy transfer (FRET) is one of the most common techniques used for studying protein-protein interactions. FRET technique is based on energy transfer from a donor fluorophore to an acceptor fluorophore in close proximity. This FRET technique has been introduced to investigate tau-tau interactions in living cells by Johnson's group (Chun & Johnson, 2007). In their study, full-length tau was conjugated with a donor fluorophore (CFP) and caspase-cleaved tau was conjugated to an acceptor fluorophore (YFP), and then co-expressed in HEK293 cells (Chun & Johnson, 2007) (Figure 6a). Energy transfer between CFP and YFP occurs only when those two tau isoforms are close enough (typically 2–6 nm). FRET microscopy showed that the two different tau isoforms bind to each other when tau phosphorylation is stimulated by GSK-3β. This FRET-based approach enables to quantify tau-tau association in cells.

However, FRET technique has several limitations for studying protein-protein interaction. First, the lifetime of donor fluorophores is only in the nanosecond range so that time is too short to measure FRET. Second, background interference arising from the fluorescence of donor can result in a poor FRET signal-to-background ratio. Third, the use of quite huge fluorescence protein tagging might interfere the interaction between the proteins of interest. Therefore, there has been effort to overcome the limitations of FRET.

4.2   Fluorescence Complementation Assays

4.2.1   Split-GFP method to investigate tau aggregation

At first, split-GFP BiFC technique was developed to quantify tau aggregation in cells

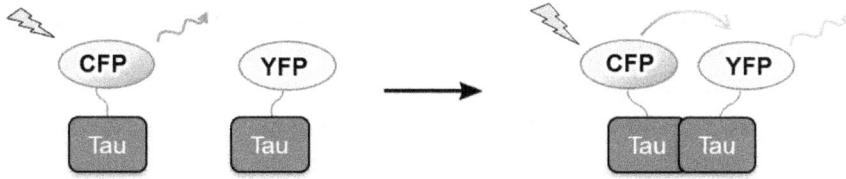

(a) FRET-based sensor to investigate tau-tau interaction.

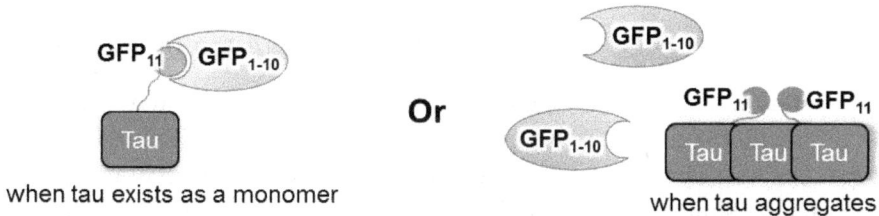

(b) Split-GFP-based sensor to investigate tau aggregation.

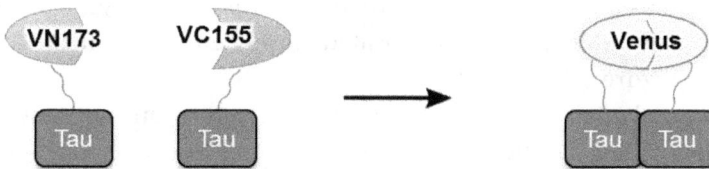

(c) Venus-based BiFC sensor to investigate tau-tau interaction.

Figure 6: Comparison of the detection of tau aggregation using fluorescence fragment. (a) FRET sensor. Tau fused to CFP or YFP. Upon tau aggregation, the FRET sensor is activated and fluorescent color is changed. (b) Split-GFP-based sensor. Tau is fused to the smaller fragment (GFP_{11}), and co-expressed in cells with larger GFP fragment (GFP_{1-10}). Active GFP is re-constituted if the two fragments re-associate; however, GFP fluorescence is decreased when tau becomes aggregate, because the tau-GFP_{11} is less accessible to the larger GFP_{1-10} fragment. (C) Venus-based BiFC. Tau is fused to VN173 and VC155. When tau becomes aggregate, VN173 and VC155 combine and turn on fluorescence.

(Chun *et al.*, 2007; 2011). In this assay, GFP is split into two non-fluorescent fragments; a small fragment containing the eleventh domain of GFP (GFP_{11}) and a large fragment containing the rest of GFP (GFP_{1-10}). Then, the small fragment (GFP_{11}) was fused to tau protein, and transiently expressed in cells with the large GFP_{1-10} fragment (Figure 6b). When tau exists as a monomer, the large fragment is accessible to the small fragment, leading to the maturation of an active GFP complex. When tau becomes aggregated, the large GFP_{1-10} fragment is not accessible to the small GFP_{11} fragment, resulting in the decrease of GFP fluorescence intensity. Actually when tau aggregation was induced by the co-expression of GSK3β, the GFP fluorescence intensity decreased significantly suggesting the increased tau aggregation in cells.

As an indirect method to measure tau aggregation, the split-GFP technique provides the overall view of tau aggregation. Even though the split-GFP assay is an innovative method to quantifying the overall tau aggregation in living cells, the resolution of split-GFP technique is not sufficient enough to distinguish tau oligomers from monomers.

4.2.2   Venus-based BiFC Method to Investigate Tau-tau Interaction

The next generation of fluorescence complementation assay overcomes the limitation of the split-GFP method and enables to monitor tau-tau interaction from the early stage of the aggregation. As a bimolecular fluorescence complementation technique, venus fluorescence protein is split into two non-fluorescent N- and C-terminal fragments; VN173 and VC155. Then, both N- and C- terminal fragments were fused to tau protein and co-expressed in cells (Tak *et al.*, 2013). Different from the split-GFP method, the N- and C-fragments do not have any intrinsic binding affinity, thus there is little fluorescence signal when tau exists as a monomer. Only when tau proteins are aggregated, the N- and C-terminal fragments of Venus could be located closely enough to form an active venus protein complex. (Figure 6c).

In the study, okadaic acid and forskolin used to turn on the Venus fluorescence protein by inducing tau assembly. Okadaic acid and forskolin are small molecules commonly used to induce tau phosphorylation (Arias *et al.*, 1993; Liu *et al.*, 2004; Tian *et al.*, 2004; Zhang & Simpkins, 2010). Forskolin promotes tau phosphorylation by the activation of tau kinase, PKA and okadaic acid protects tau phosphorylation by inhibiting tau phosphatase, PP2A. Upon the treatment of okadaic acid and forskolin, venus fluorescence intensity increased dramatically in cells (Figure 7).

As fluorescence 'turn-on' approach, tau-BiFC approach enables to achieve spatial and temporal resolution of tau aggregation in living cells (Figure 8) (Tak *et al.*, 2013). When cells were treated with okadaic acid, venus fluorescence was observed as a concentrated linear structure. In contrast, when cells were treated with forskolin, venus fluorescence was amorphously distributed in cytoplasm (Figure 8a). Forskolin and okadaic acid are small molecules commonly used to induce tau phosphorylation, however, their contribution to tau aggrega tion has not yet been clearly identified. Even though the mechanism of tau aggregation is not clearly identified, the tau-BiFC method enables to visualize diverse forms of tau aggregates in cells. In addition the spatial resolution of tau aggregation, tau-BiFC methods provide temporal resolution of tau aggregation (Figure 8b). When a higher concentration of okadaic acid (80 nM) was treated to cells, venus fluorescence was turned on within 20 minutes and the fluorescence signals become concentrated as linear structures in cells.

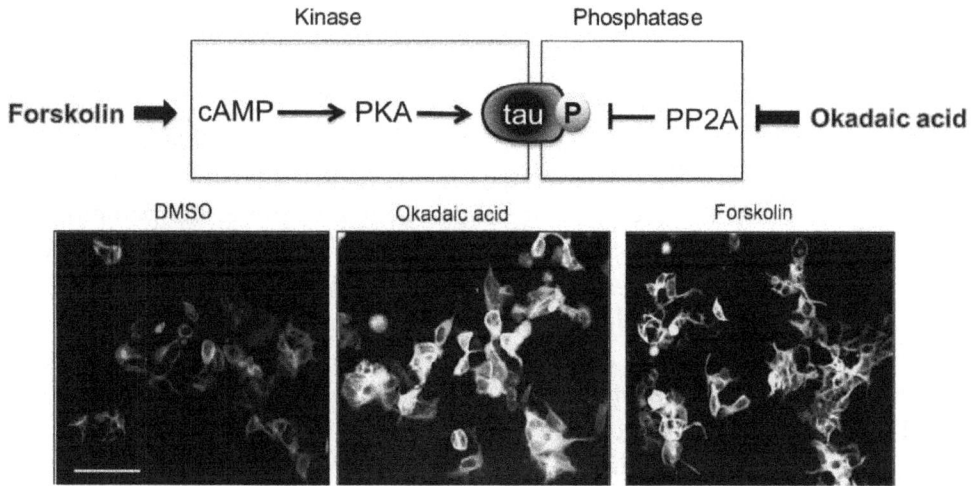

Figure 7: Maturation of tau-BiFC upon tau phosphorylation. Tau-BiFC cells were incubated with okadaic acid and forskolin to induce tau phosphorylation. Increase in tau-BiFC fluorescence indicates tau aggregation induced by hyperphosphorylation (Tak *et al.*, 2013).

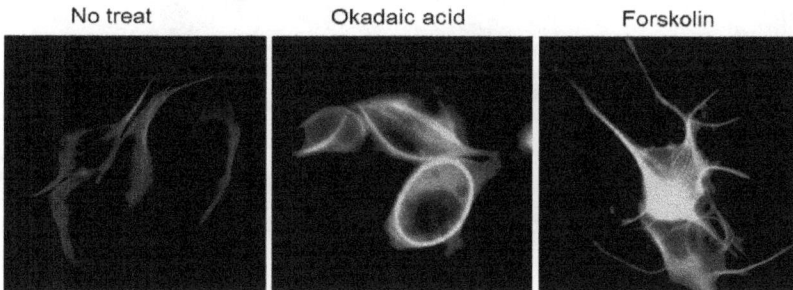

(a) Spatial resolution of tau-tau interaction.

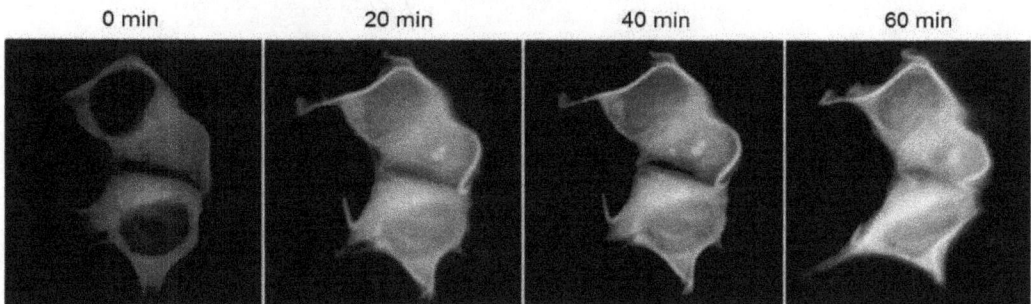

(b) Temporal resolution of tau-tau interaction.

Figure 8: Spatial and temporal resolution of tau-tau interaction in HEK293-tau-BiFC cell model (Tak *et al.*, 2013).

5   Conclusion

Tau is naturally a soluble protein that promotes microtubule assembly and stabilization. Diverse intracellular modifications make soluble tau to be a susceptible substrate for the soluble tau oligomers and insoluble filamentous aggregates. Due to the implications of tau pathology in many neuro-degenerative disorders, preventing the pathological tau aggregation become an important therapeutic strategy to halt the disease. However, tau aggregation is a multi-step process regulated by complicated cellular pathways. In tau pathology, diverse tau modifications including phosphorylation, oxidation, and truncation promote tau aggregation in a defected neuron. At the same time, the neuron activates cellular defense mechanisms such as glycosylation and ubiquitination. Here we reviewed diverse tau modifications that promote or inhibit tau aggregation, and also introduced cell-based sensors to investigate tau pathology.

Acknowledgment

The authors would like to acknowledge the financial support from the R&D Convergence Program of NST (National Research Council of Science & Technology, CRC-15-04-KIST) of Republic of Korea, and the Ministry of Health & Welfare, Republic of Korea (HI14C3344).

References

Arias, C., N. Sharma, P. Davies, & B. Shafit-Zagardo. (1993). Okadaic acid induces early changes in microtubule-associated protein 2 and tau phosphorylation prior to neurodegeneration in cultured cortical neurons. Journal of neurochemistry, 61, 673–682.

Arnold, C.S., G.V. Johnson, R.N. Cole, D.L. Dong, M. Lee, & G.W. Hart. (1996). The microtubule-associated protein tau is extensively modified with O-linked N-acetylglucosamine. The Journal of biological chemistry, 271, 28741–28744.

Augustinack, J.C., A. Schneider, E.M. Mandelkow, & B.T. Hyman. (2002). Specific tau phosphorylation sites correlate with severity of neuronal cytopathology in Alzheimer's disease. Acta neuropathologica, 103, 26–35.

Avila, J. (2006). Tau phosphorylation and aggregation in Alzheimer's disease pathology. FEBS letters, 580, 2922–2927.

Bhaskar, K., G.A. Hobbs, S.H. Yen, & G. Lee. (2010). Tyrosine phosphorylation of tau accompanies disease progression in transgenic mouse models of tauopathy. Neuropathology and applied neurobiology, 36, 462–477.

Bhat, R.V., S.L. Budd Haeberlein, & J. Avila. (2004). Glycogen synthase kinase 3: a drug target for CNS therapies. Journal of neurochemistry, 89, 1313–1317.

Brandt, R., M. Hundelt, & N. Shahani. (2005). Tau alteration and neuronal degeneration in *tauopathies: mechanisms and models. Biochimica et biophysica acta, 1739, 331–354.*

Buee, L., T. Bussiere, V. Buee-Scherrer, A. Delacourte, & P.R. Hof. (2000). *Tau protein isoforms, phosphorylation and role in neurodegenerative disorders. Brain research. Brain research reviews, 33, 95–130.*

Chen, S., B. Li, I. Grundke-Iqbal, & K. Iqbal. (2008). *I1PP2A affects tau phosphorylation via association with the catalytic subunit of protein phosphatase 2A. The Journal of biological chemistry, 283, 10513–10521.*

Chun, W., & G.V.W. Johnson. (2007). *Activation of glycogen synthase kinase 3 beta promotes the intermolecular association of tau — The use of fluorescence resonance energy transfer microscopy (vol 282, pg 23410, 2007). Journal of Biological Chemistry, 282, 28296–28296.*

Chun, W., G.S. Waldo, & G.V. Johnson. (2007). *Split GFP complementation assay: a novel approach to quantitatively measure aggregation of tau in situ: effects of GSK3beta activation and caspase 3 cleavage. Journal of neurochemistry, 103, 2529–2539.*

Chun, W., G.S. Waldo, & G.V. Johnson. (2011). *Split GFP complementation assay for quantitative measurement of tau aggregation in situ. Methods in molecular biology, 670, 109–123.*

Chung, C.W., Y.H. Song, I.K. Kim, W.J. Yoon, B.R. Ryu, D.G. Jo, H.N. Woo, Y.K. Kwon, H.H. Kim, B.J. Gwag, I.H. Mook-Jung, & Y.K. Jung. (2001). *Proapoptotic effects of tau cleavage product generated by caspase-3. Neurobiol Dis, 8, 162–172.*

Chung, S.H. (2009). *Aberrant phosphorylation in the pathogenesis of Alzheimer's disease. BMB reports, 42, 467–474.*

Cleveland, D.W., S.Y. Hwo, & M.W. Kirschner. (1977). *Physical and chemical properties of purified tau factor and the role of tau in microtubule assembly. Journal of molecular biology, 116, 227–247.*

Cohen, T.J., J.L. Guo, D.E. Hurtado, L.K. Kwong, I.P. Mills, J.Q. Trojanowski, & V.M. Lee. (2011). *The acetylation of tau inhibits its function and promotes pathological tau aggregation. Nature communications, 2, 252.*

Cripps, D., S.N. Thomas, Y. Jeng, F. Yang, P. Davies, & A.J. Yang. (2006). *Alzheimer disease-specific conformation of hyperphosphorylated paired helical filament-Tau is polyubiquitinated through Lys-48, Lys-11, and Lys-6 ubiquitin conjugation. The Journal of biological chemistry, 281, 10825–10838.*

de Calignon, A., L.M. Fox, R. Pitstick, G.A. Carlson, B.J. Bacskai, T.L. Spires-Jones, & B.T. Hyman. (2010). *Caspase activation precedes and leads to tangles. Nature, 464, 1201–1204.*

de Vrij, F.M., D.F. Fischer, F.W. van Leeuwen, & E.M. Hol. (2004). *Protein quality control in Alzheimer's disease by the ubiquitin proteasome system. Progress in neurobiology, 74, 249–270.*

Deng, Y., B. Li, Y. Liu, K. Iqbal, I. Grundke-Iqbal, & C.X. Gong. (2009). *Dysregulation of insulin signaling, glucose transporters, O-GlcNAcylation, and phosphorylation of tau and neurofilaments in the brain: Implication for Alzheimer's disease. The American journal of pathology, 175, 2089–2098.*

Dhavan, R., & L.H. Tsai. (2001). A decade of CDK5. Nat Rev Mol Cell Biol, 2, 749–759.

Dickson, D.W. (2004). Apoptotic mechanisms in Alzheimer neurofibrillary degeneration: cause or effect? The Journal of clinical investigation, 114, 23–27.

Drechsel, D.N., A.A. Hyman, M.H. Cobb, & M.W. Kirschner. (1992). Modulation of the dynamic instability of tubulin assembly by the microtubule-associated protein tau. Mol Biol Cell, 3, 1141–1154.

Fasulo, L., G. Ugolini, M. Visintin, A. Bradbury, C. Brancolini, V. Verzillo, M. Novak, & A. Cattaneo. (2000). The neuronal microtubule-associated protein tau is a substrate for caspase-3 and an effector of apoptosis. Journal of neurochemistry, 75, 624–633.

Feuillette, S., O. Blard, M. Lecourtois, T. Frebourg, D. Campion, & C. Dumanchin. (2005). Tau is not normally degraded by the proteasome. Journal of neuroscience research, 80, 400–405.

Garcia-Sierra, F., S. Mondragon-Rodriguez, & G. Basurto-Islas. (2008). Truncation of tau protein and its pathological significance in Alzheimer's disease. Journal of Alzheimer's disease : JAD, 14, 401–409.

Gong, C.X., F. Liu, I. Grundke-Iqbal, & K. Iqbal. (2005). Post-translational modifications of tau protein in Alzheimer's disease. Journal of neural transmission, 112, 813–838.

Gong, C.X., F. Liu, I. Grundke-Iqbal, & K. Iqbal. (2006). Impaired brain glucose metabolism leads to Alzheimer neurofibrillary degeneration through a decrease in tau O-GlcNAcylation. Journal of Alzheimer's disease : JAD, 9, 1–12.

Grune, T., T. Jung, K. Merker, & K.J. Davies. (2004). Decreased proteolysis caused by protein aggregates, inclusion bodies, plaques, lipofuscin, ceroid, and 'aggresomes' during oxidative stress, aging, and disease. The international journal of biochemistry & cell biology, 36, 2519–2530.

Hanger, D.P., B.H. Anderton, & W. Noble. (2009). Tau phosphorylation: the therapeutic challenge for neurodegenerative disease. Trends in molecular medicine, 15, 112–119.

Haque, M.M., D. Kim, Y.H. Yu, S. Lim, D.J. Kim, Y.T. Chang, H.H. Ha, & Y.K. Kim. (2014). Inhibition of tau aggregation by a rosamine derivative that blocks tau intermolecular disulfide cross-linking. Amyloid : the Journal of Protein Folding Disorders, 1–7.

Hong, M., D.C. Chen, P.S. Klein, & V.M. Lee. (1997). Lithium reduces tau phosphorylation by inhibition of glycogen synthase kinase-3. The Journal of biological chemistry, 272, 25326–25332.

Horiguchi, T., K. Uryu, B.I. Giasson, H. Ischiropoulos, R. LightFoot, C. Bellmann, C. Richter-Landsberg, V.M.Y. Lee, & J.Q. Trojanowski. (2003). Nitration of tau protein is linked to neurodegeneration in tauopathies. American Journal of Pathology, 163, 1021–1031.

Horowitz, P.M., K.R. Patterson, A.L. Guillozet-Bongaarts, M.R. Reynolds, C.A. Carroll, S.T. Weintraub, D.A. Bennett, V.L. Cryns, R.W. Berry, & L.I. Binder. (2004). Early N-terminal changes and caspase-6 cleavage of tau in Alzheimer's disease. The Journal of neuroscience : the official journal of the Society for Neuroscience, 24, 7895–7902.

Irwin, D.J., T.J. Cohen, M. Grossman, S.E. Arnold, S.X. Xie, V.M. Lee, & J.Q. Trojanowski. (2012). *Acetylated tau, a novel pathological signature in Alzheimer's disease and other tauopathies. Brain : a journal of neurology, 135, 807–818.*

Jung, D., D. Filliol, M. Miehe, & A. Rendon. (1993). *Interaction of brain mitochondria with microtubules reconstituted from brain tubulin and MAP2 or TAU. Cell motility and the cytoskeleton, 24, 245–255.*

Keck, S., R. Nitsch, T. Grune, & O. Ullrich. (2003). *Proteasome inhibition by paired helical filament-tau in brains of patients with Alzheimer's disease. Journal of neurochemistry, 85, 115–122.*

Kenessey, A., & S.H. Yen. (1993). *The extent of phosphorylation of fetal tau is comparable to that of PHF-tau from Alzheimer paired helical filaments. Brain Res, 629, 40–46.*

Kim, Y., Y. Kim, O. Hwang, & D.J. Kim. 2012. *Pathology of Neurodegenerative Diseases. In Tech.*

Kolarova, M., F. Garcia-Sierra, A. Bartos, J. Ricny, & D. Ripova. (2012). *Structure and pathology of tau protein in Alzheimer disease. International journal of Alzheimer's disease, 2012, 731526.*

Kopeikina, K.J., B.T. Hyman, & T.L. Spires-Jones. (2012). *Soluble forms of tau are toxic in Alzheimer's disease. Translational neuroscience, 3, 223–233.*

Korhonen, L., & D. Lindholm. (2004). *The ubiquitin proteasome system in synaptic and axonal degeneration: a new twist to an old cycle. J Cell Biol, 165, 27–30.*

Kruger, U., Y. Wang, S. Kumar, & E.M. Mandelkow. (2012). *Autophagic degradation of tau in primary neurons and its enhancement by trehalose. Neurobiology of aging, 33, 2291–2305.*

LaPointe, N.E., G. Morfini, G. Pigino, I.N. Gaisina, A.P. Kozikowski, L.I. Binder, & S.T. Brady. (2009). *The amino terminus of tau inhibits kinesin-dependent axonal transport: implications for filament toxicity. Journal of neuroscience research, 87, 440–451.*

Lasagna-Reeves, C.A., D.L. Castillo-Carranza, U. Sengupta, M.J. Guerrero-Munoz, T. Kiritoshi, V. Neugebauer, G.R. Jackson, & R. Kayed. (2012). *Alzheimer brain-derived tau oligomers propagate pathology from endogenous tau. Scientific reports, 2, 700.*

Ledesma, M.D., P. Bonay, C. Colaco, & J. Avila. (1994). *Analysis of microtubule-associated protein tau glycation in paired helical filaments. The Journal of biological chemistry, 269, 21614–21619.*

Lee, G., R. Thangavel, V.M. Sharma, J.M. Litersky, K. Bhaskar, S.M. Fang, L.H. Do, A. Andreadis, G. Van Hoesen, & H. Ksiezak-Reding. (2004). *Phosphorylation of tau by fyn: implications for Alzheimer's disease. The Journal of neuroscience : the official journal of the Society for Neuroscience, 24, 2304–2312.*

Lefebvre, T., S. Ferreira, L. Dupont-Wallois, T. Bussiere, M.J. Dupire, A. Delacourte, J.C. Michalski, & M.L. Caillet-Boudin. (2003). *Evidence of a balance between phosphorylation and O-GlcNAc glycosylation of Tau proteins — a role in nuclear localization. Biochimica et biophysica acta, 1619, 167–176.*

Li, G., H. Yin, & J. Kuret. (2004). Casein kinase 1 delta phosphorylates tau and disrupts its binding to microtubules. The Journal of biological chemistry, 279, 15938–15945.

Liu, F., J. Shi, H. Tanimukai, J. Gu, J. Gu, I. Grundke-Iqbal, K. Iqbal, & C.X. Gong. (2009). Reduced O-GlcNAcylation links lower brain glucose metabolism and tau pathology in Alzheimer's disease. Brain : a journal of neurology, 132, 1820–1832.

Liu, F., T. Zaidi, K. Iqbal, I. Grundke-Iqbal, R.K. Merkle, & C.X. Gong. (2002). Role of glycosylation in hyperphosphorylation of tau in Alzheimer's disease. FEBS letters, 512, 101–106.

Liu, S.J., J.Y. Zhang, H.L. Li, Z.Y. Fang, Q. Wang, H.M. Deng, C.X. Gong, I. Grundke-Iqbal, K. Iqbal, & J.Z. Wang. (2004). Tau becomes a more favorable substrate for GSK-3 when it is prephosphorylated by PKA in rat brain. The Journal of biological chemistry, 279, 50078–50088.

Lu, M., & K.S. Kosik. (2001). Competition for microtubule-binding with dual expression of tau missense and splice isoforms. Mol Biol Cell, 12, 171–184.

Mandelkow, E.M., K. Stamer, R. Vogel, E. Thies, & E. Mandelkow. (2003). Clogging of axons by tau, inhibition of axonal traffic and starvation of synapses. Neurobiology of aging, 24, 1079–1085.

Martin, L., X. Latypova, & F. Terro. (2011). Post-translational modifications of tau protein: implications for Alzheimer's disease. Neurochemistry international, 58, 458–471.

Martin, L., X. Latypova, C.M. Wilson, A. Magnaudeix, M.L. Perrin, & F. Terro. (2013). Tau protein phosphatases in Alzheimer's disease: the leading role of PP2A. Ageing research reviews, 12, 39–49.

Matthews-Roberson, T.A., R.A. Quintanilla, H. Ding, & G.V. Johnson. (2008). Immortalized cortical neurons expressing caspase-cleaved tau are sensitized to endoplasmic reticulum stress induced cell death. Brain Res, 1234, 206–212.

Mazanetz, M.P., & P.M. Fischer. (2007). Untangling tau hyperphosphorylation in drug design for neurodegenerative diseases. Nature reviews. Drug discovery, 6, 464–479.

Min, S.W., S.H. Cho, Y. Zhou, S. Schroeder, V. Haroutunian, W.W. Seeley, E.J. Huang, Y. Shen, E. Masliah, C. Mukherjee, D. Meyers, P.A. Cole, M. Ott, & L. Gan. (2010). Acetylation of tau inhibits its degradation and contributes to tauopathy. Neuron, 67, 953–966.

Miyata, Y., M. Hoshi, E. Nishida, Y. Minami, & H. Sakai. (1986). Binding of microtubule-associated protein 2 and tau to the intermediate filament reassembled from neurofilament 70-kDa subunit protein. Its regulation by calmodulin. The Journal of biological chemistry, 261, 13026–13030.

Morishima-Kawashima, M., M. Hasegawa, K. Takio, M. Suzuki, H. Yoshida, K. Titani, & Y. Ihara. (1995). Proline-directed and non-proline-directed phosphorylation of PHF-tau. The Journal of biological chemistry, 270, 823–829.

Morishimakawashima, M., M. Hasegawa, K. Takio, M. Suzuki, K. Titani, & Y. Ihara. (1993).

Ubiquitin Is Conjugated with Amino-Terminally Processed Tau in Paired Helical Filaments. Neuron, 10, 1151–1160.

Munoz-Montano, J.R., F.J. Moreno, J. Avila, & J. Diaz-Nido. (1997). *Lithium inhibits Alzheimer's disease-like tau protein phosphorylation in neurons. FEBS letters, 411, 183–188.*

Nonaka, T., S.T. Watanabe, T. Iwatsubo, & M. Hasegawa. (2010). *Seeded aggregation and toxicity of α-synuclein and tau: cellular models of neurodegenerative diseases. The Journal of biological chemistry, 285, 34885–34898.*

Novak, M., J. Kabat, & C.M. Wischik. (1993). *Molecular characterization of the minimal protease resistant tau unit of the Alzheimer's disease paired helical filament. The EMBO journal, 12, 365–370.*

Obulesu, M., R. Venu, & R. Somashekhar. (2011). *Tau mediated neurodegeneration: an insight into Alzheimer's disease pathology. Neurochemical research, 36, 1329–1335.*

Perry, G., H. Roder, A. Nunomura, A. Takeda, A.L. Friedlich, X. Zhu, A.K. Raina, N. Holbrook, S.L. Siedlak, P.L. Harris, & M.A. Smith. (1999). *Activation of neuronal extracellular receptor kinase (ERK) in Alzheimer disease links oxidative stress to abnormal phosphorylation. Neuroreport, 10, 2411–2415.*

Quintanilla, R.A., T.A. Matthews-Roberson, P.J. Dolan, & G.V. Johnson. (2009). *Caspase-cleaved tau expression induces mitochondrial dysfunction in immortalized cortical neurons: implications for the pathogenesis of Alzheimer disease. The Journal of biological chemistry, 284, 18754–18766.*

Reddy, P.H. (2011). *Abnormal tau, mitochondrial dysfunction, impaired axonal transport of mitochondria, and synaptic deprivation in Alzheimer's disease. Brain Res, 1415, 136–148.*

Reynolds, M.R., R.W. Berry, & L.I. Binder. (2007). *Nitration in neurodegeneration: deciphering the "Hows" "nYs". Biochemistry, 46, 7325–7336.*

Reynolds, M.R., J.F. Reyes, Y. Fu, E.H. Bigio, A.L. Guillozet-Bongaarts, R.W. Berry, & L.I. Binder. (2006). *Tau nitration occurs at tyrosine 29 in the fibrillar lesions of Alzheimer's disease and other tauopathies. The Journal of neuroscience : the official journal of the Society for Neuroscience, 26, 10636–10645.*

Robertson, L.A., K.L. Moya, & K.C. Breen. (2004). *The potential role of tau protein O-glycosylation in Alzheimer's disease. Journal of Alzheimer's disease : JAD, 6, 489–495.*

Saito, T., K. Ishiguro, T. Uchida, E. Miyamoto, T. Kishimoto, & S. Hisanaga. (1995). *In situ dephosphorylation of tau by protein phosphatase 2A and 2B in fetal rat primary cultured neurons. FEBS letters, 376, 238–242.*

Selkoe, D.J. (2004). *Cell biology of protein misfolding: the examples of Alzheimer's and Parkinson's diseases. Nature cell biology, 6, 1054–1061.*

Sergeant, N., A. Bretteville, M. Hamdane, M.L. Caillet-Boudin, P. Grognet, S. Bombois, D. Blum, A. Delacourte, F. Pasquier, E. Vanmechelen, S. Schraen-Maschke, & L. Buee. (2008). *Biochemistry of Tau in Alzheimer's disease and related neurological disorders. Expert* review of proteomics, 5, 207–224.

Shelton, S.B., & G.V. Johnson. (2004). Cyclin-dependent kinase-5 in neurodegeneration. Journal of neurochemistry, 88, 1313–1326.

Shin, R.W., T. Iwaki, T. Kitamoto, & J. Tateishi. (1991). Hydrated autoclave pretreatment enhances tau immunoreactivity in formalin-fixed normal and Alzheimer's disease brain tissues. Laboratory investigation; a journal of technical methods and pathology, 64, 693–702.

Singh, T.J., I. Grundke-Iqbal, & K. Iqbal. (1995). Phosphorylation of tau protein by casein kinase-1 converts it to an abnormal Alzheimer-like state. Journal of neurochemistry, 64, 1420–1423.

Spittaels, K., C. Van den Haute, J. Van Dorpe, H. Geerts, M. Mercken, K. Bruynseels, R. Lasrado, K. Vandezande, I. Laenen, T. Boon, J. Van Lint, J. Vandenheede, D. Moechars, R. Loos, & F. Van Leuven. (2000). Glycogen synthase kinase-3beta phosphorylates protein tau and rescues the axonopathy in the central nervous system of human four-repeat tau transgenic mice. The Journal of biological chemistry, 275, 41340–41349.

Suzuki, T., Y. Araki, T. Yamamoto, & T. Nakaya. (2006). Trafficking of Alzheimer's disease-related membrane proteins and its participation in disease pathogenesis. Journal of biochemistry, 139, 949–955.

Tak, H., M.M. Haque, M.J. Kim, J.H. Lee, J.H. Baik, Y. Kim, D.J. Kim, R. Grailhe, & Y.K. Kim. (2013). Bimolecular fluorescence complementation; lighting-up tau-tau interaction in living cells. PloS one, 8, e81682.

Tian, Q., Z.Q. Lin, X.C. Wang, J. Chen, Q. Wang, C.X. Gong, & J.Z. Wang. (2004). Injection of okadaic acid into the meynert nucleus basalis of rat brain induces decreased acetylcholine level and spatial memory deficit. Neuroscience, 126, 277–284.

Trojanowski, J.Q., & V.M. Lee. (1995). Phosphorylation of paired helical filament tau in Alzheimer's disease neurofibrillary lesions: focusing on phosphatases. FASEB journal : official publication of the Federation of American Societies for Experimental Biology, 9, 1570–1576.

Tseng, H.C., Y. Zhou, Y. Shen, & L.H. Tsai. (2002). A survey of Cdk5 activator p35 and p25 levels in Alzheimer's disease brains. FEBS letters, 523, 58–62.

Uttara, B., A.V. Singh, P. Zamboni, & R.T. Mahajan. (2009). Oxidative stress and neurodegenerative diseases: a review of upstream and downstream antioxidant therapeutic options. Current neuropharmacology, 7, 65–74.

von Bergen, M., S. Barghorn, S.A. Muller, M. Pickhardt, J. Biernat, E.M. Mandelkow, P. Davies, U. Aebi, & E. Mandelkow. (2006). The core of tau-paired helical filaments studied by scanning transmission electron microscopy and limited proteolysis. Biochemistry, 45, 6446–6457.

Walker, S., O. Ullman, & C.M. Stultz. (2012). Using Intramolecular Disulfide Bonds in Tau Protein to Deduce Structural Features of Aggregation-resistant Conformations. Journal of Biological Chemistry, 287, 9591–9600.

Wang, J.Z., I. Grundke-Iqbal, & K. Iqbal. (1996). *Glycosylation of microtubule-associated protein tau: an abnormal posttranslational modification in Alzheimer's disease. Nature medicine, 2, 871–875.*

Wang, J.Z., Y.Y. Xia, I. Grundke-Iqbal, & K. Iqbal. (2013). *Abnormal hyperphosphorylation of tau: sites, regulation, and molecular mechanism of neurofibrillary degeneration. Journal of Alzheimer's disease : JAD, 33 Suppl 1, S123–139.*

Wang, X., J. Blanchard, E. Kohlbrenner, N. Clement, R.M. Linden, A. Radu, I. Grundke-Iqbal, & K. Iqbal. (2010). *The carboxy-terminal fragment of inhibitor-2 of protein phosphatase-2A induces Alzheimer disease pathology and cognitive impairment. FASEB journal : official publication of the Federation of American Societies for Experimental Biology, 24, 4420–4432.*

Wang, Y., M. Martinez-Vicente, U. Kruger, S. Kaushik, E. Wong, E.M. Mandelkow, A.M. Cuervo, & E. Mandelkow. (2009). *Tau fragmentation, aggregation and clearance: the dual role of lysosomal processing. Human molecular genetics, 18, 4153–4170.*

Zambrano, C.A., J.T. Egana, M.T. Nunez, R.B. Maccioni, & C. Gonzalez-Billault. (2004). *Oxidative stress promotes tau dephosphorylation in neuronal cells: the roles of cdk5 and PP1. Free radical biology & medicine, 36, 1393–1402.*

Zhang, Z., & J.W. Simpkins. (2010). *An okadaic acid-induced model of tauopathy and cognitive deficiency. Brain Res, 1359, 233–246.*

Zhao, Y., & B. Zhao. (2013). *Oxidative stress and the pathogenesis of Alzheimer's disease. Oxidative medicine and cellular longevity, 2013, 316523.*

Chapter 10

Proteins from Halophilic Bacteria: Purification and Their Applications

Beste Çalımlıoğlu[1] and Kazim Yalcin Arga[2]

1 General overview on Halophilic Organisms and Proteins

Extremophiles are organisms that can survive in different extreme conditions, and fall into a number of various classes including thermophiles, acidophiles, alkalophiles, psychrophiles, halophiles, metalophiles, barophiles and others. They have great potential withstand harsh conditions in industrial applications over the past decade. Due to their industrial potential, the research on extreme microorganisms and their products, such as proteins and polymers, have led to greater understanding of stability factors involved in their adaptations to unusual environmental conditions (Demirjan et al., 2001).

A distinct class of extremophiles is halophiles. The name "Halophile" comes from the Greek roots "hals", meaning salt, and "phil", meaning friendly with, so halophily means that salt is required for survive (Madern et al., 2000). Halophilic behavior was observed in three domains; Archaea, Eukarya, and Bacteria (Kamekura, 1998; Oren, 2013).

Halophiles, themselves, are also categorized according to salt concentration wherein they show optimal growth. According to Kushner and Kamekura (1988), four different categories were defined: (1) non-halophilic organisms, (2) slight halophiles, (3) moderate halophiles, and (4) extreme halophiles. *Non-halophilic organisms* are defined as those requiring less than 1% NaCl. Although they do not need high salt concentration, if they can tolerate, they are considered as halotolerant microorganisms (de Lourdes Moreno et al., 2013). With respect to halophilic microorganisms, *slight halophiles* (for

[1] Department of Bioengineering, Faculty of Engineering and Architecture, Istanbul Medeniyet University, Turkey
[2] Department of Bioengineering, Faculty of Engineering, Marmara University, Turkey

example, marine Bacteria) grow best in media with 1% to 6% NaCl, whereas the optimal salt concentrations for *moderate halophiles* range between 7% and 15% NaCl; on the other hand, *extreme halophiles* show optimal growth in media containing 15% to 30% NaCl (Madigan & Martinko, 2006).

Owing to high salt content of growth medium, fermentation with halophilic microorganisms have a significant advantage in prevention of possible contamination risk with undesired microorganisms. Another advantage served by halophilic microorganisms is diversity and characteristics of their products. Halophilic microorganisms produce enzymes, metabolites, exopolysaccharides, pigments and compatible solutes (Brown, 1976), which have high commercial value. Since halophilic organisms have ability to live under extreme conditions, biomolecules produced by them are stable and unique (Oren, 2013). Therefore, they exhibit significant potential or actual use in different industries such as cosmetic, pharmaceutical, environmental, chemical, etc.

As a eukaryotic halophile, genus *Dunaliella* is motile, rod to ovoid shaped, unicellular green alga, which is responsible for most of the primary production in hypersaline environments. The commercial cultivation of *Dunaliella* for the production of β-carotene is one of the success stories of halophile-based biotechnology. β-carotene is a valuable chemical, in high demand as a natural food coloring agent, as pro-vitamin A (retinol), as additive to cosmetics, and as a health food. First pilot plant was established in USSR in 1966. In addition, *Dunaliella* has become a convenient model organism for the study of salt adaptation in eukaryotic cells (Oren, 2005).

Genus *Haloarchaean*, *Halobacterium*, *Haloferax*, and *Haloarcula* are well-known examples of halophilic Archaea (Litchfield, 2011). There are various potential applications of the halophilic Archaea due to their capability of living in extreme conditions. Unique compound such as bacteriorhodopsin is synthesized, though they are not directly connected with their life in high salt environments but synthesized by halophiles (e.g., in *Halobacterium salinarum*). The retinal protein bacteriorhodopsin in their membranes may use light energy for the direct generation of the proton electrochemical gradient, so it can be used in photochemical processes, biocomputing, production of pigments for food coloring and compatible solutes as stress protectants (Oren, 2006; Kerkar *et al.*, 2004). There are also various protein molecules and industrially important enzymes produced by haloarchaea. One of the oldest enzyme purification studies is on nicotinamide adenine dinucleotide-linked malic acid dehydrogenase from *Halobacterium salinarium* (Holmes & Halvorson, 1965). The first amylase from haloarchaea was reported in 1969 since then, different types of α-amylases were reported from *Halobacterium salinarum* (Good & Hartman, 1970), *Natronococcus* sp. strain Ah-36 (Kobayashi *et al.*, 1992), *Haloferaxmediterranei* (Perez-Pomares *et al.*, 2003), and *Haloarculahispanica* (Hutcheon *et al.*, 2005). Beside amylases, the endo-β-xylanase and the β–xylosidases from the haloarchaeon *Halorhabdus utahensis* have been partially purified (Wainø & Ingvorsen, 2003). Cellulase activity in extremely halophilic Archaea was first reported by Birbir and coworkers (2004). Extracellular lipase and esterase activities are also quite common among halophilic Archaea including *Natronococcus* sp. showing lipase activity (Kobayashi *et al.*, 1992) and *Haloarcula marismortui* showing both lipase and esterase activities (Camacho *et al.*, 2009).

Halophilic prokaryotes are isolated from a wide range of habitats such as saline lakes, saltern ponds, hypersaline soils, and fermented foods; however, the habitats for Bacteria are limited with respect to halophilic Archaea. On the other hand, moderately halophilic Bacteria may be existed in unusual environments, like on desert plants and desert animals (Ventosa *et al.*, 1998).

The halophilic Bacteria include Gram-negative species from different genera such as *Halomonas, Flavobacterium, Paracoccus, Pseudomonas, or Chromobacterium, Kushneria* (Sanchez-Porro *et al.*, 2009a), *Cobetia* (Kim *et al.*, 2010) and Gram-positive species from the genera such as *Halobacillus, Marinococcus, Salinicoccus, Nesterenkonia,* and *Tetragenococcus*. These halophiles are typically non-sporing rods or cocci. Their sizes and shapes may be influenced by the concentration of the salt present in surrounding environment (Ventosa *et al.* 1998). The cell wall glycoproteins are endowed with unusually high acidic amino acids contents (Fukuchi *et al.* 2003).

There are promising studies on halophilic Bacteria, since halophilic Bacteria are also capable of producing biochemicals, which exhibit significant potential or actual use in various industries. For instance, organic osmotic solutes within moderately halophilic Bacteria, i.e. ectoine, hydroxyectoine, are commercially valuable products. Ectoine synthesized from *Halomonas* and other moderately halophilic Bacteria are used for protecting and stabilizing enzymes, DNA, membranes, and even whole cells against stress factors such as high salinity, thermal denaturation, desiccation and freezing, and used as a moisturizer in the cosmetic industry. The compatible solute ectoine from *Halomonas elongata* is currently produced at large scale by Bitop AG (Germany) (Ma *et al.*, 2010). Development of producer strain, fermentation and purification process, current and future applications of ectoine were all described in detailed (Kunte *et al.*, 2014). Ectoine from *H. elongata* and β-carotene from *Dunaliella* are two commercial products from halophiles reported until now. Halophiles are also assigned in bioremediation processes in environmental industry. Organic pollutants are biologically degraded by halophilic Bacteria and Archaea, which are good candidates for the bioremediation of hypersaline environments and treatment of saline effluents. These include phenol, 2,4-dichlorophenoxyacetic acid, aromatic acids, sulfur compounds and azo dyes (Le Borgne *et al.*, 2008). Petroleum compounds are problems in hypersaline environments therefore halophilic microorganisms provide a solution for biodegradation of crude oil, aliphatic hydrocarbons, polycyclic aromatic hydrocarbons, phenolics and benzoates (Fathepure, 2014). Fermented foods are another application area for halophilic Bacteria, since large amounts of salt are used in the preparation of certain types of traditionally fermented foods, especially in those popular in the Far-East (Oren, 2010). Halophilic Bacteria are also capable of producing biopolymers of industrial and medical interest. One of the *Halomonas, Halomonas boliviensis* LC1 is used for production of PHB (Quillaguamán *et al.*, 2008). Besides, levan is an extracellular biopolymer produced by *Halomonas smyrnensis* AAD6, which is a moderately halophilic bacterium (Poli *et al.*, 2009).

There are also different studies on purification of halophilic proteins which lead to understand their osmoregulation capacity and the other unique features. Enhanced hydrophobic interactions, increased hydration of ions, decreased availability of free water are caused to protein aggregation and directly, intra and inter-molecular electrostatic interactions are prevented because of aggregation (Detkova & Boltyanskaya, 2007).

A statistical analysis of a dozen halophilic proteins confirms the nature of the halophiles and the results showed that proteins from halophiles are abundant in acidic amino acids (Tokunaga *et al.*, 2008). The relationship between acidic residues and salt binding was suggested by a stabilization model proposed for the tetrameric malate dehydrogenase (MalDH) from *Haloarcula marismortui*. Moreover, the amino acid residues located at the protein surface have been proposed to bind in a network of hydrated salt ions that cooperatively contribute to the stabilization. Relatively low hydrophobicity at the core of the protein is observed. Aspartic acid, lysine, asparagine, alanine, and threonine significantly contributed to the compositional differences of halophiles from meso- and thermophiles (Fukuchi *et al.*, 2003). The amino acid compositions of halophilic proteins show an increased usage of glutamic and aspartic acids relative to their nonhalophilic counterparts (Lanyi, 1974). Therefore, it is possible to generalize common characteristics of a halophilic protein: high content of acidic residues possess significant roles in binding of essential water molecules and salt ions, preventing protein aggregation, coping with salting-out effects of high-salt conditions at neutral pH and providing flexibility to structure of the protein through electrostatic repulsion (Mevarech *et al.*, 2000; Siddiqui &Thomas, 2008; Tokunaga *et al.*, 2010).Enzymes from the halophilic Archaea tend to be more thermostable than expected from the organisms' growth temperatures. The large number of salt bridges, plus an increased number of negative charges at the N-termini of the helices (counteracting the helix dipoles) and an increased alanine helical content, are all viewed (Karan *et al.*, 2012).

Proteins from halophilic Bacteria are mentioned as acidic amino acid abundant which confers to the extensive negatively charged at neutral pH and high aqueous solubility, as well. This negative charge prevents protein aggregation when denatured and leads to highly efficient protein refolding (Tokunaga *et al.*, 2010). These properties enable function in solutions of low water activity, including organic solvent/water mixtures (Ma *et al.*, 2010). Since halophiles thrive in environments with low water activity, it is predicted that many of their enzymes are functional in organic, hydrophobic solvents (Litchfield, 2011). According to their location as mentioned intracellular, membrane bound or extracellular proteins, salt requirements are changed. For instance, enzymatic activities of moderately halophilic are changed their location which is mentioned related to salt concentration. Three distinct categories of activities are discriminated: (i) intracellular enzymes, which are not exposed to the salt concentration of the medium but sense the "true" intracellular environment—in most cases characterized by low ion concentrations and the presence of organic osmotic solutes; (ii) membrane-bound activities, including transport proteins, which sense both the intracellular environment and the outer medium; and (iii) extracellular enzymes, exposed to the external hypersaline conditions (Ventosa *et al.* 1998).

2   Proteins from Halophilic Bacteria

In biotechnology research, an important part of effort is spent in usage of protein engineering techniques to modify or design proteins with optimized properties for specific industrial applications. In order to ensure this, scientists must be able to isolate and purify proteins of interest, so their conformations, substrate specificities, reactions with other ligands, and specific activities can be studied. The required degree of purity depends on the intended end use of the protein. There are conventional methods to purify proteins. Whereas the separation of one protein from all others depends on the protein features such as protein size, physicochemical properties such as charge, solubility, binding affinity and biological activity. Purification methods include steps such as extraction, precipitation, ultrafiltration and chromatography. If the desired enzyme is extracellular, extraction step can be omitted. Precipitation is one of the easy and cheap options to concentrate the sample. Most of the enzymes are extracellular in halophilic Bacteria that make the purification relatively easy comparing to intracellular proteins which needs cell disruption. Crude preparations of extracellular proteins can be obtained simply by removing the cells using centrifugation.

Source	Bacteria	Gram +/–	Enzyme	Localization
Extremely halophilic Bacteria	*Salicola marasensis* sp. IC10	Gram (–)	Lipase Protease	Extracellular Extracellular
Moderately halophilic Bacteria	*Marinobacter lipolyticus*	Gram (–)	Lipase	Intracellular
	Chromohalobacter sp. TVSP101	Gram (–)	Protease	Extracellular
	Pseudoalteromonas ruthenica	Gram (–)	Haloprotease	Extracellular
	Halomonas sp. AAD21	Gram (–)	α-amylase	Extracellular
	Halobacillus karajensis	Gram (+)	Protease	Extracellular
	Nesterenkonia sp. strain F	Gram (+)	α-amylase	Extracellular
	Thalassobacillus sp. LY18	Gram (+)	α-amylase	Extracellular

Table 1: General examples of enzymes from halophilic Bacteria and their localization.

Isolation and characterization of novel industrially important enzymes from halophiles with unique properties of salt, thermal, alkaline and organic solvent stability may supply the current demand of industrially stable enzymes in different processes (Souza, 2010). However, salt tolerant enzymes are not exploited industrially yet. Halophilic Bacteria are involved in the production of fish sauce or soy sauce, in the form of mixed cultures (Oren, 2002).

Researchers have applied to stabilize enzyme by variety of techniques like immobilization, chemical modification, mutagenesis and enzyme engineering. In this manner, enzymes produced by extremophiles are naturally stable under their native conditions which are extreme conditions for mesophiles. The advantages for halophilic enzyme technology are increased salt and heat tolerance, constitution of a catalytic environment which enables use of less polar educts, and potential reversal of hydrolytic reactions, all of which make them strong candidates for industrial biocatalysts (Ma *et al.*, 2010). They are not only salt stable but also can resist and carry out reactions under extreme conditions like harsh operational conditions in industrial processes (Kumar *et al.*, 2012). There are halophilic examples along with properties of thermophilic or alkaliphilic microorganisms. Because of these reasons, halophiles and their enzymes are potentially useful candidates for variety of applications such as food, agricultural, environmental and medical industries (DasSarma *et al.*, 2010).

2.1 Amylases

α-amylases (E.C.3.2.1.1) are enzymes which catalyze the hydrolysis of glycosidic linkages in starch and form low molecular weight polymers composed of units of glucose, maltose and maltotriose (Gupta *et al.*, 2003).

Amylases are favorite industrial enzymes with widespread potential applications in various processes in concern with food, fermentation, textile, paper, energy and pharmaceutical industries. In food industry, amylase is mainly used in starch liquefaction process that converts starch into fructose and glucose syrups (Couto & Sanroman, 2006). Besides production of syrups, it is employed in processed-food industry concerning with processes such as baking, brewing, preparation of digestive aids and fruit juices (Souza, 2010). To enhance detergents ability to clear the residues of starch contained foods (such as potatoes, custard, chocolate) to smaller oligosaccharides, amylases are one of the enzymes widely used in liquid detergents for laundry and automatic dishwashing (Gupta *et al.*, 2003; Souza, 2010). Amylases are also used in bioethanol production, since starch is the most widely used substrate due to its low price and ease of availability in almost every geographic region. Amylases are used to convert starch to fermentable sugar such as glucose for ethanol production in saccharification stepof bioethanol production by yeasts (Sanchez & Cordona, 2008). In textile industry, amylases are used for desizing process since starch is used for sizing agent (Souza, 2010).Each application of enzymes requires different optimal conditions. For instance, amylases with activity at low pH are preferred in starch industry. On the other hand, activity at lower temperatures and higher pH, and the oxidative stability are significant criteria for preference of amylases in detergents, whereas activity at higher temperatures is required to shorten the duration of desizing process (Saravanan *et al.*, 2011).

Amylases produced by halophilic microorganisms are able to be active at high salinities and could therefore be used in harsh process conditions of detergent industry and starch hydrolysis (Karan *et al.*, 2012). Early researches on halophilic amylases were studied in *Halobacterium halobium* (Good &Hartman 1970), but then amylases have been studied in many organisms including halophilic Bacteria. Halophilic amylases have been characterized from halophilic Bacteria including *Chromohalobacter* sp.(Prakash *et al.*, 2009), *Halobacillus* sp.(Amoozegar *et al.*, 2003), *Halomonas meridiana* (Coronado *et al.*, 2000a), *Streptomyces* sp. (Chakraborty *et al.*, 2011), *Marinobacter* sp.(Kumar & Khare,2012), *Bacillus dipsosauri* (Deutch, 2002), and some other amylases isolated from halophilic Bacteria are summarized in Table 2. All amylases in Table 2 are α-amylase with a single exception: β-amylase from *Salimicrobium halophilum strain* LY20.

The optimum pH for enzyme activity for amylases from halophilic Bacteria varies in the range of pH 6.5–7.5 with a few exceptions. The optimum pH of *Salimicrobium halophilum* strain LY20, *Thalassobacillus* sp.LY18and *Chromohalobacter* sp. TVSP 101 appears at pH 9 and even higher (Prakash *et al.*, 2009; Li &Yu 2011; Li &Yu 2012). Moreover, *Saccharopolyspora* sp. A9 can tolerate up to pH 12 (Chakraborty *et al.*, 2011), *Streptomyces* sp. D1 and *Marinobacter* sp. EMB8 tolerate up to pH11(Kumar & Khare, 2012; Chakraborty *et al.*, 2009). The optimum temperature for amylases from halophilic Bacteria varies between 45 °C to 65 °C. On the other hand, *Marinobacter* sp. EMB8 has the activity at 80 °C, which is relatively higher for halophilic Bacteria. Molecular weight of halophilic amylases produced by Bacteria ranges from 31 kDa in *Thalassobacillus* sp.LY18 to 100 kDa in *Nesterenkonia* sp. strain F. However, the molecular weight of rest of the halobacterial amylases varies between 50 kDa and 65 kDa.

Recombinant productions of halophilic amylases are also achieved. The amylase gene, *amyA*, from *Halothermothrix orenii* has been cloned, overexpressed, and purified. The results showed that the recombinant enzyme can tolerate salt up to 25% NaCl, although optimum salt concentration is 5% NaCl (Mijts & Patel, 2002). A halophilic α-amylase (*EAMY*) gene from *Escherichia coli* JM109 was overexpressed in another *E. coli* strain, and the recombinant protein was purified and characterized. Although *E.coli* is not halophilic, extraordinarily the activity of the *EAMY* was depended on the presence of both Na+ and Cl-ions. Its maximum activity was in 2 M NaCl at 55 °C and pH 7.0, and it has been reported as the first study on identification of a halophilic α-amylase with high specific activity from non-halophilic Bacteria (Wei *et al.*, 2013).

There are also few studies on revealing the crystal structures of halophilic amylases. The crystal structure of AmyA from *Halothermothrix orenii* indicated a conserved acidic surface, which is considered essential for protein stability at high salinity (Sivakumar *et al.*, 2006). In addition, the crystal structure of a membrane-bound, halophilic, and thermostable alpha-amylase, AmyB, from *Halothermothrix orenii* has also been reported (Tan *et al.*, 2008).

2.2   Proteases

Proteases cleave proteins into smaller polypeptides or amino acids in aqueous media.

Contrarily, in low water or solvent medium, reverse reaction occurs, since most of the proteases are generally inactive. Different types of proteases are preferred in various industries such as detergents, leather, food and pharmaceutical (Rao *et al.*, 1998; Karan *et al.*, 2012).

Serine proteases are characterized by the presence of serine group in active site and divided into different groups inside. Serine alkaline proteases hydrolyze a peptide bond which has tyrosine, phenylalanine, or leucine and indicate optimum activity at high pH. Subtilisin is *Bacillus* origin serine protease with a commercially important type subtisilin Carlsberg. Metalloproteases are the most diverse of the catalytic types of proteases with requirement for a divalent metal ion for activity. In addition to these proteases, there are several other types including aspartic proteases (Rao *et al.*, 1998).

Commercial proteases are purified mostly from mesophilic organisms, especially *Bacillus*; however, proteases from halophiles have different advantages besides being stable at high salinities and broad alkaliphilic pH range (Karan *et al.*, 2012). Industrially valuable proteases are expected to be stable in solvent medium. Most of the known proteases are inactivated or present low catalytic activities in organic solvents. Recently, halophilic serine metalloprotease from *Salinivibrio* sp.strain AF-2004 (Karbalaei-Heidari *et al.*, 2007), halophilic serine proteases from *Geomicrobium* sp.EMB2 (Karan & Khare, 2010) and *Virgibacillus* sp.SK33 (Sinsuwan *et al.*,2009) were reported as stable in organic solvents. Moreover, serine proteases from *Geomicrobium* sp.EMB2 (Karan & Khare, 2010), *Haloalkaliphilic Bacillus* sp., (Gupta *et al.*, 2005) and *Bacillus mojavensis* A21 (Haddar *et al.*, 2009) has been reported as detergent stable which serves a chance to use in detergent industry.

Halophilic proteases have been characterized from halophilic Bacteria such as *Chromohalobacter* sp.(Vidyasagar *et al.*, 2009), *Halobacillus* sp. (Yang *et al.*, 2013; Xin *et al.*, 2011; Namwong *et al.*, 2006), *Bacillus* sp. (Sinha & Khare, 2013), and *Pseudoalteromonas ruthenica* (Sanchez-Porro *et al.*, 2009b). Besides halobacteria, there are also purification attempts from halotolerant microorganisms. For instance, Ates and colleagues (2007) reported an alkaline protease producer halotolerant *Bacillus licheniformis* strain BA17.

Some of potential proteases from halophilic Bacteria are listed in Table 3. It is seen that optimum pH for enzyme activity varies in the range of pH 8–11 as alkaline environment with a single exception. Only the optimum pH of protease from *Virgibacillus* sp.SK33 is pH 7.5 (Sinsuwan *et al.* 2009), indicating that most of the halobacterial proteases also present alkaliphilic features. These properties of halobacterial proteases make them suitable for use in the detergent industry. The optimum temperature varies between 50 °C to 60 °C. *Salimicrobium halophilum* strain LY20has the activity at 80 °C, which is relatively higher temperature for halophilic Bacteria. Molecular weight of halophilic proteases produced by Bacteria ranges from 15.5 kDa for BM2 sourced from *Bacillus mojavensis* A21 (Haddar *et al.*, 2009) to 69 kDa (Xin *et al.*, 2011). However, the molecular weight of the halobacterial proteases was distributed between 30–45 kDa. There are also halophilic proteases isolated from Archaea such as *Halobacterium mediterranei* (Stepanov *et al.*, 1992) and *Halobacterium halobium* (Izotova *et al.*, 1983). Their activity range is between 2–5M NaCl which is higher than moderately halophiles. It was reported that their activity is reversibly lost under 2M NaCl. It means that during their purification process, minimum NaCl concentration should be around 2 M NaCl at least. This may explain why ammonium sulphate precipitation and ion exchange can be applied for purification of proteases from moderately halophiles as seen in many studies comparing to archeal proteases. These two processes are quite affected at high salt concentrations since dissolution of ammonium sulphate will be reduced and column charge will be affected negatively at high NaCl concentrations. Comparing to Archaea, protein purification from moderately halophiles is similar to mesophilic proteins.

Recombinant productions of halophilic proteases were also achieved in a limited number of studies. The *rapT* gene was cloned to produce protease, and 3D structure of an extracellular SDS-resistant alkaline protease (VapT) from *Vibrio metschnikovii* strain RH530 was characterized (Kwon *et al.*, 1995). More recently, Karan and coworkers (2011) cloned and sequenced a halophilic serine protease gene from *Geomicrobium* sp. EMB2.

2.3   Lipases and Esterases

Esterases (EC 3.1.1.X) catalyze the hydrolysis of esters into an acid or an alcohol, and synthesis of ester bonds. Lipases (E.C. 3.1.1.3) are carboxyl ester hydrolases of esterase enzyme group and catalyze the cleavage and formation of long-chain acylglycerols. Lipases are produced by many different microorganisms such as various eukaryotes and prokaryotes (Salameh & Wiegel, 2007). Lipases are mainly active against water-insoluble substrates, as well as triglycerides composed by long-chain fatty acids, whereas esterases preferentially catalyze simple esters (Lopes *et al.*, 2011).

The ability of lipases to perform very specific chemical or bio-transformation has make them increasingly popular in the food, detergent, paper, cosmetic, organic synthesis, agrochemical, fuel and pharmaceutical industries and also in pollution control (Thakur, 2012; Verma *et al.*, 2012). In environmental management, cold-adapted lipases have great potential in the field of wastewater treatment, bioremediation in fat contaminated cold environment and production of active compounds. Due to similar reasons, lipases have also been useful ingredients in laundry detergents for the removal of oil/grease stains (DasSarma *et al.*, 2010). On the other hand, lipases have a significant potential in esterification of fatty acids in biodiesel production (Fan *et al.*, 2012). Biotechnological potential of microbial lipases are derived by their stability in organic solvents, adapted to different temperatures and being active without the aid of cofactors (Verma *et al.*, 2012).There are interesting features that distinguishes the lipase from other types of esterases, which generally hydrolyze water-soluble shorter-chain acylesters. In general, esterase reactions with soluble substrates exhibit Michaelis-Menten kinetics. They have low activities toward insoluble glycerides and the maximum reaction rate is reached well before the saturation point (the maximum concentration of dissolved monomer). Contrarily, triacylglycerol lipases are activated at the water-lipid interface, they exhibit low activity when the substrate is in the monomeric form, and their activity increases dramatically above the solubility limit where lipids start to form emulsions (Salameh & Wiegel, 2007; Schreck & Grunden, 2014).

There are not so much examples of halophilic esterases, especially lipases produced by Bacteria yet. Sanchez-Porro and collegues (2003) screened 892 environmental isolates; 122 strains were randomly selected for further characterization of hydrolase produced by moderately halophilic and halotolerant eubacteria from Spanish salterns. Only 23% of the 892 strains showed extracellular lipolytic activity. Lipolytic enzyme activity has also been reported in *B.halodurans*, *B. alcalophilus* and *B. licheniformis* strains isolated from a Kenyan alkaline soda lake (Vargas *et al.*, 2004). 50 halophilic Bacteria from various environments in Iran were isolated and characterized to assay extracellular lipolytic activity, and only a single strain from the genus *Salinivibrio*, SA-2, was identified for further study. It is able to produce an extracellular lipase that exhibited optimum activity at a salt concentration, pH, and temperature of 0.5 M NaCl, pH 7.5, and 50 °C, respectively (Amoozegar *et al.*, 2008).

There are also some molecular studies on production of halophilic lipases. For example, a lipase and lipase activator protein from *Vibrio vulnificus* CKM-1 were cloned and characterized (Su *et al.*, 2004). A lipolytic enzyme was observed in halophilic bacterium *M. lipolyticus*, which has excellent properties to be used in the food industry, especially in the enrichment process of omega-3 PUFAs (Perez *et al.*, 2011).Therefore, a lipolytic enzyme LipBL from the moderate halophile *Marinobacter lipolyticus* SM19 was cloned into *E. coli*, overexpressed and purified as the recombinant lipase. Surprisingly, maximal activity of this enzyme was found to be in the absence of NaCl. Addition of 0.5 M NaCl inhibited activity by 80%, yet the enzyme showed 20% activity at NaCl concentrations up to 4M.

It should be noted the fact that halophilic lipases and enzymes are interesting for biotechnological applications stems from their ability to retain activity in the presence of low water conditions. These adaptations are useful in harsh industrial environments where enzymatic reactions may need to be carried out in an organic solvent such as DMSO (Sana *et al.*, 2007).

2.4   Other Enzymes from Halophilic Bacteria

Number of the screening studies, which belong to moderately halophilic Bacteria, are increasing gradually (Sanchez-Porro *et al.*, 2003; Cojoc *et al.*, 2009; Dang *et al.*, 2009; Rohban *et al.*, 2009; Kumar *et al.*, 2012; Jayachandra *et al.*,2012). Moderately halophilic Bacteria establish the most versatile group of microorganisms that can be used as a source of salt-adapted enzymes. This is an advantage over extreme halophiles, since halophilic Bacteria do not have a strict salt requirement and grow in wide salt range. Solvent stability of amylase, lipase and protease from these halophilic isolates make them potentially useful for application in non-aqueous enzymology for synthesis of oligosaccharides, esters and peptides (Kumar *et al.*, 2012).

231 moderately halophilic Bacteria were isolated from Howz Soltan playa, a hypersaline lake in the central desert zone of Iran, to screen enzyme activity of lipases, amylases, proteases, inulinases, xylanases, cellulases, pullulanases, DNases, and pectinases(Sanchez-Porro *et al.*, 2003). As a result, the Gram-positive halophilic rods showed more hydrolytic activities in comparison with Gram-negative Bacteria. Halophilic Bacteria were isolated from deep-sea sediments of the Southern Okinawa Trough and re-

sults showed more than 72.4% of the isolates showed extracellular hydrolytic enzyme activities, such as amylases, proteases, lipases and DNases, and nearly 59.2% were cold-adapted exoenzyme producers (Dang *et al.*, 2009). In another study, Bacteria belonging to the genera *Salinicoccus* were shown to have potential to produce the extracellular enzymes such as amylase, protease, inulinase and gelatinase, but not lipase (Jayachandra *et al.*, 2012).

Nucleases consisting of both RNase and DNase were isolated from halophilic *Bacillus* sp. (Onishi *et al.*, 1983) and *Micrococcus varians* (Kamekura & Onishi, 1974). Their purifications were obtained with the conventional purification cascade, which includes alcohol pre-precipitation, chromatography and gel filtration. The optimum pH of halophilic *Bacillus* sp. and *M. varians* were similar, i.e. 8 and 8.5, respectively. However, the optimum temperature of halophilic *Bacillus* sp. was 50 °C for DNase activity and 60 °C for RNase activity, whereas the optimum temperature of *M. varians* was lower, i.e., 43 °C.

Halophilic microorganisms are also promising industrial PHA producers. Polyhydroxyalkanoates (PHAs) are a group of microbial intracellular biopolymers which have wide potential applications in the plastics industry. The PHA synthase genes (*phaC1* and *phaC2*) from two *Halomonas* strains (a new isolate, *Halomonas* sp. O-1, and the genome-sequenced strain, *Halomonas elongata* DSM2581) were recently cloned and characterized (Ilham *et al.*,2014). The cloned *phaC1*HO1 and *phaC1*He genes were found to be functional when expressed in *Escherichia coli* JM109 and *Ralstonia eutropha* PHB-4. In this manner, this PHA synthase enzyme is first halophilic and polymer producing enzyme reported until now.

Various debranching enzymes, such as pullulanases and xylanases, as well as several lipolytic enzymes have been characterized from non-halophilic microorganisms, and the corresponding genes have been cloned (Sanchez-Porro *et al.*, 2003).On the other hand, studies on halophilic debranching enzymes should be encouraged.

Xylanases are enzymes degrading xylan in the hemicellulose complex, which represents a huge reserve of utilizable biomass (Enache & Kamekura, 2010). Two extremely halotolerant endo-xylanases Xyl1 and Xyl2 from a novel halophilic bacterium, strain CL8, has been purified and characterized for the first time (Wejse *et al.*, 2003). Purification of enzymes was conducted by anion exchange and hydrophobic interaction chromatography. The enzymesXyl1 and Xyl2 had relative molecular masses of 43 kDa and 62 kDa, respectively. Enzyme activity was stimulated by Ca^{2+}, Mn^{2+}, Mg^{2+}, Ba^{2+}, Li^{2+}, NaN_3 and isopropanol. Optimal activity was observed at 1 M NaCl, but substantial activity remained at 5 M NaCl for both enzymes. In another screening study, 87 Bacterial isolates were obtained from evaporator ponds and divided into groups according to their characteristic features. Isolates were screened for xylanase, mannanase and cellulase activities. *Nesterenkonia* sp. Sua-BAC020 was found as a halophilic xylanase producer when cultivated at pH 8 in 10% NaCl (Govender *et al.*, 2009). An aerobic xylanolytic *Gracilibacillus* sp. TSCPVG was reported with unique wide range stability profile which can survive at slight to extreme salinity (1–30%) and neutral to alkaline pH (6.5–10.5). Xylanase was partially purified by three precipitation cascades which includes acetone, ethanol and ammonium sulphate. This was the first report on hemi-cellulose degrading both halo-alkali-thermotolerant enzyme from *Gracilibacillus* species (Giridhar & Chandra, 2010).Haloalkaline xylanase from marine *Bacillus pumilus* strainGESF-1 has been also reported (Menon *et al.*, 2010). Enhancement of enzyme activity with ions (Ca^{2+}, Mn^{2+}, Mg^{2+}, Na$^+$), organic reagents (β-mercaptoethanol, EDTA), and heavy metals (Hg^{2+},Fe^{3+}, Cu^{2+}, Cd^{2+}, and Zn^{2+}) strongly inhibited its activity. In another study, an extreme halophilic xylanase was purified from cultures of *Chromohalobacter* sp. TPSV 101 by ultrafiltration, hydroxylapatite and gel filtration chromatography (Prakash *et al.*, 2012).Molecular weight of xylanase was reported as 15 kDa, the lowest among xylanases reported in literature. The xylanase had a maximum activity at pH 9.0 and 65 °C, whereas it was stable in the presence of 15–25% NaCl, in the pH range of 7.0–9.0, and temperatures between 50 °C to 70 °C. The xylanase from *Chromohalobacter* sp. TPSV 101 was completely inhibited by Hg^{2+} ions and was partially inhibited by Ca^{2+}, Cu^{2+} and Pb^{2+} ions, whereas Zn^{2+}, Mn^{2+} and Co^{2+} ions enhanced its activity (Prakash *et al.*, 2012). This enzyme is different with being partially inhibited by Ca^{2+} ion which mostly stimulates other xylanases (Wejse *et al.*, 2003; Menon *et al.*, 2010). There are also recombinant productions of halophilic xylanases. The gene, *xyn40* from *Bacillus subtilis* cho40 was cloned and expressed in *E. coli* (Khandeparker *et al.*, 2011) as similar as the gene *xynFCB* from *Thermoanaerobacterium saccharolyticum* NTOU1, which was expressed in *E. coli* BL21(DE3) pLys (Hung *et al.*, 2011).

Cellulases are hydrolytic enzymes catalyzing the hydrolysis of cellulose into sugars, which can in turn be fermented to generate energy as bioethanol and bio-based products (Wang *et al.*, 2009). Several studies on cellulase isolated from halophilic or halotolerant Bacteria have been reported. Examples include halostable cellulase from *Salinivibrio* sp. strain NTU-05 (Wang *et al.*, 2009); alkali-halotolerant cellulase from *Bacillus flexus* isolated from green seaweed *Ulva lactuca* (Trivedi *et al.*, 2011a);organic solvent stable alkaline cellulase from marine bacterium *Bacillus aquimaris* (Trivedi *et al.*, 2011b) and carboxymethyl cellulase from *Artemia salina* (Zin *et al.*, 2014). An alternative solvent, called ionic liquids (ILs), has been used for pretreatment of lignocelluloses. However, ILs exhibit an inhibition on cellulases activity because of salt, thus directly, make the saccharification inefficient. In recent work, halophilic cellulases produced from *Aspergillus terreus* UniMAP AA-6 have been reported with higher tolerance to ILs and enhanced thermo stability in the hypersaline environments (Gunny *et al.*, 2014).

Two different cytoplasmic glutamate dehydrogenase (GDHI and GDHII) activities from *Salinibacter ruber* were reported (Bonete *et al.*, 2003). GDHII depended on high salt concentrations for both activity and stability, whereas GDHI presented a strong dependence on high salt concentrations for stability, but not for activity, displaying maximal activity in the absence of salts.

Bacterial glycine-betaine-synthesizing enzymes have become a major target in the creation of stress-resistant transgenic plants with the goal of genetically engineering stress tolerance, nowadays. As mentioned previously, compatible solutes are valuable for water deficient conditions. Glycine-betaine is catalyzed with oxidation of choline by choline dehydrogenase (EC 1.1.99.1) via a betaine-aldehyde intermediate. For this reason, the *betA* gene from the moderate halophile *Halomonas elongata* which codes for a hypothetical choline dehydrogenase cloned and expressed in *E.coli* because its purification has been hampered by instability of the enzyme *in vitro* (Gadda & McAllister-Wilkins, 2003).

Alkaline phosphatase (ALP) is the enzyme responsible for dephosphorylation of many types of molecules, including nucleotides, proteins, and alkaloids as well as a well-studied periplasmic enzymes. Compared to halophilic Archaea, the reports on the ALP from moderately halophilic Bacteria are almost limited to *Vibrio* species. Alkaline phosphatase gene (*HaALP*) from moderate halophile *Halomonas* sp. 593was efficiently expressed in *E.coli* BL21Star (DE3) pLysS, but in an inactive form (Ishibashi *et al.*, 2011).The purified recombinant HaALP was separated into fourfractions by gel filtration, but they were still inactivated. Then, fractions were dialyzed against 50 mM Tris–HCl (pH 8.0)/2 mM MgCl$_2$ buffer containing 3 M NaCl, as a consequence one of these four fractions was activated to almost full activity.

β–lactamases are major cause of Bacterial resistance to β-lactam antibiotics and localized to the periplasmic space in Gram-negative Bacteria. β-lactamases were reported as heat stable; however, a halophilic β-lactamase from the moderately halophilic bacterium *Chromohalobacter* sp. 560 was highly stable against heat inactivation, i.e. it retained 75% of its activity after boiling for 5 min in the presence of 0.2 M NaCl (Tokunaga *et al.*, 2004). This study indicated that halophilic β–lactamase has high aqueous solubility and highly efficient structural reversibility from denaturation. Because of this reason, β-lactamase was chosen as a new fusion tag protein with enhancement of protein solubility, folding and expression of the "difficult-to-express" heterologous target proteins. Human IL1α was successfully expressed in *E. coli* and processed and elicited the biological activity (Tokunaga *et al.*, 2010).

3   Future Perspective

Until now, the potentials of halophiles and their products such as haloenzymes, halophilic proteins and other biomolecules such as bacteriorhodopsin have been extensively reviewed (Ventosa *et al.* 1998; Madern *et al.* 2000; Oren 2002, 2010; Ma *et al.*, 2010; DasSarma *et al.*, 2010; Karan *et al.*, 2012).Bacterial strain selection is an important question to be answered. Recently, Uratani and coworkers (2014) have studied the different systematic approaches for decision of halophilic microbial sources according to halophilic bioprocess. Besides general features and industrial application of halophiles and halophilic proteins, Vargas and Nieto (2004) reported genetic tool for manipulation of moderately halophilic Bacteria of the family *Halomonadaceae* (*Halomonas, Chromohalobacter*, and *Zymobacter*) with promising applications in biotechnology.

Halophilic enzymes are potential candidates to be used in biotransformation reactions at high salt concentrations. The potential of halophilic enzymes is high to be used in harsh industrial environments which require addition of organic solvents, relatively high temperatures, low water level, high salt concentration, alkali pH levels, etc. As mentioned, hydrolytic enzymes able to perform biotransformations which make them increasingly popular and each enzyme has various potential applications in different industries such as textile, cosmetic, detergent, agrochemical, fuel, paper, energy and pharmaceutical industries. They are also used in bioremediation of toxic compounds, decontamination of saline industrial for pollution control.

Halophilic proteins, such as ferrodoxin, and ribosomes are good candidates to explore the structure-function rules, protein folding and stability in high saline and low water environments. Because of this reason, structural studies are necessary to exhibit their three-dimensional structures in order to understand structural differences and metabolic functions of haloproteins compared to their non-halophilic homologs.

As a result of natural and man-made global changes, hypersaline environments are increasing day by day. Therefore, halophiles and their enzymes may also be utilized in bioremediation of saline wastes produced by many modern day industries. To decrease the production cost of halophilic proteins, seawater may be used in fermentations, potentially.

Availability of halophilic genomes will provide an opportunity for increasing efficiency of characterizing the targeted extremozymes and identifying promising biocatalysts for polysaccharide degradation at individual genome level (Sogutcu *et al.*, 2012). This will also provide a chance to conduct comparative genomic analyses which help reveal novel commercially important enzymes that can be used at large scale and recombinant studies andin enhancement of halophilic proteins with unique properties. Especially, applied genetic engineering approaches such as mutations, recombinations on halophilic enzymes and their production in mesophilic heterologous host may result in larger yields. Moreover, systems biology studies should be applied for halophilic microorganisms with whole genome sequence to explore metabolic interactions which affect production of haloproteins (Ates *et al.*, 2011; 2013).

Despite many studies were already performed on halophilic proteins, halophiles are still untapped resource to fulfill future biotechnological and industrial demands. There are still many halophilic candidates producing desirable biocatalysts and biomolecules. Isolation and characterization of novel halophilic species from new saline environments may provide better opportunities for the future.

Acknowledgements

Financial support to authors by The Scientific and Technological Research Council of Turkey (TUBITAK) through grant MAG/110M613, and by Marmara University Research Fund through grant FEN-C-YLP-101013-0403 are greatly acknowledged.

References

Amoozegar, M. A., Malekzadeh, F., & Malik, K. A. (2003). *Production of amylase by newly isolated moderate halophile, Halobacillus sp. strain MA-2. Journal of microbiological methods, 52(3), 353–359.*

Amoozegar, M. A., Salehghamari, E., Khajeh, K., Kabiri, M., & Naddaf, S. (2008). *Production of an extracellular thermohalophilic lipase from a moderately halophilic bacterium, Salinivibrio sp. strain SA-2. Journal of basic microbiology,48(3), 160–167.*

Ates, Ö., Arga, K. Y., & Toksoy Öner. E. (2013) .*The stimulatory effect of mannitol on levan biosynthesis: lessons from metabolic systems analysis of Halomonas smyrnensis AAD6. Biotechnology Progress, 29(6), 1386–1397.*

Ates, Ö., Oner, E. T., Arikan, B., Denizci, A. A., & Kazan, D. (2007). *Isolation and identification of alkaline protease producer halotolerantBacillus licheniformis strain BA17. Annals of microbiology, 57(3), 369–375.*

Ates, Ö., Toksoy Öner, E., & Arga, K. Y. (2011). *Genome-scale reconstruction of metabolic network for a halophilic extremophile, Chromohalobacter salexigens DSM 3043. BMC Systems Biology, 5, 12.*

Awad, H. M., Mostafa, E. S. E., Saad, M. M., Selim, M. H., & Hassan, H. M. (2013). *Partial purification and characterization of extracellular protease from a halophilic and thermotolerant strain Streptomyces pseudogrisiolus NRC-15. Indian Journal of Biochemistry & Biophysics, 50; 305–311.*

Birbir, M., Ogan, A., Calli, B., & Mertoglu, B. (2004). *Enzyme characteristics of extremely halophilic archaeal community in Tuzkoy Salt Mine, Turkey. World Journal of Microbiology and Biotechnology, 20(6), 613–621.*

Bonete, M. J., Pérez-Pomares, F., Díaz, S., Ferrer, J., & Oren, A. (2003). *Occurrence of two different glutamate dehydrogenase activities in the halophilic bacterium Salinibacter ruber. FEMS microbiology letters, 226(1), 181–186.*

Brown, A. D. (1976). *Microbial water stress. Bacteriol. Rev. 40(4), 803–846.*

Camacho, R. M., Mateos, J. C., González-Reynoso, O., Prado, L. A., & Córdova, J. (2009). *Production and characterization of esterase and lipase from Haloarcula marismortui. Journal of industrial microbiology & biotechnology, 36(7), 901–909.*

Chakraborty, S., Khopade, A., Biao, R., Jian, W., Liu, X. Y., Mahadik, K., ...& Kokare, C. (2011). *Characterization and stability studies on surfactant, detergent and oxidant stable α-amylase from marine haloalkaliphilicSaccharopolysporasp. A9. Journal of Molecular Catalysis B: Enzymatic,68(1), 52–58.*

Chakraborty, S., Khopade, A., Kokare, C., Mahadik, K., & Chopade, B. (2009). *Isolation and characterization of novel α-amylase from marine Streptomycessp. D1. Journal of Molecular Catalysis B: Enzymatic, 58(1), 17–23.*

Cojoc, R., Merciu, S., Oancea, P., Pincu, E., Dumitru, L., & Enache, M. (2009). *Highly thermostable exopolysaccharide produced by the moderately halophilic bacterium isolated from a man-made young salt lake in Romania. Polish Journal of Microbiology, 58(4), 289-294.*

Coronado, M., Vargas, C., Hofemeister, J., Ventosa, A. & Nieto, J. J. (2000). *Production and biochemical characterization of an α-amylase from the moderate halophile Halomonas meridiana. FEMS Microbiol Lett 183, 67–71.*

Couto, S. R., & Sanromán, M. A. (2006). *Application of solid-state fermentation to food industry — a review. Journal of Food Engineering, 76(3), 291–302.*

Dang, H., Zhu, H., Wang, J., & Li, T. (2009). Extracellular hydrolytic enzyme screening of culturable heterotrophic bacteria from deep-sea sediments of the Southern Okinawa Trough. World Journal of Microbiology and Biotechnology, 25(1), 71–79.

DasSarma, P., Coker, J.A.,Huse, V. & DasSarma, S. (2010) Halophiles, Biotechnology. In: Flickinger M.C. (ed) Encyclopedia of Industrial Biotechnology: Bioprocess, Bioseparation, and Cell Technology, 2769–2777,

de Lourdes Moreno, M., García, M. T., Ventosa, A., & Mellado, E. (2009). Characterization of Salicola sp. IC10, a lipase-and protease-producing extreme halophile. FEMS microbiology ecology, 68(1), 59–71.

Demirjian, D. C., Morís-Varas, F., & Cassidy, C. S. (2001). Enzymes from extremophiles. Current opinion in chemical biology, 5(2), 144–151.

Detkova, E. N., & Boltyanskaya, Y. V. (2007). Osmoadaptation of haloalkaliphilic bacteria: role of osmoregulators and their possible practical application. Microbiology, 76(5), 511–522.

Deutch, C. E. (2002). Characterization of a salt-tolerant extracellular a-amylase from Bacillus dipsosauri.Letters in applied microbiology, 35(1), 78–84.

Dodia, M. S., Rawal, C. M., Bhimani, H. G., Joshi, R. H., Khare, S. K., & Singh, S. P. (2008). Purification and stability characteristics of an alkaline serine protease from a newly isolated Haloalkaliphilic bacterium sp. AH-6. Journal of industrial microbiology & biotechnology, 35(2), 121–131.

Enache, M.,& Kamekura, M. (2010). Hydrolytic enzymes of halophilic microorganisms and their economic values. Rom. J. Biochem, 47, 47–59.

Fan, X., Niehus, X., & Sandoval, G. (2012). Lipases as biocatalyst for biodiesel production. In Lipases and Phospholipases (471–483). Humana Press.

Fathepure, B.Z. (2014) Recent studies in microbial degradation of petroleum hydrocarbons in hypersaline environments. Front. Microbiol. 5, 173.

Fukuchi, S., Yoshimune, K., Wakayama, M., Moriguchi, M., & Nishikawa, K. (2003). Unique amino acid composition of proteins in halophilic bacteria. Journal of molecular biology, 327(2), 347–357.

Gadda, G.,& McAllister-Wilkins, E. E. (2003). Cloning, expression, and purification of choline dehydrogenase from the moderate halophile Halomonas elongata. Applied and environmental microbiology, 69(4), 2126–2132.

Giridhar, P. V.,& Chandra, T. S. (2010). Production of novel halo-alkali-thermo-stable xylanase by a newly isolated moderately halophilic and alkali-tolerant Gracilibacillussp. TSCPVG. Process Biochemistry, 45(10), 1730–1737.

Good, W. A. & Hartman, P. A. (1970). Properties of the amylase from Halobacterium halobium. J Bacteriol 104, 601–603.

Govender, L., Naidoo, L., & Setati, M. E. (2009). Isolation of hydrolase producing bacteria from Sua pan solar salterns and the production of endo-1, 4-bxylanase from a newly isolated haloalkaliphilic Nesterenkonia sp. African Journal of Biotechnology, 8(20).

Gunny, A. A. N., Arbain, D., Gumba, R. E., Chyan, J. B., & Jamal, P. (2014). Potential halophilic cellulases for in situenzymatic saccharification of ionic liquids pretreated lignocelluloses. Bioresource technology. 155, 177–181.

Gupta, A., Roy, I., Patel, R. K., Singh, S. P., Khare, S. K., & Gupta, M. N. (2005). One-step purification and characterization of an alkaline protease from haloalkaliphilic Bacillus sp. Journal of chromatography A, 1075(1), 103–108.

Gupta, R., Gigras, P., Mohapatra, H., Goswami, V. K., & Chauhan, B. (2003). Microbial α-amylases: a biotechnological perspective. Process Biochemistry, 38(11), 1599–1616.

Haddar, A., Bougatef, A., Agrebi, R., Sellami-Kamoun, A., & Nasri, M. (2009). A novel surfactant-stable alkaline serine-protease from a newly isolated Bacillus mojavensisA21. Purification and characterization. Process Biochemistry, 44(1), 29–35.

Hiraga, K., Nishikata, Y., Namwong, S., Tanasupawat, S., Takada, K., & Oda, K. (2005). Purification and characterization of serine proteinase from a halophilic bacterium, Filobacillus sp. RF2-5. Biosci Biotechnol Biochem, 69(1), 38–44.

Holmes, P. K.,& Halvorson, H. O. (1965).Properties of a purified halophilic malic dehydrogenase. Journal of bacteriology, 90(2), 316–326.

Hung, K. S., Liu, S. M., Tzou, W. S., Lin, F. P., Pan, C. L., Fang, T. Y., ...& Tang, S. J. (2011). Characterization of a novel GH10 thermostable, halophilic xylanase from the marine bacteriumThermoanaerobacterium saccharolyticum NTOU1.Process Biochemistry, 46(6), 1257–1263.

Hutcheon, G. W., Vasisht, N., & Bolhuis, A. (2005). Characterisation of a highly stable α-amylase from the halophilic archaeon Haloarcula hispanica. Extremophiles, 9(6), 487–495.

Ilham, M., Nakanomori, S., Kihara, T., Hokamura, A., Matsusaki, H., Tsuge, T., Mizuno, K. (2014). Characterization of polyhydroxyalkanoate synthases from Halomonas sp. O-1 and Halomonas elongata DSM2581: Site-directed mutagenesis and recombinant expression. Polymer Degradation and Stability, in press.

Ishibashi, M., Oda, K., Arakawa, T., & Tokunaga, M. (2011). Cloning, expression, purification and activation by Na ion of halophilic alkaline phosphatase from moderate halophile Halomonas sp. 593. Protein expression and purification, 76(1), 97–102.

Izotova, L. S., Strongin, A. Y., Chekulaeva, L. N., Sterkin, V. E., Ostoslavskaya, V. I., Lyublinskaya, L. A., ... & Stepanov, V. M. (1983). Purification and properties of serine protease from Halobacterium halobium. Journal of bacteriology, 155(2), 826–830.

Jayachandra, S. Y., Kumar, A., Merley, D. P., & Sulochana, M. B. (2012). Isolation and characterization of extreme halophilic bacterium Salinicoccus sp. JAS4 producing extracellular hydrolytic enzymes. Recent Research in Science and Technology, 4(4).

Jiang, X., Huo, Y., Cheng, H., Zhang, X., Zhu, X., & Wu, M. (2012). Cloning, expression and characterization of a halotolerant esterase from a marine bacterium Pelagibacterium halotolerans B2T. Extremophiles, 16(3), 427–435.

Kamekura, M. (1998). Diversity of extremely halophilic bacteria. Extremophiles, 2(3), 289–295.

Kamekura, M.,& Onishi, H. (1974). Protease formation by a moderately halophilic Bacillus strain.Applied microbiology, 27(4), 809–810.

Karan, R., Kumar, S., Sinha, R., & Khare, S. K. (2012). Halophilic Microorganisms as Sources of Novel Enzymes. In Microorganisms in Sustainable Agriculture and Biotechnology. 555–579. Springer Netherlands.

Karan, R., Singh, S. P., Kapoor, S., & Khare, S. K. (2011). A novel organic solvent tolerant protease from a newly isolated Geomicrobium sp. EMB2 (MTCC 10310): production optimization by response surface methodology. New biotechnology, 28(2), 136–145.

Karan, R.,& Khare, S. K. (2010). Purification and characterization of a solvent-stable protease from Geomicrobium sp. EMB2. Environmental technology,31(10), 1061–1072.

Karbalaei-Heidari, H. R., Amoozegar, M. A., Hajighasemi, M., Ziaee, A. A., & Ventosa, A. (2009). Production, optimization and purification of a novel extracellular protease from the moderately halophilic bacterium Halobacillus karajensis.Journal of industrial microbiology &biotechnology, 36(1), 21–27.

Karbalaei-Heidari, H. R., Ziaee, A. A., & Amoozegar, M. A. (2007). Purification and biochemical characterization of a protease secreted by the Salinivibrio sp. strain AF-2004 and its behavior in organic solvents. Extremophiles, 11(2), 237–243.

Kerkar, S. (2004).Ecology of hypersaline microorganisms. Marine Microbiology: Facets & Opportunities; Ramaiah, N (Ed.), 37–47.

Khandeparker, R., Verma, P., & Deobagkar, D. (2011). A novel halotolerant xylanase from marine isolate Bacillus subtilis cho40: gene cloning and sequencing. New biotechnology, 28(6), 814–821.

Kim, M.S., Roh, S.W. &Bae, J.W. (2010). Cobetia crustatorum sp. nov., a novel slightly halophilic bacterium isolated from traditional fermented seafood in Korea. International Journal of Systematic andEvolutionary Microbiology. 60, 620–626.

Kiran, K.K.,&Chandra, T.S. (2008). Production of surfactant and detergent-stable, halophilic,and alkalitolerant alpha-amylase by a moderately halophilic Bacillus sp. strain TSCVKK. Appl. Microbiol. Biotechnol., 77, 1023–1031.

Kobayashi, T., Kanai, H.., Hayashi, T., Akiba, T., Akaboshi, R., & Horikoshi, K. (1992). Haloalkaliphilic maltotriose-forming alpha-amylase from the archaebacterium Natronococcus sp. strain Ah-36. Journal of bacteriology, 174(11), 3439–3444.

Kumar, S., Karan, R., Kapoor, S., Singh, S. P., & Khare, S. K. (2012). Screening and isolation of halophilic bacteria producing industrially important enzymes. Brazilian Journal of Microbiology, 43(4), 1595–1603.

Kumar, S.,& Khare, S.K. (2012) Purification and characterization of maltooligosaccharide-forming a-amylase from moderately halophilic Marinobacter sp. EMB8. Bioresource Technology, 116, 247–251.

Kunte, H. J., Lentzen, G., & Galinski, E.A. (2014) Industrial Production of the Cell Protectant

Ectoine: Protection Mechanisms, Processes and Products. Current Biotechnology, 3, 10–25

Kushner, D. J. & Kamekura, M. (1988). *Physiology of halophilic eubacteria. In Halophilic Bacteria, vol. 1, 109–140. Edited by F. Rodriguez-Valera. Boca Raton, FL: CRC Press.*

Kwon, Y. T., Kim, J. O., Moon, S. Y., Yoo, Y. D., & Rho, H. M. (1995). *Cloning and characterization of the gene encoding an extracellular alkaline serine protease from Vibrio metschnikovii strain RH530. Gene, 152(1), 59–63.*

Lanyi, J. K. (1974). *Salt-dependent properties of proteins from extremely halophilic bacteria.Bacteriological Reviews, 38(3), 272.*

Le Borgne, S., Paniagua, D., & Vazquez-Duhalt, R. (2008). *Biodegradation of organic pollutants by halophilic bacteria and archaea. Journal of molecular microbiology and biotechnology, 15(2–3), 74–92.*

Li, X., Yu, H. Y., & Lin, Y. F. (2012). *Purification and characterization of an extracellular esterase from a moderately halophilic bacterium, Halobacillus sp. strain LY 5. African Journal of Biotechnology, 11(23), 6327–6334.*

Li, X.,& Yu, H. Y. (2011). *Extracellular production of beta-amylase by a halophilic isolate, Halobacillus sp. LY9. Journal of industrial microbiology & biotechnology, 38(11), 1837–1843.*

Li, X.,& Yu, H. Y. (2012). *Purification and characterization of novel organic-solvent-tolerant β-amylase and serine protease from a newly isolated Salimicrobium halophilum strain LY20. FEMS microbiology letters, 329(2), 204–211.*

Litchfield, C. D. (2011). *Potential for industrial products from the halophilic Archaea.Journal of industrial microbiology & biotechnology, 38(10), 1635–1647.*

Lopes, D. B., Fraga, L. P., Fleuri, L. F., & Macedo, G. A. (2011). *Lipase and esterase: to what extent can this classification be applied accurately? Food Science and Technology (Campinas), 31(3), 603–613.*

Ma, Y., Galinski, E. A., Grant, W. D., Oren, A., & Ventosa, A. (2010). *Halophiles 2010: life in saline environments. Applied and environmental microbiology, 76(21), 6971–6981.*

Madern, D., Ebel, C., & Zaccai, G. (2000). *Halophilic adaptation of enzymes. Extremophiles, 4(2), 91–98.*

Madigan, M.& Martinko, J. 2006. *Brock biology of Microorganisms. Pearson Prentice Hall, New Jersey, 167.*

Maruthiah, T., Esakkiraj, P., Prabakaran, G., Palavesam, A., & Immanuel, G. (2013). *Purification and characterization of moderately halophilic alkaline serine protease from marine Bacillus subtilis AP-MSU 6. Biocatalysis and Agricultural Biotechnology, 2(2), 116–119.*

Menon, G., Mody, K., Keshri, J., & Jha, B. (2010). *Isolation, purification, and characterization of haloalkaline xylanase from a marine Bacillus pumilus strain, GESF-1. Biotechnology and Bioprocess Engineering, 15(6), 998–1005.*

Mesbah, N. M.,& Wiegel, J. (2014). *Purification and biochemical characterization of halophilic,* alkalithermophilic protease AbCP fromAlkalibacillussp. NM-Fa4. *Journal of Molecular Catalysis B: Enzymatic,105, 74–81.*

Mevarech, M., Frolow, F., & Gloss, L. M. (2000). *Halophilic enzymes: proteins with a grain of salt. Biophysical Chemistry,86(2), 155–164.*

Mijts, B. N.,& Patel, B. K. (2002). *Cloning, sequencing and expression of an α-amylase gene, amyA, from the thermophilic halophile Halothermothrix orenii and purification and biochemical characterization of the recombinant enzyme. Microbiology, 148(8), 2343–2349.*

Namwong, S., Hiraga, K., Takada, K., Tsunemi, M., Tanasupawat, S., & Oda, K. (2006). *A Halophilic Serine Proteinase from Halobacillus sp. SR 5–3 Isolated from Fish Sauce: Purification and Characterization. Bioscience, biotechnology, and biochemistry, 70(6), 1395–1401.*

Onishi, H., Mori, T., Takeuchi, S., Tani, K., Kobayashi, T., & Kamekura, M. (1983). *Halophilic nuclease of a moderately halophilic Bacillus sp.: production, purification, and characterization. Applied and environmental microbiology, 45(1), 24–30.*

Onishi, H.,& Hidaka, O. (1978). *Purification and properties of amylase produced by a moderately halophilic Acinetobacter sp. Canadian journal of microbiology, 24(9), 1017–1023.*

Onishi, H.,& Sonoda, K. (1979). *Purification and some properties of an extracellular amylase from a moderate halophile, Micrococcus halobius. Applied and environmental microbiology, 38(4), 616–620.*

Oren, A. (2002). *Biotechnological applications and potentials of halophilic microorganisms.Halophilic Microorganisms and their Environments, 357–388.*

Oren, A. (2005). *A hundred years of Dunaliella research: 1905–2005. Saline systems, 1(2), 1–14.*

Oren, A., (2006). *Life at High Salt Concentrations. In: The Prokaryotes, Vol. 2., Dworkin, M., S. Falkow, E. Rosenberg, K. Schleifer and E. Stackebrandt (Eds.). Springer, New York, USA., 263–282.*

Oren, A. (2010). *Industrial and environmental applications of halophilic microorganisms. Environmental technology, 31(8–9), 825–834.*

Oren, A. (2013). *Life at high salt concentrations,intracellular KCl concentrations,and acidic proteomes. Frontiers in Microbiology, 4, 1–6.*

Pérez, D., Martín, S., Fernández-Lorente, G., Filice, M., Guisán, J. M., Ventosa, A., ...& Mellado, E. (2011). *A novel halophilic lipase, LipBL, showing high efficiency in the production of eicosapentaenoic acid (EPA). PloS one,6(8), e23325.*

Pérez-Pomares, F., Bautista, V., Ferrer, J., Pire, C., Marhuenda-Egea, F. C., & Bonete, M. J. (2003). *α-Amylase activity from the halophilic archaeon Haloferax mediterranei. Extremophiles, 7(4), 299–306.*

Poli, A., Kazak, H., & Gürleyendag, B., et al. (2009). *High level synthesis of levan by a novel Halomonas species growing on defined media. Carbohydrate Polymers, 78, 651–657.*

Prakash, B., Vidyasagar, M., Jayalakshmi, S. K., & Sreeramulu, K. (2012). *Purification and some properties of low-molecular-weight extreme halophilic xylanase from Chromohalobacter sp. TPSV 101. Journal of Molecular Catalysis B: Enzymatic, 74(3), 192–198.*

Prakash, B., Vidyasagar, M., Madhukumar, M. S., Muralikrishna, G., & Sreeramulu, K. (2009). *Production, purification, and characterization of two extremely halotolerant, thermostable, and alkali-stable α-amylases from Chromohalobacter sp. TVSP 101. Process Biochemistry, 44(2), 210–215.*

Quillaguamán, J., Doan-Van, T., Guzmán, H., Guzmán, D., Martín, J., Everest, A., & Hatti-Kaul, R. (2008). *Poly (3-hydroxybutyrate) production by Halomonas boliviensis in fed-batch culture. Applied microbiology and biotechnology, 78(2), 227–232.*

Rao, M. B., Tanksale, A. M., Ghatge, M. S., & Deshpande, V. V. (1998). *Molecular and biotechnological aspects of microbial proteases. Microbiology and molecular biology reviews, 62(3), 597–635.*

Rohban, R., Amoozegar, M. A., & Ventosa, A. (2009). *Screening and isolation of halophilic bacteria producing extracellular hydrolyses from Howz Soltan Lake, Iran. Journal of industrial microbiology & biotechnology, 36(3), 333–340.*

Salameh, M., & Wiegel, J. (2007). *Lipases from extremophiles and potential for industrial applications.Adv Appl Microbiol, 61, 253–283.*

Sana, B., Ghosh, D., Saha, M., & Mukherjee, J. (2007). *Purification and characterization of an extremely dimethylsulfoxide tolerant esterase from a salt-tolerant Bacillus species isolated from the marine environment of the Sundarbans. Process Biochemistry, 42(12), 1571–1578.*

Sánchez, O. J., & Cardona, C. A. (2008). *Trends in biotechnological production of fuel ethanol from different feedstocks. Bioresource technology, 99(13), 5270–5295.*

Sánchez-Porro, C., Martin, S., Mellado, E., & Ventosa, A. (2003). *Diversity of moderately halophilic bacteria producing extracellular hydrolytic enzymes. Journal of Applied Microbiology, 94(2), 295–300.*

Sánchez-Porro, C., de la Haba, R.R.,Soto-Ramırez, N., Márquez, M.C., Montalvo-Rodrıguez, R. & Ventosa, A. (2009a). *Description of Kushneria aurantia gen. nov., sp. nov., a novel member of the family Halomonadaceae, and a proposal for reclassification of Halomonas marisflavi as Kushneria marisflavi comb. nov., of Halomonas indalinina as Kushneria indalinina comb. nov. and of Halomonas avicenniae as Kushneria avicenniae comb. nov. International Journal of Systematic and Evolutionary Microbiology. 59, 397–405.*

Sánchez-Porro, C., Mellado, E., Pugsley, A. P., Francetic, O., & Ventosa, A. (2009). *The haloprotease CPI produced by the moderately halophilic bacterium Pseudoalteromonas ruthenica is secreted by the type II secretion pathway. Applied and environmental microbiology, 75(12), 4197–4201.*

Saravanan, D., Arul Prakash, A., Jagadeeshwaran, D., Nalankilli, G., Ramachandran, T., & Prabakaran, C. (2011). *Optimization of thermophile Bacillus licheniformis α-amylase desizing of cotton fabrics. Indian Journal of Fibre and Textile Research, 36(3), 253.*

Schreck, S. D., & Grunden, A. M. (2014). *Biotechnological applications of halophilic lipases and thioesterases. Applied microbiology and biotechnology, 98, 1001–1021.*

Shafiei, M., Ziaee, A. A., & Amoozegar, M. A. (2011). Purification and characterization of an organic-solvent-tolerant halophilic α-amylase from the moderately halophilic Nesterenkonia sp. strain F. Journal of industrial microbiology & biotechnology, 38(2), 275–281.

Shahbazi, M.,& Karbalaei-Heidari, H. R. (2012). A novel low molecular weight extracellular protease from a moderately halophilic bacterium Salinivibrio sp. strain MS-7: production and biochemical properties. Molecular Biology Research Communications, 1(2), 45–56.

Shanmughapriya, S., Kiran, G. S., Selvin, J., Thomas, T. A., & Rani, C. (2010). Optimization, purification, and characterization of extracellular mesophilic alkaline cellulase from sponge-associated Marinobacter sp. MSI032. Applied biochemistry and biotechnology, 162(3), 625–640.

Siddiqui, K. S.,& Thomas, T. (Eds.). (2008). Protein Adaptation in Extremophiles. Nova Publishers.

Sinha, R.,& Khare, S. K. (2013). Characterization of detergent compatible protease of a halophilicBacillus sp. EMB9: Differential role of metal ions in stability and activity. Bioresource technology, 145, 357–361.

Sinsuwan, S., Rodtong, S., & Yongsawatdigul, J. (2009). Purification and characterization of a salt-activated and organic solvent-stable heterotrimer proteinase from Virgibacillus sp. SK33 isolated from Thai fish sauce. Journal of agricultural and food chemistry, 58(1), 248–256.

Sivakumar, N., Li, N., Tang, J.W.,Patel, B.K.C. & Swaminathan, K. (2006). Crystal structure of AmyA lacks acidic surface and provide insights into protein stability at poly-extreme conditions. FEBS Letters, 580, 2646–2652.

Sogutcu, E., Emrence, Z., Arikan, M., Cakiris, A., Abaci, N., Toksoy Öner, E., Üstek, D. & Arga, K. Y. (2012). Draft genome sequence of Halomonas smyrnensis AAD6. J. Bacteriology, 194(20), 5690.

Souza, P. M. D. (2010). Application of microbial α-amylase in industry-A review.Brazilian journal of microbiology, 41(4), 850–861.

Stepanov, V. M., Rudenskaya, G. N., Revina, L. P., Gryaznova, Y. B., Lysogorskaya, E. N., Filippova, I. Y. U., & Ivanova, I. I. (1992). A serine proteinase of an archaebacterium, Halobacterium mediterranei. A homologue of eu subtilisins. Biochem. J, 285, 281–286.

Su, J. H., Chang, M. C., Lee, Y. S., Tseng, I. C., & Chuang, Y. C. (2004). Cloning and characterization of the lipase and lipase activator protein fromVibrio vulnificus CKM-1. Biochimica et Biophysica Acta (BBA)-Gene Structure and Expression, 1678(1), 7–13.

Suthindhiran, K., Jayasri, M. A., Dipali, D., & Prasar, A. (2013). Screening and characterization of protease producing actinomycetes from marine saltern. Journal of basic microbiology. doi: 10.1002/jobm.201300563.

Tan, T. C., Mijts, B. N., Swaminathan, K., Patel, B. K., & Divne, C. (2008). Crystal Structure of the Polyextremophilic α-Amylase AmyB from Halothermothrix orenii: Details of a Productive Enzyme–Substrate Complex and an NDomain with a Role in Binding Raw Starch. Journal of molecular biology, 378(4), 852–870.

Thakur, S. (2012). Lipases, its sources, properties and applications: A review. International Journal of Scientific and Engineering Res, 3(7), 1–29.

Tokunaga, H., Arakawa, T., & Tokunaga, M. (2008). Engineering of halophilic enzymes: Two acidic amino acid residues at the carboxy terminal region confer halophilic characteristics to Halomonas and Pseudomonas nucleoside diphosphate kinases. Protein Science, 17(9), 1603–1610.

Tokunaga, H., Ishibashi, M., Arakawa, T., & Tokunaga, M. (2004). Highly efficient renaturation of β-lactamase isolated from moderately halophilic bacteria. FEBS letters, 558(1), 7–12.

Tokunaga, H., Saito, S., Sakai, K., Yamaguchi, R., Katsuyama, I., Arakawa, T., ...& Tokunaga, M. (2010). Halophilic β-lactamase as a new solubility-and folding-enhancing tag protein: production of native human interleukin 1α and human neutrophil α-defensin. Applied microbiology and biotechnology, 86(2), 649–658.

Trivedi, N., Gupta, V., Kumar, M., Kumari, P., Reddy, C. R. K., & Jha, B. (2011a). An alkali-halotolerant cellulase fromBacillus flexus isolated from green seaweed Ulva lactuca. Carbohydrate Polymers, 83(2), 891–897.

Trivedi, N., Gupta, V., Kumar, M., Kumari, P., Reddy, C. R. K., & Jha, B. (2011b). Solvent tolerant marine bacteriumBacillus aquimaris secreting organic solvent stable alkaline cellulase. Chemosphere, 83(5), 706–712.

Uratani, J.M., Kumaraswamy, R. & Rodrıguez, J. (2014). A systematic strain selection approach for halotolerant and halophilic bioprocess development: a review Extremophiles, 18, 629–639

Uzyol, K. S., Akbulut, B. S., Denizci, A. A., & Kazan, D. (2012). Thermostable a-amylase from moderately halophilic Halomonas sp. AAD21. Turkish Journal of Biology, 36(3), 327–338.

Vargas, C.,& Nieto, J. J. (2004). Genetic tools for the manipulation of moderately halophilic bacteria of the family Halomonadaceae. In Recombinant Gene Expression (183–208). Humana Press.

Vargas, V. A., Delgado, O. D., Hatti-Kaul, R., & Mattiasson, B. (2004).Lipase-producing microorganisms from a Kenyan alkaline soda lake. Biotechnology letters, 26(2), 81–86.

Ventosa, A., Nieto, J. J., & Oren, A. (1998). Biology of moderately halophilic aerobic bacteria. Microbiology and Molecular Biology Reviews, 62(2), 504–544.

Verma, N., Thakur, S., & Bhatt, A. K. (2012). Microbial Lipases: Industrial Applications and Properties (A Review). Int Res J Biol Sci, 1(8), 88–92.

Vidyasagar, M., Prakash, S., Mahajan, V., Shouche, Y. S., & Sreeramulu, K. (2009). Purification and characterization of an extreme halothermophilic protease from a halophilic bacterium Chromohalobacter sp. TVSP101. Brazilian Journal of Microbiology, 40(1), 12–19.

Wainø M,& Ingvorsen K. (2003). Production of beta-xylanaseand beta-xylosidase by the extremely halophilic archaeon Halorhabdus utahensis. Extremophiles,7(2): 87–93.

Wang, C. Y., Hsieh, Y. R., Ng, C. C., Chan, H., Lin, H. T., Tzeng, W. S., & Shyu, Y. T. (2009). Purification and characterization of a novel halostable cellulase from Salinivibrio sp. strain

NTU-05. *Enzyme and Microbial Technology, 44(6), 373–379.*

Wei, Y., Wang, X., Liang, J., Li, X., Du, L., & Huang, R. (2013). *Identification of a halophilic α-amylase gene from Escherichia coli JM109 and characterization of the recombinant enzyme. Biotechnology letters, 35(7), 1061–1065.*

Wejse, P. L., Ingvorsen, K., & Mortensen, K. K. (2003). *Purification and characterisation of two extremely halotolerant xylanases from a novel halophilic bacterium. Extremophiles, 7(5), 423–431.*

Xin, L., Hui-Ying, Y., Xiao-Xue, L., & Xiao, S. (2011). *Production and characterization of a novel extracellular metalloproteinase by a newly isolated moderate halophile, Halobacillus sp. LY6.Folia microbiologica, 56(4), 329–334.*

Yang, J., Li, J., Mai, Z., Tian, X., & Zhang, S. (2013). *Purification, characterization, and gene cloning of a cold-adapted thermolysin-like protease fromHalobacillus sp. SCSIO 20089. Journal of bioscience and bioengineering, 115(6), 628–632.*

Zin, H.W., Park K.H., &Choi, T.J. (2014) *Purification and characterization of a carboxymethyl cellulase from Artemia salina. Biochem Biophys Res Commun. 443(1),194–9.*

Chapter 11

The *Clostridium Difficile* Toxins: Mechanism of Action and Immunopathogenesis

Charles Darkoh[1] and Chioma Odo[2]

1   Introduction

Clostridium difficile infection (CDI) is now the most common definable cause of hospital-acquired and antibiotic-associated diarrhea in the United States, with the total cost of treatment estimated between 1 to 4.8 billion U.S. dollars annually (Dubberke and Olsen, 2012; DuPont, 2011; Kyne et al., 2002; Magill et al., 2014; O'Brien et al., 2007; Wilkins and Lyerly, 2003). This bacterium is responsible for 10–25% of the cases of antibiotic-associated diarrhea, 50–75% of antibiotic-associated colitis, and 90–100% of pseudo-membranous colitis (Bartlett, 2002; Elliott et al., 2007). Morbidity and mortality resulting from CDI-associated diseases have also increased significantly over the past ten years, making C. difficile the most common emerging pathogen in the US (Ananthakrishnan, 2011; McDonald et al., 2005; O'Brien et al., 2007; Redelings et al., 2007). C. difficile over-populates the colon after the normal gut microbiota has been altered by antibiotic therapy. Therefore, the highest risk factor for CDI is previous antibiotic therapy (Bartlett and Perl, 2005). Treatment of CDI has been hampered by increased virulence of the causative strains, sporulation, recurrence of the infection, and antibiotics used in treatment that further alter the composition and colonization resistance of the normal colonic microbiota. Moreover, treatment with antimicrobials is, in as many as 25% of cases, ineffective resulting in recurrence of the infection (Burke and Lamont, 2013; Hansen et al., 2013).

---

[1] School of Public Health, Division of Epidemiology, Human Genetics, and Environmental Sciences, Center For Infectious Diseases, Houston, The University of Texas Health Science Center at Houston, Texas, USA

[2] The University of Texas School of Biomedical Informatics, Houston, Texas, USA

Pathogenic strains of C. difficile possess a 19.6 kb pathogenicity locus, which is composed of tcdR, tcdB, tcdE, tcdA, and tcdC. This locus is responsible for the production of toxin A and toxin B, encoded by tcdA and tcdB, respectively. These toxins are essential in C. difficile pathogenesis to the extent that only strains that are able to produce either of these toxins cause disease (Geric et al., 2004; Kuehne et al., 2010; Lyerly et al., 1985; Rupnik et al., 2001; Voth and Ballard, 2005). This section specifically discusses recent data on the properties of the C. difficile toxins A and B, their mechanism of action, and the immunopathogenesis of these toxins.

2   The History of C. difficile

Clostridium difficile was first isolated in 1935 by Hall and O'Toole (Hall, 1935), who were investigating the development of normal bacterial flora in neonates. They collected feces of new-born babies from sterile diapers, suspended the feces in sterile water, and examined prepared slides microscopically using the Gram's method (Bass *et al.*, 2013) and methylene blue staining. Primary cultures were prepared and tested for the presence of aerobic bacteria on blood agar and eosin methylene blue lactose agar plates. The presence of anaerobic Bacilli was also tested using dextrose broth constricted tubes and deep iron brain medium. Different bacterial species were isolated and identified from the feces of these neonates including various species of *Streptococcus*, *Micrococcus*, *Lactobacillus*, and anaerobic Bacilli. The most interesting among them was an obligate anaerobic Bacillus (Figure 1) that was observed to be an actively motile, heavy-bodied rod with elongated sub-terminal or nearly terminal spores of about the same diameter as the rods (Hall, 1935). This obligate anaerobic Bacillus was associated with *Kopfchenbacterien* in feces from three of the infants. Both bacteria appeared and disappeared at about the same time under similar conditions. According to Hall and O'Toole (Hall, 1935), the isolation of each of the two was complicated when both were present, but this anaerobic Bacillus was more difficult to isolate than the *Kopfchenbacterien*. This bacterium was also much more difficult to study, due to its slower growth and lack of distinctive morphological properties.

Based on Hall and O'Toole's account (Hall, 1935), the colonies of this anaerobic Bacillus generally emerged in deep agar after 48 hours of incubation and initially appeared minute, flat, and opaque. After 3 days, the colonies appeared lobulated in shape with a diameter of about 1 mm. Single colonies on blood agar slants under alkaline pyrogallol were irregular in form, flat, and non-hemolytic.

Dextrose broth cultures of 13 isolated strains of this new anaerobic Bacillus were incubated for 48 hours under anaerobic conditions at 37 °C and subcutaneously inoculated into guinea pigs. Following inoculation, the guinea pigs refused to eat and exhibited moderate to marked edema on the belly, breasts, and at the site of inoculation. Postmortem observation showed marked subcutaneous edema with or without congestion, but with no emphysema. Smears from the subcutaneous site of inoculation in one animal that died within 4 hours showed numerous Gram-positive rods, but no spores or leukocytes were observed (Hall, 1935). In all the animals, no evidence of septicemia was

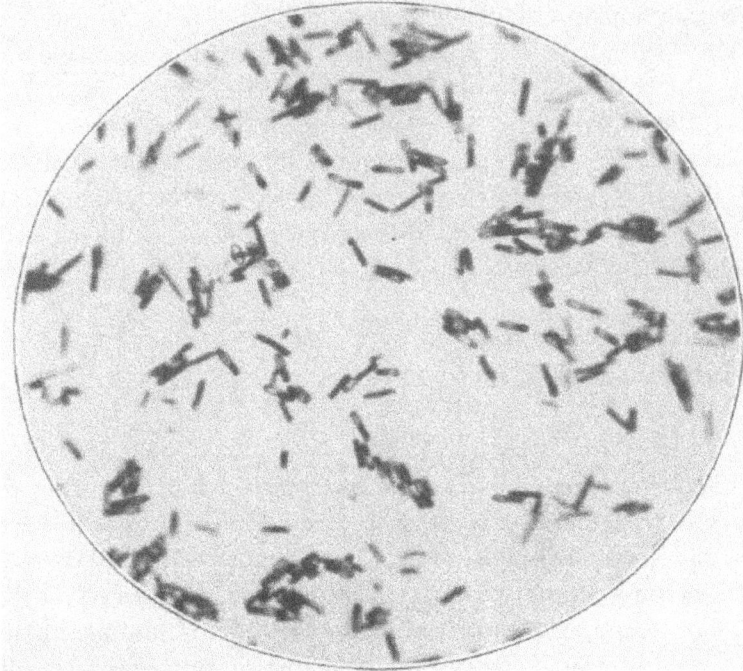

Figure 1: *Bacillus difficilis* (now *Clostridium difficile*) grown for 48 hours on a blood agar slant under alkaline pyrogallol. The Gram stain (Bass *et al.*, 2013) showed vegetative rods and spores (Hall, 1935). Kingdom: Bacteria; Phylum: Firmicutes; Class: Clostridia; Order: Clostridiales; Family: Clostridiaceae; Genus: *Clostridium*; Species: *Clostridium difficile* (Hall, 1935).

apparent, but phagocytic leukocytes were found with few free bacteria. A guinea pig injected with a culture filtrate died within 24 hours, whereas boiling of the culture filtrate for one minute completely destroyed the toxicity. These observations indicated that the new anaerobic Bacillus produced and released soluble exotoxins into the medium. Hall and O'Toole (Hall, 1935) thus, named this new anaerobic bacterium *Bacillus difficilis* (now called *Clostridium difficile*), due to the difficulties in its isolation and culture.

3   The Life Cycle of C. difficile

C. difficile exist either as actively dividing vegetative cells or as spores. The vegetative cells are obligate anaerobes and are sensitive to oxygen. In order to survive under aerobic conditions, *C. difficile* forms oxygen-resistant spores. Thus, the vegetative cells of *C. difficile* excreted in feces must transform into spores to survive aerobically (Jump *et al.*, 2007). It is therefore, widely acknowledged that the *C. difficile* spores initiate the infection process by serving as the disseminating form of this obligate anaerobic pathogen.

As a result, germination of the spores into vegetative cells inside the gastrointestinal tract is essential in *C. difficile* pathogenesis. This is because only the vegetative cells cause disease.

Little is known about sporulation and germination in Clostridial species. However, the physiological and morphological changes that occur during sporulation in the well-studied Bacillus species are similar to that of Clostridial species (Lofland *et al.*, 2013). Sporulation is initiated under conditions of nutrient limitation or other unfavorable conditions, when the cells can no longer maintain vegetative growth. When *C. difficile* initiates sporulation, an asymmetrically placed division septum is formed that divides the cell into two unequal compartments (the mother cell and a forespore). Each of these two compartments contains one copy of the chromosome. The larger mother cell compartment engulfs the forespore leading to maturation (Hilbert and Piggot, 2004). The process of maturation involves addition of a peptidoglycan cortex and several layers of proteins that coat around the forespore. The mother cell finally lyses and the spore is released into the environment (Henriques and Moran, 2007).

The spore is metabolically dormant when released from the mother cell, but resistant to various harsh environmental conditions, including high temperature, oxygen, pH, alcohols, among others. The spores germinate and grow as vegetative cells under suitable conditions such as the presence of germinants, abundance of nutrients, and anaerobic conditions. In *B. subtilis*, germination can be induced by different compounds such as L-alanine or a mixture of asparagine, glucose, fructose, and potassium ions (Kelly *et al.*, 2012). The *B. subtilis* receptors that have been identified to be involved in sensing these environmental signals are GerA, GerB, and GerK. A large amount of calcium dipicolinate is released subsequent to sensing of the germinant, leading to hydration of the core, degradation of the cortex, and resumption of metabolism (Setlow, 2003). Homologs of GerA, GerB, and GerK have been identified in many Clostridial species except *C. difficile*. This suggests that *C. difficile* spores respond to a different kind of environmental signal for germination (Sebaihia, Wren *et al.* 2006).

Cholate derivatives of bile salts, such as taurocholate and the amino acid glycine, act as co-germinants of *C. difficile* spores (Sorg and Sonenshein, 2010) and improve the germination of *C. difficile* spores from environmental surfaces and stool samples (Bliss *et al.*, 1997; Weese *et al.*, 2000). Lysozyme and thioglycolate also improve the colony formation of *C. difficile* spores (Kamiya *et al.*, 1989). However, the exact mechanism by which these molecules stimulate germination of *C. difficile* spores is unknown. Patients infected with *C. difficile* shed dormant spores in their stools. These spores remain viable on hospital surfaces for months and facilitate the spread of CDI and recurrence (Gerding *et al.*, 2008; Rupnik *et al.*, 2009). Thus, the formation of spores by *C. difficile* is a significant impediment in overcoming hospital-acquired *C. difficile*-associated diseases and recurrence. The spores contribute to the survival of this bacterium after treatment of surfaces with antiseptics and disinfectants as well as antibiotic therapy, which disrupts the colonic microflora and precipitates *C. difficile* infection, colonization, and overgrowth in the intestinal tract (Montoya and Detorres, 2013). As a result, there is a growing interest in utilizing agents that inhibit germination as a therapeutic strategy for *C. difficile* infections. For instance, Howerton *et al.* (2013) have demonstrated that a bile salt analog, CamSA, inhibits *C. difficile* spore germination *in vitro*. They further demonstrated that a single dose of CamSA (50-mg/kg) protected mice from *C. difficile* infection and that lower doses of CamSA resulted in delayed onset of the infection and less severe disease symptoms (Howerton *et al.*, 2013).

4   Epidemiology of C. difficile Infection

The incidence of *C. difficile* infections in acute care hospitals in the United States during the early 1990s was maintained at stable rate of 30 to 40 cases per 100,000 population (McDonald *et al.*, 2005). By 2001, the incidence of CDI had risen to almost 50 per 100,000 population. The incidence rate in 2005 (84 per 100,000) was almost triple that of 1996 (31 per 100,000) with concomitant increases in the severity and fatality of this infection (Ji *et al.*, 1997; Loo *et al.*, 2005). Currently, the number of cases of CDI in hospitals in the United States exceeds 250,000 per year (over 80 cases per 100,000), with the total cost of treatment estimated between 1 billion and 4.8 billion U.S. dollars annually (Dubberke and Olsen, 2012; DuPont, 2011). The number of cases occurring in the community and non-hospital healthcare facilities appears to make CDI the most common form of bacterial diarrhea in the United States. Morbidity and mortality resulting from CDI in recent years have increased significantly as a result of changes in the virulence of the causative strains, the expanding number of the elderly and immunocompromised patients in the population, improved diagnostics, and antibiotic usage patterns (Gould *et al.*, 2013; Longtin *et al.*, 2013; McDonald *et al.*, 2005; O'Brien *et al.*, 2007; Redelings *et al.*, 2007; Zilberberg *et al.*, 2008).

It is generally felt that antibiotic therapy allows *C. difficile* to overcome the normal gut microbiota colonization resistance mechanisms against CDI, which include occupying the space required for *C. difficile* proliferation, direct impairment of *C. difficile* growth or germination, siphoning nutrients or germinants from *C. difficile*, and shaping the host's innate and adaptive immune responses. CDI predominantly affects the elderly and immunocompromised patients in hospitals and nursing homes (Ji *et al.*, 1997; McDonald *et al.*, 2005). It is a frequent cause of morbidity and mortality among elderly hospitalized patients. Nevertheless, other populations are also at risk of the infection, such as young and healthy individuals who have not undergone antimicrobial therapy or were not exposed to a health care environment. Severe CDI that results in either death or colectomy has also been described in young women.

Asymptomatic carriage of *C. difficile* in children is estimated to be about 50% or higher (Schutze and Willoughby, 2013; Viscidi *et al.*, 1981). Interestingly, infants have been reported to have high levels of toxigenic *C. difficile* and toxins in their stools, but exhibit no clinical symptoms (Jafari *et al.*, 2013; Karadsheh and Sule, 2013; Rogers *et al.*, 2013). Although, it is not known why neonates are unusually refractory to CDI, several theories have been proposed. First, the membrane receptors required for toxin binding in the colon may be absent in neonates. Secondly, mucins directly inactivate or neutralize the *C. difficile* toxins (Vyas *et al.*, 2013). Third, the thick layer of colonic mucus in neonates may mask the toxin receptors. Fourth, the intestinal epithelial cells in neonates have reduced sensitivity to intoxication than adult cells, and this may contribute to the asymptomatic carriage. In fact, infant hamsters are also insensitive to CDI (Deshpande *et al.*, 2013; Lyerly *et al.*, 1988).

The emergence of hypervirulent high toxin producing strains of *C. difficile* has contributed to the increasing incidence of CDI. *C. difficile* isolates collected between 2000 and 2003 from eight health care facilities in six states (Illinois, Pennsylvania, Maine, Georgia, New Jersey, and Oregon) during CDI outbreaks and analyzed by McDonald *et al.* (2005) showed that a single strain accounted for half of the isolates from five of the facilities (McDonald *et al.*, 2005; Warny *et al.*, 2005). Moreover, 82% of the stool samples from another outbreak in Quebec, Canada were positive for the same strain (McDonald *et al.*, 2005). In the 1980s, this epidemic strain was initially identified by restriction endonuclease analysis and named BI, but it is currently referred to as North American Pulsed Field Type 1 (NAP1) and PCR ribotype 027 (i.e., BI/NAP1/027, or NAP1/027) (McDonald *et al.*, 2005). The unique characteristics of this virulent NAP1/027 strain are increased toxins A and B production, fluoroquinolone resistance, and production of the binary toxin. Also, high-level of gatifloxacin and moxifloxacin resistance has been reported in recent isolates, but not in the original NAP1 strains. Resistant strains may have a competitive advantage in the hospital environment where fluoroquinolone use is widespread (Khodaverdian *et al.*, 2013).

5   The *C. difficile* Pathogenicity Island

The main virulence factors of *C. difficile* essential for disease are two large toxins that are chromosomally encoded by the genes *tcdA* (toxin A) and *tcdB* (toxin B). The toxin genes together with the genes that encode the proteins TcdR, TcdE, and TcdC (Figure 2) are located within a 19.6 kb pathogenicity locus (PaLoc) in the *C. difficile* genome (Braun *et al.*, 1996; Hammond and Johnson, 1995). Toxin A (308 kDa) is known to function as an enterotoxin causing gastrointestinal damage, whereas toxin B (269 kDa) is a highly potent cytotoxin (Lyerly *et al.*, 1985).

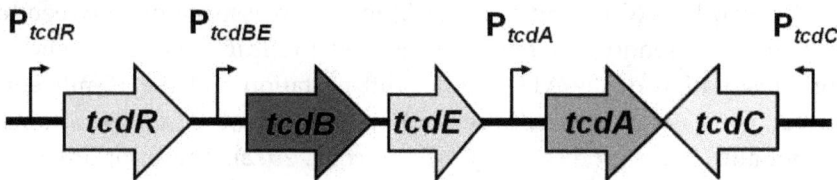

Figure 2: The pathogenicity locus of *C. difficile*. The *tcdA* and *tcdB* genes encode toxins A and B, respectively. The *tcdR* gene encodes a sigma factor that controls the transcription of the toxin genes, whereas the *tcdC* encodes a protein that has been proposed to play a negative role in toxin gene regulation by antagonizing TcdR. *TcdE* codes for a protein similar to holin, which is suggested to be involved in the release of the toxins.

The *tcdR* gene, which is located upstream of *tcdB* in the pathogenicity locus, encodes an RNA polymerase sigma factor that regulates transcription from the toxin promoters and from its own promoter (Mani & Dupuy, 2001; Mani *et al.*, 2002). TcdR is homologous to transcriptional activators of several Clostridium species and families of RNA polymerase sigma factors found in many organisms (Moncrief, Barroso *et al.* 1997). Proteins that have been found in other pathogenic Clostridia similar to TcdR include the sigma factors that control the tetanus neurotoxins (*TetR*) in *Clostridium tetani*, botulinum toxin (*BotR*) in *Clostridium botulinum,* and UV-inducible bacteriocin (*UviA*) in *Clostridium perfringens* (Dupuy *et al.*, 2005; Raffestin *et al.*, 2005). The first evidence for the role of TcdR in *C. difficile* toxin regulation was reported by Moncrief (Moncrief *et al.*, 1997) and his co-workers using *E. coli* as a surrogate host. These results were supported by similar experiments using *C. perfringens* as a surrogate host and later in *C. difficile* (Mani & Dupuy, 2001; Mani *et al.*, 2002). Biochemical and genetic evidence suggest that the role of TcdR is indispensable for initiation of transcription from the *tcdA* and *tcdB* promoters. Furthermore, the expression of TcdR and the toxin genes are both influenced in parallel by the growth phase, growth temperature, and the composition of the growth medium (Karlsson *et al.*, 2003). The same expression pattern is observed for all the genes in the pathogenicity locus except *tcdC*, which is highly expressed during the rapid exponential growth phase and less expressed during the stationary phase (Hundsberger *et al.*, 1997).

Genetic evidence suggests that TcdC negatively regulates toxin production by disrupting the capability of TcdR-containing RNA polymerase to recognize the *tcdA* and *tcdB* promoters (Mani & Dupuy, 2001; Mani *et al.*, 2002). Thus, it has been proposed that *tcdC* encodes a negative regulator of toxin production (Hundsberger *et al.*, 1997) and this concept has been supported by qualitative functional genetics and *in vitro* protein interaction studies (Carter *et al.*, 2011; Matamouros *et al.*, 2007). Evidence to support this hypothesis includes the inverse transcription pattern of *tcdC* in relation to the toxin genes, and the emergence of epidemic strains (NAP1/027 strains) with deletions or frame-shift mutations in the *tcdC* gene that produce high toxin levels (Carter *et al.*, 2011; Curry *et al.*, 2007; Hundsberger *et al.*, 1997; Matamouros *et al.*, 2007; McDonald *et al.*, 2005; Warny *et al.*, 2005). Moreover, all NAP1/027 isolates from the 1980s and 1990s, like those from recent outbreaks, carry *tcdC* mutations (Loo *et al.*, 2005; McDonald *et al.*, 2005). These reports highlight the importance of *tcdC* in the pathogenesis of *C. difficile*. However, Cartman and co-workers (Cartman *et al.*, 2012) found no association between toxin production and the *tcdC* genotype when they deleted the *tcdC* gene by allelic exchange. Furthermore, restoration of the Δ117 frame-shift mutation and the 18-nucleotide deletion that occur naturally in the *tcdC* gene of some virulent *C. difficile* strains such as R20291 did not alter toxin production (Cartman *et al.*, 2012). These reports suggest that the regulation of *C. difficile* toxin synthesis is more complex than previously thought and that the mechanism may involve other key regulatory elements.

Indeed, our laboratory recently reported that *C. difficile* toxin synthesis is regulated by an accessory gene regulator quorum signaling system (Darkoh *et al.*, 2015). Using an unbiased biochemical and genetic approach and a classic quorum signaling bioassay, our laboratory determined that *C. difficile* toxin synthesis is regulated by a novel cyclic quorum-signaling thiolactone peptide. The thiolactone was purified from the stationary phase supernatant by acetone precipitation, anion exchange chromatography, and HPLC. The purified thiolactone induced early transcription of the *C. difficile* toxin genes and stimulated elevated toxin production. Furthermore, the thiolactone was detected in stools from *C. difficile*-infected patients, but not in *C. difficile*-negative stools from patients with diarrhea. This underscores the clinical relevance of the cyclic thiolactone in *C. difficile* pathogenesis during infection. An isogenic toxin synthesis mutant was generated by Himar-based random mutagenesis, which was determined to contain an insertion in the accessory gene regulator (Agr) response regulator gene, *agrA*. This mutant is able to generate the thiolactone, but does not respond to the thiolactone. Response to the thiolactone and toxin synthesis was restored by complementation with the wild-type *C. difficile agrA* gene. These findings provide direct evidence that *C. difficile* toxin synthesis is regulated by an Agr quorum signaling system and offers new avenues for both rapid CDI detection and development of quorum signaling-based non-antibiotic therapies to combat this life-threatening emerging pathogen.

Between the toxin genes is a small open reading frame, *tcdE*, which encodes a putative holin, a protein whose activity is thought to allow the release of the toxins from the cell (Tan *et al.*, 2001). The *tcdE* open reading frame encodes a small, hydrophobic protein with 166 amino acids comprising a short hydrophilic stretch at the N-terminus and a series of charged residues at the C-terminus. TcdE is predicted to contain three transmembrane domains with structural features and a primary sequence similar to class I holins. Holins are small membrane proteins encoded by double-stranded DNA phages required for lysis of host cells following completion of intracellular phage development (Wang *et al.*, 2000; Young *et al.*, 2000). Holins oligomerize in the plasma membrane of the host cell forming a disruptive lesion, which enables the transport of prophage-encoded endolysin (a muralytic enzyme) across the membrane (Desvaux *et al.*, 2009). The prophage-encoded endolysin hydrolyzes the murein of the host cell leading to cell lysis and release of the phage particles. Even though, most holins are associated with terminal lysis of phage-infected bacteria, some holin-like proteins are known to be involved in the release of proteins from uninfected bacteria (Desvaux *et al.*, 2009).

TcdE was initially suggested to play a role in the secretion of *C. difficile* toxins due to its homology to holins. Govind and Dupuy (Govind and Dupuy, 2012) demonstrated empirically that TcdE is required for efficient secretion of the *C. difficile* toxins and facilitates release of toxins without inducing cell lysis or general membrane permeability. On the other hand, Olling *et al.* insertionally inactivated the *tcdE* gene and observed no delay or inhibition of toxin release (Olling *et al.*, 2012). Olling, *et al.* further stated that inactivation of TcdE did not either alter the kinetics of toxin release or the absolute level of secreted toxins A and B, suggesting that TcdE does not account for the pathogenicity of *C. difficile*. Moreover, no significance difference was observed between the wild-type and *tcdE*-deficient *C. difficile* when the secretome was analyzed by mass spectrometry, thus, excluding the proposed secretory role of TcdE. In *C. difficile*, *tcdE* encodes a 19-kDa protein but when expressed in *E. coli*, TcdE appears as a 19 and 16-kDa protein. The truncated 16-kDa protein was associated with bacterial cell death, suggesting that TcdE does not exhibit pore-forming function in *C. difficile*, since only the non-lytic full length 19-kDa protein is present (Olling *et al.*, 2012).

6   The Large *C. difficile* Toxins

The toxins A and B are the essential virulence factors in *C. difficile* pathogenesis and belong to a family of the large Clostridial glucosylating toxins (Geric *et al.*, 2004; Lyerly *et al.*, 1985; Rupnik *et al.*, 2001; Voth and Ballard, 2005). Strains that do not produce either of these toxins are not associated with disease (Elliott *et al.*, 2007; Voth and Ballard, 2005). Both toxins have similar enzymatic cleavage activities (Dillon *et al.*, 1995; Just *et al.*, 1995a; Just *et al.*, 1995b) and are cytotoxic to cultured cells; however, toxin B is 100-1,000-fold more potent than toxin A (Just and Gerhard, 2004; von Eichel-Streiber *et al.*, 1996; Voth and Ballard, 2005). *C. difficile* toxins A and B share high amino acid sequence identity and similar in structure (Pruitt *et al.*, 2010). These toxins are structurally similar to each other (Figure 3) with an N-terminal enzymatic domain composed of a glucosyltransferase domain and an autocatalytic cysteine proteinase domain, a central translocation domain encompassing a hydrophobic region, and a C-terminal receptor binding domain made up of Clostridial repetitive oligopeptides (CROPs) (Jank and Aktories, 2008; von Eichel-Streiber *et al.*, 1996).

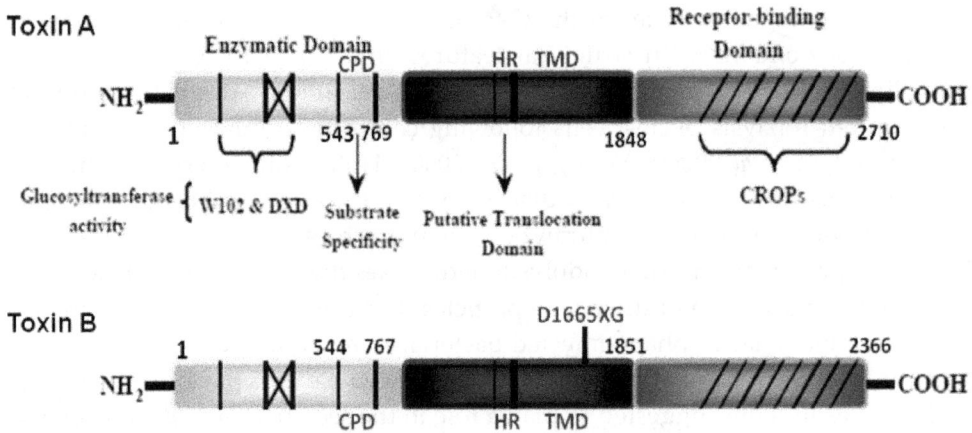

Figure 3: Structural comparison of *C. difficile* toxins A and B. These toxins have three domains: an N-terminal enzymatic domain consisting of a glucosyltransferase domain and an autocatalytic cysteine protease domain (CPD); a central translocation domain (TMD) encompassing a hydrophobic region (HR); and a C-terminal receptor binding domain containing the Clostridial repetitive oligopeptides (CROPs). The DXD (Asp-X-Asp) motif and a conserved tryptophan (W102) present in the glucosyltransferase domain are involved in Mn^{2+} and UDP-glucose binding. The DXG (Asp-X-Gly) motif in the TMD region of TcdB has an aspartate protease activity, which may be involved in toxin cleavage (Sun *et al.*, 2010).

The N-terminus of the toxins harbors the glucosyltransferase activity, which is the biologically active domain, and a domain with conserved catalytic triad (Asp587-

His653-Cys698) of a cysteine protease, which mediates toxin autocleavage during internalization in the host cell (Sun *et al.*, 2010).

The crystal structure of the TcdB glucosyltransferase domain has been determined and the essential amino acid residues involved in the glucosyltransferase reaction or substrate binding have been identified (Reinert *et al.*, 2005). The Asp-X-Asp (DXD) motif and a conserved tryptophan (W102) play a role in Mn^{2+} and UDP-glucose binding (Reinert *et al.*, 2005). There is limited information concerning the transmembrane domain and its function. The transmembrane domain comprises more than 50% of the total amino acid content of the toxins. It also includes a hydrophobic region whose role may be for membrane insertion.

The CROPs of the receptor binding domain has 21-, 30-, and 50- repetitive amino acid residues. The CROPS of TcdA contains between 30 and 38 contiguous repeats, whereas that of TcdB has between 19 and 24 repeats (Greco *et al.*, 2006; Ho *et al.*, 2005). The CROPs may be involved in the initial target cell interaction and receptor binding by the toxins. The crystal structure of the receptor binding domain of TcdA showed a solenoid-like structure that has been proposed to increase the surface area of proteins and enable protein-protein or protein- carbohydrate interactions (Greco *et al.*, 2006; Ho *et al.*, 2005). TcdA has been reported to bind to the trisaccharide, Galα1-3Galβ1-4GlcNAc, carbohydrate antigens, components in human milk, and glycosphingolipids (Krivan *et al.*, 1986; Rolfe and Song, 1993; Teneberg *et al.*, 1996; Tucker and Wilkins, 1991). The crystal structure of TcdA was solved in complex with the synthetic carbohydrate, Gal-α1-3Gal-β1-4GlcNAc (Greco *et al.*, 2006). On the contrary, a functional α-galactosyltransferase does not exist in humans, suggesting that Gal-α1-3Gal-β1-4GlcNAc cannot be an intestinal receptor in human (Jank *et al.*, 2007). The disaccharide Gal-β1-4GlcNAc, which is present in humans, has therefore been suggested to be part of the host receptor (Jank *et al.*, 2007). Little is known about the TcdB receptor, but it has been suggested that the TcdB receptor appears to be at the basolateral sites, whereas the TcdA receptor is on the apical sites on the host intestinal cells (Stubbe *et al.*, 2000). However, researchers have been unsuccessful in identifying the actual host receptor for the toxins. The interaction between the receptor binding domain of the toxins and the host cell receptors initiates receptor-mediated endocytosis (Florin and Thelestam, 1983; Karlsson, 1995; Tucker and Wilkins, 1991).

7   The *C. difficile* Binary Toxins

Some *C. difficile* isolates including the epidemic NAP1/027 strain also produce a third toxin that is unrelated to the pathogenicity locus called the *C. difficile* binary toxin (CDT). The binary toxin was first isolated by Popoff *et al.* in a patient with severe pseudomembranous colitis (Popoff *et al.*, 1988). This toxin is detected in 17% to 23% of *C. difficile* strains in the general population (Eckert *et al.*, 2013) and encoded by two genes, *cdtA* and *cdtB*, located on the CDT locus. *C. difficile* strains carrying the CDT locus have been grouped into specific toxinotypes; e.g. toxinotypes III, IV, V and XI, or more rarely, to strains for which the pathogenicity locus is absent (Geric *et al.*, 2003).

The binary toxin is a two-component ADP ribosyltransferase comprising the enzymatic component (CDTa) and binding component (CDTb) and its genes were first sequenced in 1997 (Perelle *et al.*, 1997). It has emerged that the CDT locus is present either as a whole or as a truncated version (Stare *et al.*, 2007). There is a unique 68 bp sequence in the chromosomal location of the CDT locus in strains that lack the whole or truncated CDT (Gerding *et al.*, 2014). The mature enzymatic component (CDTa) has two domains with a mass of ~48 kDa (Gerding *et al.*, 2014). Both domains exhibit analogous folding and this has been suggested to be due to duplication of an ancient ADP-ribosyltransferase gene (Han *et al.*, 1999). The N-terminal region of mature CDTa consists of residues 1–215 and has 5 α-helices and 8 β-strands, probably involved in the interaction with the binding component (CDTb). The C-terminal region covers residues 224–420 and houses the ADP-ribosyltransferase activity. The binding component CDTb has 4 domains and consists of 876 amino acids with a molecular mass of about 98.8 kDa and expressed with a signal sequence of 42 amino acids (Gerding *et al.*, 2014).

The role of the binary toxin in *C. difficile* pathogenesis is not clear. Toxins A- and B-negative binary toxin-positive strains cause fluid accumulation in rabbit ileal loops, but no diarrhea or death in hamster models (Doder *et al.*, 2013). Moreover, *C. difficile* strains that produce the binary toxin in the absence of toxins A and B do not appear to cause disease. The production of the binary toxin by NAP1/027 epidemic strains has renewed speculation that this toxin may act synergistically with toxins A and B in causing severe colitis (Loo, Poirier *et al.* 2005; McDonald, Killgore *et al.* 2005).

8   The Mechanism of *C. difficile* Toxins A and B Entry into the Host Cell

During infection, toxins A and B are released into the intestinal lumen where they bind to surface receptors on colonic epithelial cells via their receptor-binding domain (Figure 4). They are then internalized by the host cell by receptor-mediated endocytosis (Dingle *et al.*, 2008; Ho *et al.*, 2005). The acidic environment within the endosomes activates the cysteine protease activity of the toxins, which cleaves and releases the glucosyltransferase domain located at the N-terminus into the cytosol of the mammalian host (Egerer *et al.*, 2007; Hofmann *et al.*, 1997; Pfeifer *et al.*, 2003; Reineke *et al.*, 2007; Rupnik *et al.*, 2005). A host cofactor, inositol hexakisphosphate, has been suggested to serves as a trigger of the cysteine protease-mediated autocatalytic cleavage of the toxins (Reineke *et al.*, 2007).

Small GTPases (8–28 kDa) are characterized by their C-termini that are polyisoprenylated, and an intrinsic ability to bind to guanine nucleotides. In addition, they serve as molecular relays that transmit signals when bound to GTP and discontinue signal transmission when bound to GDP (Sun *et al.*, 2010). Small GTPases are subdivided into the subfamilies of Rho, Rab, Ras, Ran and Arf, and Ran. The Rho subfamily members (Rho GTPases or Rho proteins) such as RhoA, Rac1, and Cdc42 are the major known intracellular targets of TcdA and TcdB (Just and Gerhard, 2004). Once in the cytosol, the glucosyltransferase effector domain of the toxins mono-O-glucosylates low molecular weight GTPases of the Rho family (RhoA, Rac1, and CDC42) using cellular

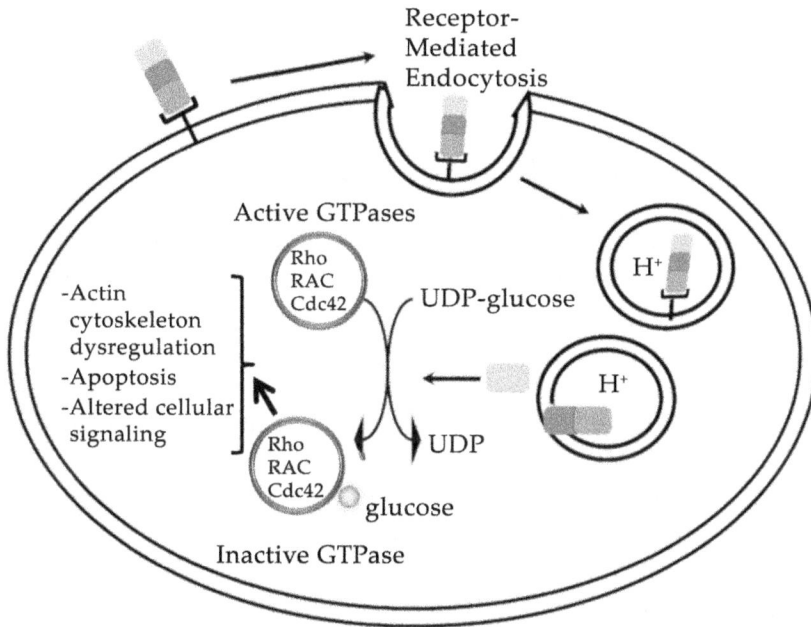

Figure 4: Mechanism of *C. difficile* toxins entry into host cells. The toxins bind to unknown host cell receptors and are subsequently internalized by receptor-mediated endocytosis (Reineke *et al.*, 2007). The low pH within the endosomes stimulates the autocatalytic cysteine protease activity of the N-terminally located enzymatic domain, resulting in the release of the glucosyltransferase domain. The released glucosyltransferase inactivates small molecular weight GTPases by monoglucosylation (Voth and Ballard, 2005).

uridine diphosphoglucose (UDP-glucose) as the glucose donor (Just and Gerhard, 2004; Just *et al.*, 1995a). In the GDP-bound form, Rho GTPases are inactive and associate with guanine nucleotide dissociation inhibitors, which keep the GTPases in the cytosol. Rho GTPases interact with different effectors to control several signaling processes upon activation by guanine nucleotide exchange factors (Sun *et al.*, 2010). They regulate many host cell functions, such as epithelial barrier functions, adhesion, phagocytosis, cytosecretion, immune cell migration, and immune cell signaling (Jank and Aktories, 2008; Just and Gerhard, 2004).

Monoglucosylation of the Rho GTPases by the toxins interrupts their normal functions leading to various deleterious effects including massive fluid secretion, apoptosis, cell rounding, actin cytoskeleton dysregulation, loss of tight junction integrity, acute inflammation and necrosis of the colonic mucosa, and altered cellular signaling (Genth *et al.*, 2008; Hofmann *et al.*, 1997; Huelsenbeck *et al.*, 2009; Just and Gerhard, 2004; Just *et al.*, 1995a). Cellular intoxication by the toxins also induces the release of various immunomodulatory mediators from epithelial cells, phagocytes, and mast cells resulting in inflammation and accumulation of neutrophils (Pothoulakis, 2000; Thelestam and Chaves-Olarte, 2000). The clinical manifestations of *C. difficile* infections are highly variable: ranging from asymptomatic carriage, mild self-limiting diarrhea, to severe and mostly fatal pseudomembranous colitis.

9   Characterization of Toxin A and B Activity

Purified toxins A and B were tested for their ability to cleave p-nitrophenyl-β-D-glucopyranoside (PNPG), a substrate similar to the native substrate of the toxins, uridine diphosphoglucose (UDP). From this analysis, the PNPG substrate was established to be useful for the detection of the *C. difficile* toxin A and B activity (Darkoh *et al.*, 2011). To confirm the cleavage of the PNPG substrate by each of the toxins, Western immunoblot analysis was used. Sodium dodecyl sulfate polyacrylamide gel electrophoresis (SDS-PAGE) were performed on purified PNPG-active toxins A and B and transferred onto a membrane. Monoclonal antibodies specific for each toxin were used to probe the membrane for the presence of each toxin. Single bands were observed in each of the samples that had PNPG activity and contained either purified toxin A or toxin B due to their specific reactivity with monoclonal antibodies that recognize toxin A or B, respectively. These results demonstrate that both toxins A and B cleave the PNPG substrate, and consistent with the reported *in vivo* activity of the toxins, in that they both cleave the same cellular substrate, UDP-glucose (Just and Gerhard, 2004; Just *et al.*, 1995a; Just *et al.*, 1995b).

Both toxins A and B demonstrate optimal PNPG cleavage activities within a pH range of 7–9 (Figure 5A). In contrast to toxin A, which showed significant activity within the pH range of 6 to 12, toxin B displays a more narrow range of PNPG cleavage activity within the pH range of 7 to 10. This is consistent with the pathophysiological environment of the colon, where *C. difficile* causes disease. The pH of the colon varies from 6.4 ± 0.6 to 7.5 ± 0.4 (Khan *et al.*, 2010). Both toxins shows activity optima at a temperature range of 35–40 °C, with toxin A showing a broader range of activity than toxin B (Figure 5B) (Darkoh *et al.*, 2011).

Based on the ProtParam analysis (Gasteiger E., 2005) of the amino acid sequences of the toxins, toxin A has a total of 588 charged residues out of 2710 residues, of which 54% and 46% are negatively and positively charged, respectively. Toxin B has more charged residues (597 out of a total of 2366 residues); 66% and 34% are negatively and positively charged, respectively. These data support the lower isoelectric point (IEP) of 4.42 estimated for toxin B compared to that of toxin A (5.51). The implication of this lower IEP for toxin B is a wide pH range for the maintenance of its overall negative charge at physiological pH. Toxin A is computed to be more stable with an instability index (Guruprasad *et al.*, 1990) of 29.6 compared to that of 36.5 for toxin B. However, both toxins are estimated to have relatively long *in vitro* half-lives based on the N-terminal end rule (Bachmair *et al.*, 1986; Gonda *et al.*, 1989; Tobias *et al.*, 1991) of 30 hours. These computational data suggest that toxin A should function in and tolerate a wider range of physiological and environmental conditions than toxin B (Darkoh *et al.*, 2011).

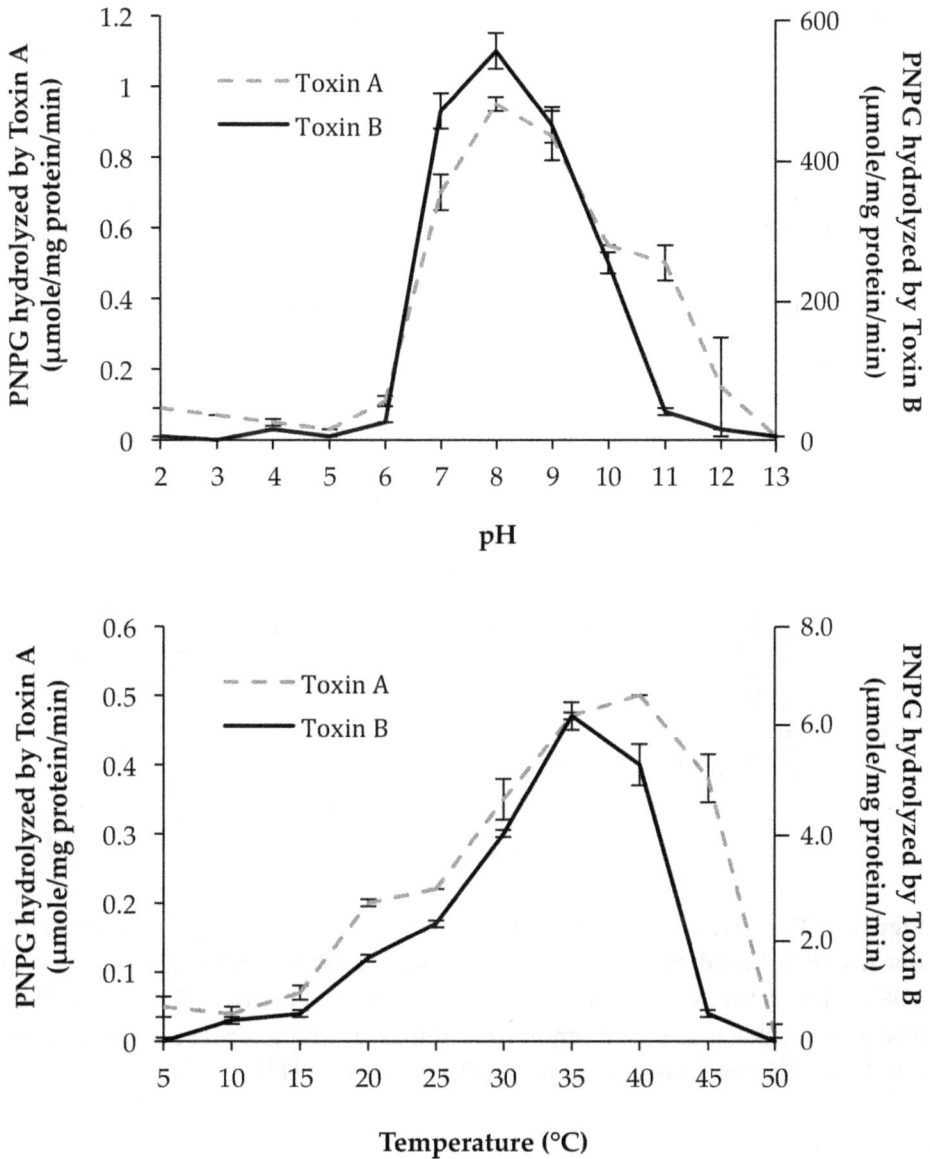

Figure 5: Effect of pH (A) and temperature (B) on the PNPG cleavage activities of toxins A and B. For the pH experiment, the toxin activity assay was performed by incubating 100 μg of toxin A or B with 3 mM PNPG at 37 °C for 4 hrs in buffers at the various pH values shown. For the temperature experiment, the toxin activity assay was performed by incubating 100 μg of toxin A or B in 50 mM Tris-HCl containing 50 mM NaCl (pH 7.4) with 3 mM PNPG at the temperatures indicated for 4 hrs. The assay was monitored by absorbance at 410 nm. Error bars represent standard deviation between two replicate experiments (Darkoh *et al.*, 2011).

The activity of both toxins follow the Michaelis-Menten curve (Figure 6), indicating that the toxins have a single active site. The Michaelis-Menten constant (Km) values of the toxins for the PNPG substrate as determined by the non-linear regression are 1.04 mM for toxin A and 0.24 mM for toxin B. The maximum velocity (Vmax) for toxin A for the PNPG substrate is 1.5 μmoles/mg/min, whereas that for toxin B is 6.4 μmoles/mg/min. These data indicate that the affinity of toxin B for the PNPG substrate is more than 4-fold higher than toxin A. Moreover, the rate of cleavage of the PNPG substrate was 4.3-fold faster for toxin B than toxin A. These results agree with assays of the relative damage by toxins A and B to tissue culture cells, in which toxin B was found to be more potent than toxin A (Just *et al.*, 1995a; von Eichel-Streiber *et al.*, 1996; Voth and Ballard, 2005).

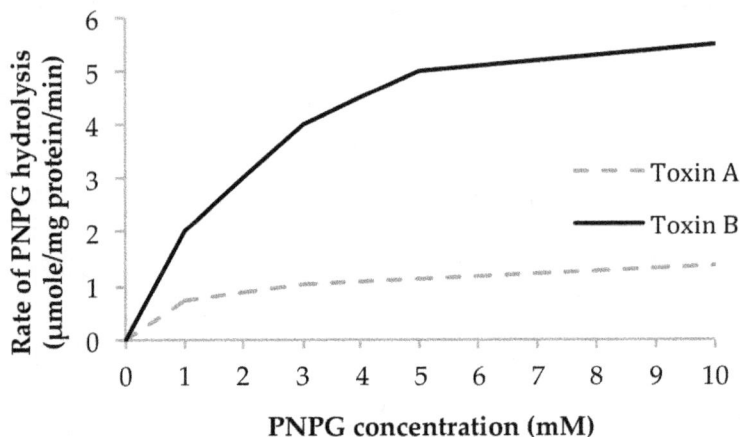

Figure 6: The Michaelis-Menten plot for the PNPG cleavage by *C. difficile* toxins A and B based on non-linear regression method. For toxin A: Km = 1.04 ± 0.06 mM and Vmax = 1.50 ± 0.03 μmoles/mg/min. For toxin B: Km = 0.24 ± 0.02 mM and Vmax = 6.40 ± 0.12 μmoles/mg/min. Error bars represent standard deviation from four replicate experiments (Darkoh *et al.*, 2011).

10   Inhibition of the *C. difficile* Toxins A and B Activity

To further characterize the toxin-substrate interactions, our laboratory has identified bile salts and their derivatives as potent inhibitors of the *C. difficile* toxin activity. For instance, the addition of 300 mM of sodium taurocholate reduced the activities of toxins A and B within one hour of incubation by 71% and 86%, respectively (Figure 7). Interestingly, taurocholate and phosphatidylserine (both negatively charged lipids) have been reported to inhibit β-glucosidases in a non-competitive manner (Choy and Davidson, 1980; Grabowski *et al.*, 1984; Holleran *et al.*, 1992; Peters *et al.*, 1976). These results support the idea that the cleavage of the PNPG substrate is due to the glucosyltransferase/hydrolase activities of the toxins (Darkoh *et al.*, 2011).

Toxin A

Toxin B

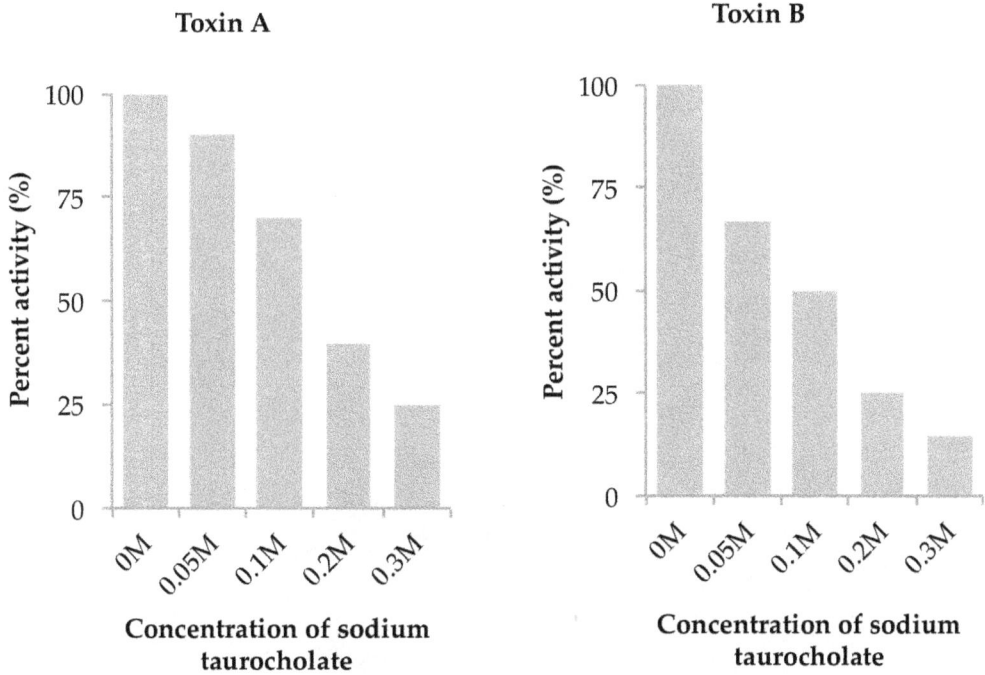

Figure 7: Dose-response inhibition by sodium taurocholate of toxin A and B PNPG cleavage activities. These experiments were performed by incubating 55 μg of each toxin for 1 hr with the amount of sodium taurocholate indicated at 37 °C in 30 mM Tris-HCl buffer (pH 7.4) containing 50 mM NaCl, and 10 mM of the PNPG. Error bars indicate standard deviation from three different experiments (Darkoh et al., 2011).

Treatment of C. difficile infections has been hampered by the recurrence of the infection, multi-drug resistance, emergence of strains with increased toxin production, and the indiscriminate use of antibiotics that further alter the colonization resistance of the gut microbiota. As a result, there is an urgent need for non-antibiotic treatments, either as stand-alone therapies or as therapies designed to augment the efficacy of currently used antibiotic regimens. An important potential treatment approach is to inhibit the activities of toxins A and B, which are directly responsible for the intestinal damage and subsequent inflammation associated with the infection. This approach, which targets the toxins without affecting bacterial cell growth, may be ideal since it is unlikely to impose selective pressure on the intestinal microbiome, thereby minimizing the risk of developing resistance.

Physiologic concentration of taurocholate (5 mM) was able to protect human colonic epithelial Caco-2 cells from C. difficile toxin B-mediated damage (Darkoh et al., 2013). When taurocholate and toxin B (16 μg) are added simultaneously to confluent Caco-2 cell monolayers, toxin-mediated cytopathic effects is prevented (Figure 8).

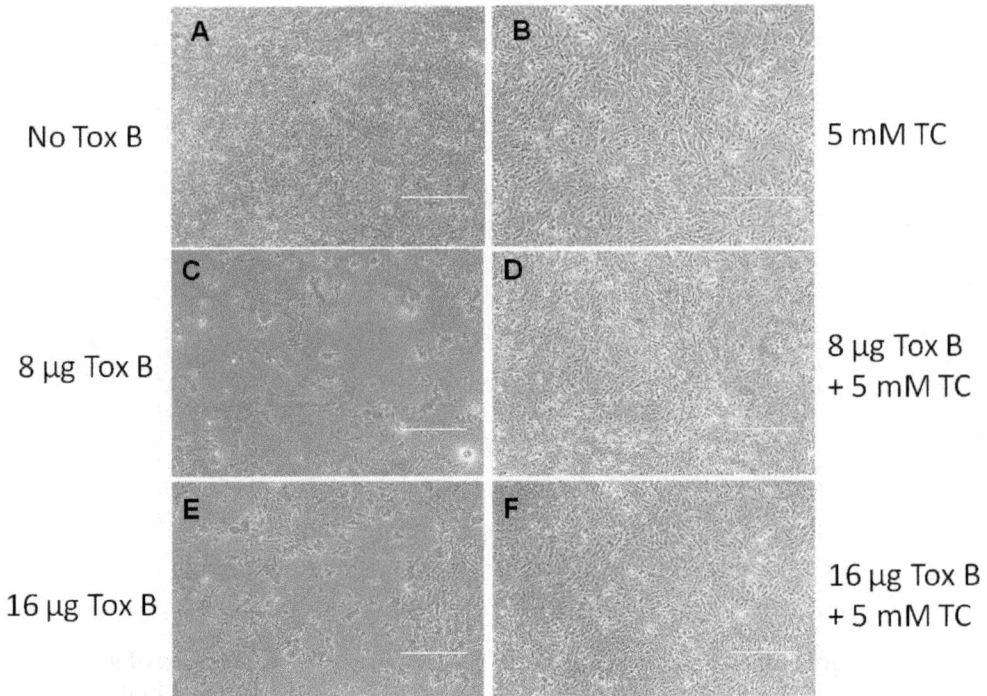

Figure 8: **Effect of *C. difficile* toxin B and taurocholate on Caco-2 Cells**. Conflu-ent Caco-2 cell monolayers were incubated with 8 and 16 µg of toxin B in the presence or absence of 5 mM taurocholate in a total medium volume of 2 ml in 24-well plates for 24 hrs. Images were captured using an EVIS XL microscope. Magnification 10X. Tox B, purified toxin B; TC, taurocholate (Darkoh *et al.*, 2013).

One of the mechanisms by which *C. difficile* toxins mediate cell damage is by in-ducing apoptosis. Specifically, toxin A has been reported to induce cell death in human epithelial cells *ex vivo* by activating caspases (Brito *et al.*, 2002; Carneiro *et al.*, 2006; Gerhard *et al.*, 2008). Toxin B also induces caspase-3 production in Caco-2 cells in a dose-dependent manner (Figure 9) (Darkoh *et al.*, 2013). Moreover, taurocholate re-duced caspase-3 production in the presence of lethal toxin B concentrations.

The mechanism of taurocholate-mediated inhibition of *C. difficile* toxin activity remains to be determined. Brandes *et al.* (Brandes *et al.*, 2011) reported that taurour-sodeoxycholic acid, a modified conjugated bile acid, affect the host cell by inducing phosphorylation of Rac1/Cdc42 that inhibited *C. difficile* toxin B-mediated monogluco-sylation of this GTPase. Taurocholate may also function through hydrophobic interac-tions to saturate the Caco-2 cell membranes, thereby inhibiting toxin entry and/or toxin activity. Other inhibitory mechanisms may involve direct effects of taurocholate on tox-ins such as alterations to toxin structure leading to loss of activity, or binding of tau-rocholate to the toxins leading to the prevention of entry into the host cell. Further re-search is on-going to identify the mechanism of taurocholate action.

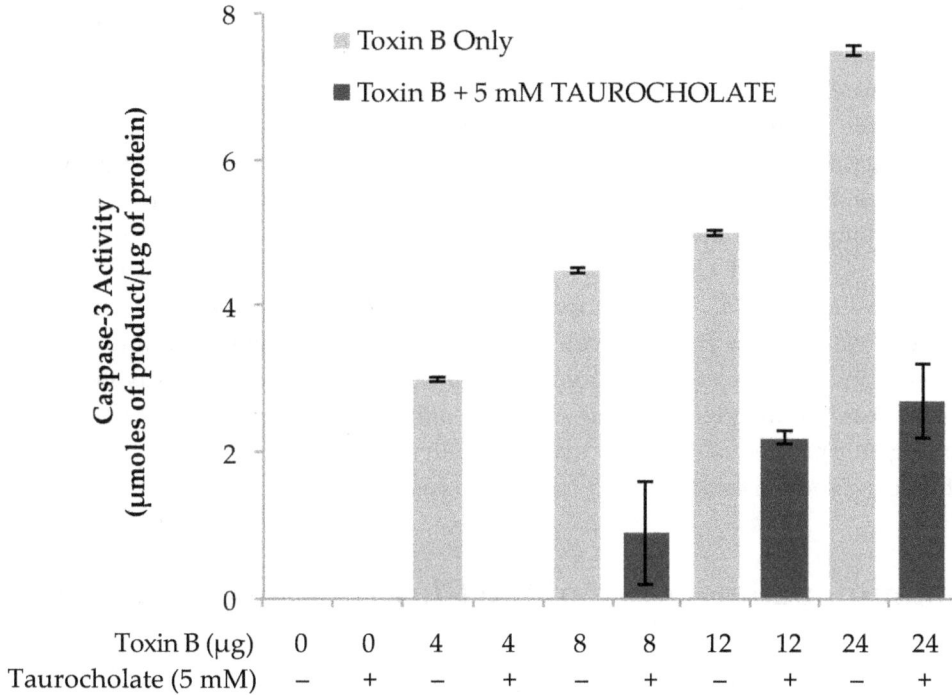

Figure 9: Effect of *C. difficile* toxin B and taurocholate on caspase-3 activity in Caco-2 cells. Caco-2 cells were incubated for 48 h with 0, 4, 8, 12 and 24 μg of toxin B in the presence or absence of 5 mM taurocholate. Cell monolayers were scraped from the bottoms of wells of a 24-well plate and lysed to obtain crude protein lysates. Caspase-3 activity was determined using Caspase-3 Colorimetric Kit (Invitrogen, Carlsbad, CA). Crude protein lysates (75 μg) were incubated with DEVD-NA caspase-3 substrate reagent for 8 h at 37 °C and absorbance at 410 nm was measured. A molar extinction coefficient for *p*-nitrophenol of $\varepsilon = 17700$ $M^{-1}cm^{-1}$ was used in the calculations (Shikita *et al.*, 1999). The error bars represent the standard deviation from three different experiments.

The majority of nutrient absorption in the gastrointestinal tract occurs in the small intestine, where bile salts are at much higher concentrations compared to the colon. This difference in bile salts concentration is due to the reabsorption of more than 95% of the total human bile via the enterohepatic circulation in the ileum (Dowling, 1973), which is directly proximal to the colon. Clearly, only a small amount of bile salts enter the colon where *C. difficile* most frequently colonizes. An intriguing explanation for the *C. difficile* pathology being mostly limited to the bile salt-deficient colon and the associated sparing of the bile salt-rich small intestine is that toxin activity may be inhibited in the small intestine by the high bile salt concentrations. The *C. difficile* toxins may be active in the colon because of its low bile salt concentrations and not active in the small intestine due to its high bile salt concentration. Thus, bile salt concentration may represent a host-mediated mechanism that naturally protects the absorptive surfaces of the small intestine from deleterious microbial products produced by pathogens such as *C. difficile* and acts to inhibit bacterial growth. Moreover, the lack of bile salts in the small intestine in diseased states (such as cirrhosis of the liver) may lead to bacterial overgrowth and result in competition for the essential nutrients required for normal human growth and function. The therapeutic benefits of bile salts are well documented; they prevent hepatocyte injury and cholestasis (Heuman *et al.*, 1991a; Heuman *et al.*, 1991b; Poupon *et al.*, 1991), drug-induced cholestasis (Queneau *et al.*, 1993), and endotoxin absorption (Bailey, 1976; Gouma *et al.*, 1986). Uncovering a mechanism to deliver higher concentrations of bile salts and/or their derivatives, perhaps in conjunction with antibiotics into the colon of individuals suffering from recurrent *C. difficile* infections may help protect the colon from the damaging effects of the *C. difficile* toxins and facilitate clearance of the pathogen. This line of research may result in a novel treatment of *C. difficile* infections that can produce recurrent and chronic disease or death.

11 Immunopathogenesis of the *Clostridium difficile* Toxins A and B

Major gaps still remain in our understanding of the immunopathogenesis of *C. difficile* infections (CDI), despite its increasing prevalence rates and poor patient outcomes. Our laboratory evaluated the relative amounts of 36 major biomarkers from stools collected from *C. difficile* infected- and non-*C. difficile*-infected patients. The data demonstrate that the immunopathogenesis of *C. difficile* infections is complex and elicits both Th1 and Th2 response, with an increased expression of pro-inflammatory proteins (Figure 10) (Darkoh *et al.*, 2014).

Interleukin- 8 (IL-8) and IL-23 appear to be important in the immunopathogenesis of CDI. These two cytokines were detected in the majority of the CDI-positive stools compared to the CDI-negative stools. The average concentration of IL-8 in the CDI-positive stools was significantly ($p < 0.05$) higher than that of the stools from CDI-negative and hospitalized controls without diarrhea. IL-8 is a chemoattractant involved in the recruitment of neutrophils to sites of infection and has been implicated to play a key role in the pathogenesis of CDI (Tixier *et al.*, 2005). Increased levels of IL-8 is associated with more severe forms of CDI (Steiner *et al.*, 1997). Moreover, a single nucleotide polymorphism (SNP) in the promoter region of the IL-8 gene that increases its expression is associated with susceptibility to CDI (Jiang *et al.*, 2007). These reports are consistent with our data showing high levels of IL-8 in the majority of CDI-positive stools compared to the stools from the CDI-negative and hospitalized controls without diarrhea.

The average concentration of IL-23 in the CDI-positive stools was lower than that of the CDI-negative and hospitalized controls without diarrhea, even though IL-23 was present in a larger number of the CDI-positive stools. IL-23 is produced by activated macrophages and dendritic cells and plays an important role in host defense against

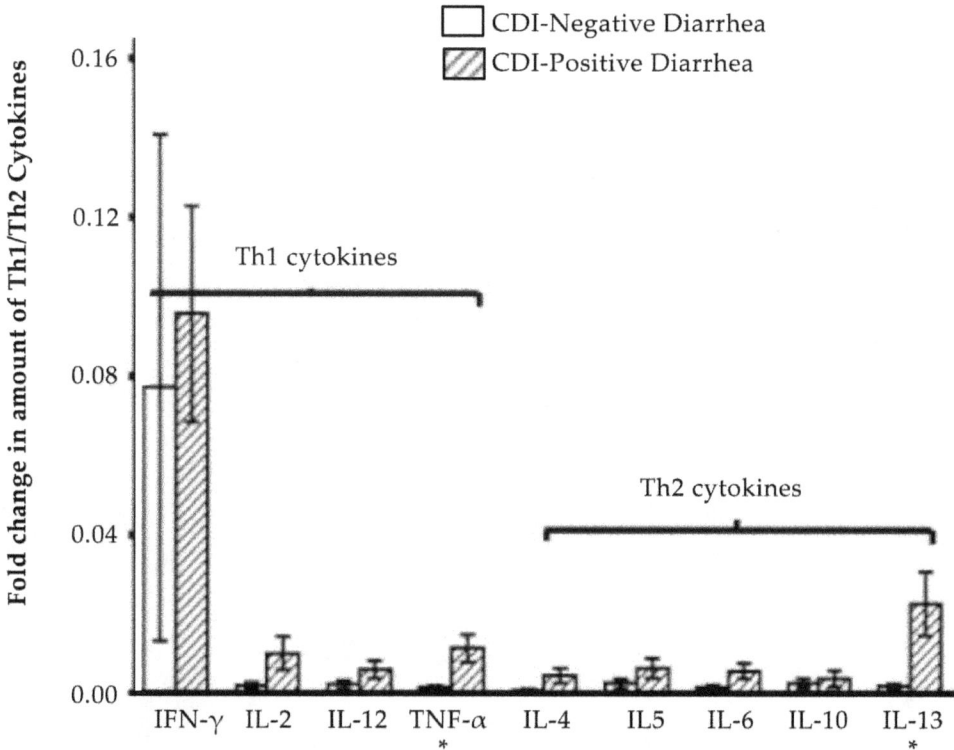

Figure 10 (A): Comparison of Th1 and Th2 cytokines in CDI-positive and CDI-negative stools. Fold change in amount of Th1 (IFN-γ, IL-2, IL-12, TNF-α) and Th2- (IL-4, IL-5, IL-6, IL-10, IL-13) cytokines obtained using Proteome Profiler Human Cytokine Array assay (R&D Systems, Minneapolis, MN). Stools (300 mg) from 100 antibiotic-associated diarrheal patients (50 CDI-positive and 50 CDI-negative) were evaluated for the presence of 36 inflammatory proteins using the Proteome Profiler Human Cytokine Array Panel A kit (R&D Systems, Minneapolis, MN). Data expressed as the mean of the relative band intensity of each cytokine. Stools from the hospitalized controls without diarrhea were not evaluated by the initial assay, but were included retrospectively in the quantitative ELISA for comparison. Error bars represent the standard error of measurement between two replicates per sample. * = $P < 0.05$.

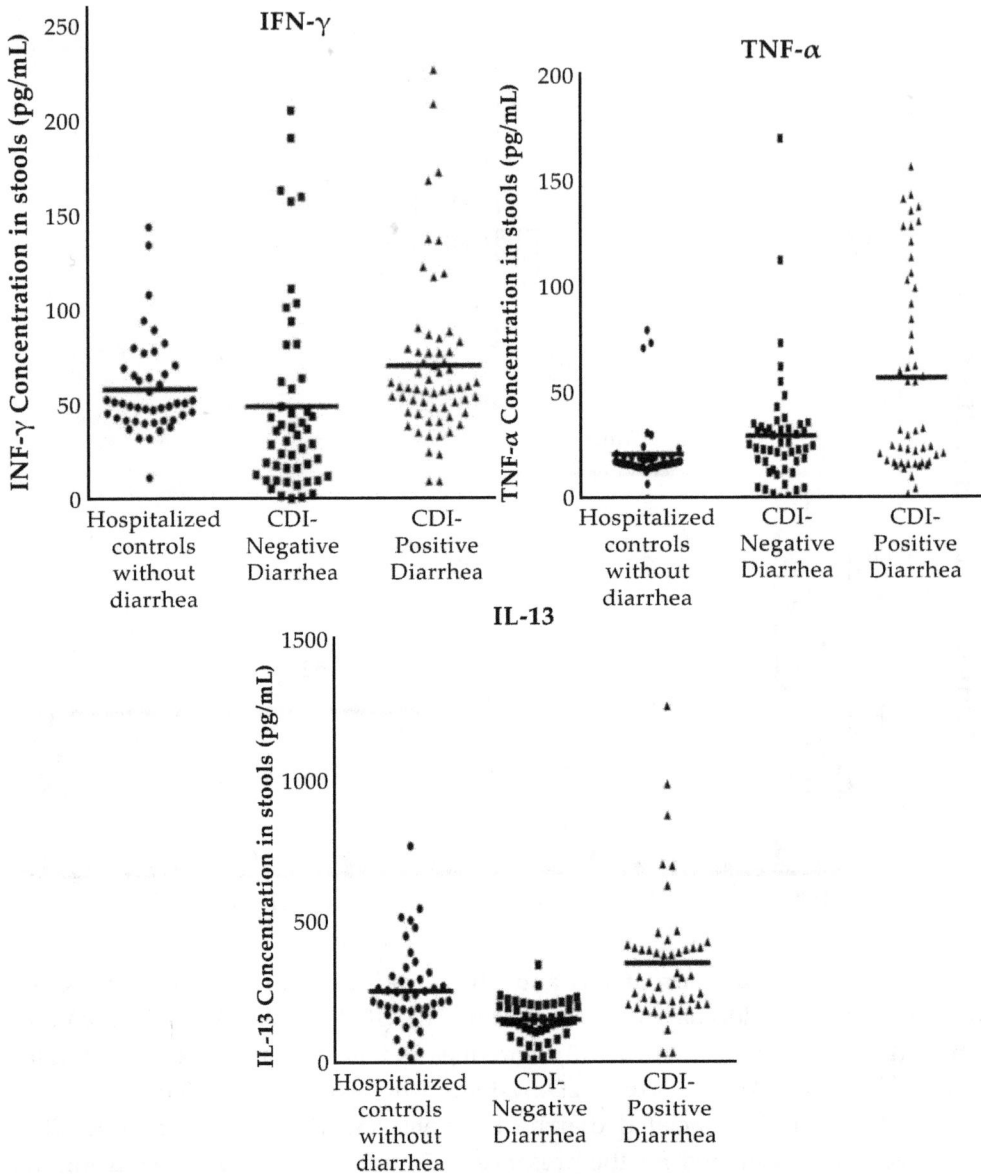

Figure 10 (B): Comparison of Th1 and Th2 cytokines in CDI-positive and CDI-negative stools. Concentrations of IFN-γ, TNF-α, and IL-13 in CDI-positive stools and stools from CDI-negative diarrheic patients and hospitalized controls without diarrhea, determined by quantitative ELISA (R&D Systems, Minneapolis, MN). The Krustal-Wallis test showed significant differences between the means (p< 0.0001). Horizontal bar = mean concentration in μg/ml. Key: IFN-γ, interferon-gamma; IL-2, interleukin-2; IL-12, interleukin-12; TNF-α, tumor necrosis factor-alpha; IL-4, interleukin-4; IL-5, interleukin-5; IL-6, interleukin-6; IL-10, interleukin-10; IL-13, interleukin-13.

bacterial infections and development of chronic inflammation (Iwakura and Ishigame, 2006). During bacterial infection, antigen-stimulated dendritic cells and macrophages produce IL-23 that promotes the development of Th17 cells leading to enhanced priming of memory T cells (Iwakura and Ishigame, 2006; Yen *et al.*, 2006). This results in induction and production of a variety of inflammatory mediators that triggers potent inflammatory responses. IL-23 also stimulates generation of pro-inflammatory cytokines such as IL-1, IL-6, IFN-γ, and TNF-α through its effects on dendritic cells and macrophages (Lankford and Frucht, 2003; Oppmann *et al.*, 2000; Parham *et al.*, 2002). The average fecal concentration of IL-23 in the stools of CDI-positive patients was significantly ($P<0.05$) lower than that of hospitalized controls without diarrhea and CDI-negative patients. This suggests that the amount of IL-23 produced during CDI may be inadequate to sustain the cellular immunity conferred by this cytokine in promoting the induction and proliferation of effector memory T cells. Thus, decreased production of IL-23 may explain the lack of robust immunological response exhibited by a proportion of CDI patients and may also relate to recurrence. Perhaps, boosting the level of IL-23 may help activate the cellular immune response required for a robust response to CDI.

The average concentrations of lactoferrin and calprotectin in healthy adults range between 1.45–4.6 µg/ml (Joshi *et al.*, 2010; Kane *et al.*, 2003) and ≤ 10 µg/ml (Dolwani *et al.*, 2004), respectively. This is consistent with the concentrations obtained from our study; 6.8+/−0.85 µg/ml (for lactoferrin) and 10.2+/−0.92 µg/ml (for calprotectin). Elevated levels of lactoferrin and calprotectin in stools is associated with colonic inflammation (Konikoff and Denson, 2006). Our data shows that 88% and 80% of the CDI-positive stools had average lactoferrin and calprotection concentrations, respectively, higher than the hospitalized controls without diarrhea. These results agree with that of Shastri *et al.* (Shastri *et al.*, 2008), in which 85.1% and 82.8% of CDI patients stools had higher levels of lactoferrin and calprotectin, respectively, than healthy adults. Lactoferrin and calprotectin serve as part of the innate inflammatory response and so their overexpression during CDI may provide insight into the extent of inflammation associated with this infection.

The differentiation of naïve CD4[+] helper T-cells into either Th1 or Th2 cells is critical in the development of adaptive immune response (Murphy and Reiner, 2002). Th1 inflammatory response usually induces IFN-γ production leading to activation of phagocytes, whereas Th2 response results in humoral immunity, allergic inflammation, and stimulates host resistance to intracellular infections or agents (Abbas *et al.*, 1996; Finkelman *et al.*, 2004). The patterns of Th1- and Th2-associated cytokines found in the CDI-positive stools were not distinct from that of the CDI-negative stools (Darkoh *et al.*, 2014). However, the concentrations of TNF-α and IL-13 in the stools of CDI-positive patients were significantly higher than that of the CDI-negative and hospitalized controls without diarrhea. This suggests a mixed Th1/Th2 response during CDI and infers that the host response to CDI is complex, pro-inflammatory, and encompasses both the innate and the adaptive arms of the immune system. These results may also denote a probable intracellular response to the toxins and an extracellular response to the bacterium.

12 Conclusion Remarks

Our understanding of the immunopathogenesis of the *C. difficile* toxins and their mechanisms of action has advanced as a result of the various exciting developments in the field. However, many important questions remain unanswered in spite of the progress made to date. These include the respective roles of toxins A and B in the host inflammatory response, a thorough understanding of the host immune response to the toxins, the exact function of the binary toxins in pathogenesis, identification of the specific host receptors for toxins A and B, generation of anti- toxin vaccines, and the development of non-antibiotic therapeutics for the treatment of the infection. With the increasing importance of *C. difficile* infections in public health, considerable research is warranted to fill these gaps in our knowledge of the immunopathogenesis in order to better prevent and treat the disease to reduce its public health burden.

References

Abbas, A.K., K.M. Murphy, and A. Sher. 1996. *Functional diversity of helper T lymphocytes. Nature. 383:787–793.*

Ananthakrishnan, A.N. 2011. *Clostridium difficile infection: epidemiology, risk factors and management. Nature reviews. Gastroenterology & hepatology. 8:17–26.*

Bachmair, A., D. Finley, and A. Varshavsky. 1986. *In vivo half-life of a protein is a function of its amino-terminal residue. Science. 234:179–186.*

Bailey, M.E. 1976. *Endotoxin, bile salts and renal function in obstructive jaundice. The British journal of surgery. 63:774–778.*

Bartlett, J.G. 2002. *Clinical practice. Antibiotic-associated diarrhea. N Engl J Med. 346:334–339.*

Bartlett, J.G., and T.M. Perl. 2005. *The new Clostridium difficile – what does it mean? N Engl J Med 353:2503–2505.*

Bass, S.N., S.R. Bauer, E.A. Neuner, and S.W. Lam. 2013. *Comparison of treatment outcomes with vancomycin alone versus combination therapy in severe Clostridium difficile infection. The Journal of hospital infection. 85:22–27.*

Bliss, D.Z., S. Johnson, C.R. Clabots, K. Savik, and D.N. Gerding. 1997. *Comparison of cycloserine-cefoxitin-fructose agar (CCFA) and taurocholate-CCFA for recovery of Clostridium difficile during surveillance of hospitalized patients. Diagn Microbiol Infect Dis. 29:1–4.*

Brandes, V., I. Schelle, S. Brinkmann, F. Schulz, J. Schwarz, R. Gerhard, and H. Genth. 2011. *Protection from C. difficile Toxin B-catalysed Rac/Cdc42 glucosylation by tauroursodeoxycholic acid-induced Rac/Cdc42 phosphorylation. Biol. Chem.*

Braun, V., T. Hundsberger, P. Leukel, M. Sauerborn, and C. von Eichel-Streiber. 1996. *Definition of the single integration site of the pathogenicity locus in Clostridium difficile. Gene. 181:29–38.*

Brito, G.A., J. Fujji, B.A. Carneiro-Filho, A.A. Lima, T. Obrig, and R.L. Guerrant. 2002. *Mechanism of Clostridium difficile toxin A-induced apoptosis in T84 cells. J. Infect. Dis.* 186:1438–1447.

Burke, K.E., and J.T. Lamont. 2013. *Fecal Transplantation for Recurrent Clostridium difficile Infection in Older Adults: A Review. J. Am. Geriatr. Soc.* 61:1394–1398.

Carneiro, B.A., J. Fujii, G.A. Brito, C. Alcantara, R.B. Oria, A.A. Lima, T. Obrig, and R.L. Guerrant. 2006. *Caspase and bid involvement in Clostridium difficile toxin A-induced apoptosis and modulation of toxin A effects by glutamine and alanyl-glutamine in vivo and in vitro. Infect. Immun.* 74:81–87.

Carter, G.P., G.R. Douce, R. Govind, P.M. Howarth, K.E. Mackin, J. Spencer, A.M. Buckley, A. Antunes, D. Kotsanas, G.A. Jenkin, B. Dupuy, J.I. Rood, and D. Lyras. 2011. *The anti-sigma factor TcdC modulates hypervirulence in an epidemic BI/NAP1/027 clinical isolate of Clostridium difficile. PLoS Pathog.* 7:e1002317.

Cartman, S.T., M.L. Kelly, D. Heeg, J.T. Heap, and N.P. Minton. 2012. *Precise manipulation of the Clostridium difficile chromosome reveals a lack of association between the tcdC genotype and toxin production. Appl. Environ. Microbiol.* 78:4683–4690.

Choy, F.Y., and R.G. Davidson. 1980. *Gaucher's disease II. Studies on the kinetics of beta-glucosidase and the effects of sodium taurocholate in normal and Gaucher tissues. Pediatr. Res.* 14:54–59.

Curry, S.R., J.W. Marsh, C.A. Muto, M.M. O'Leary, A.W. Pasculle, and L.H. Harrison. 2007. *tcdC genotypes associated with severe TcdC truncation in an epidemic clone and other strains of Clostridium difficile. J Clin Microbiol.* 45:215–221.

Darkoh, C., E.L. Brown, H.B. Kaplan, and H.L. DuPont. 2013. *Bile salt inhibition of host cell damage by Clostridium difficile toxins. PLoS One.* 8:e79631.

Darkoh, C., H.L. DuPont, S.J. Norris, and H.B. Kaplan. 2015. *Toxin Synthesis by Clostridium difficile Is Regulated through Quorum Signaling. MBio.* 6:e02569–02514.

Darkoh, C., H.B. Kaplan, and H.L. DuPont. 2011. *Harnessing the glucosyltransferase activities of Clostridium difficile for functional studies of toxins A and B. Journal of clinical microbiology.* 49:2933–2941.

Darkoh, C., B.P. Turnwald, H.L. Koo, K.W. Garey, Z.D. Jiang, S.L. Aitken, and H.L. DuPont. 2014. *Colonic immunopathogenesis of Clostridium difficile infections. Clin Vaccine Immunol.* 21:509–517.

Deshpande, A., S. Kundrapu, V.C. Sunkesula, J.L. Cadnum, D. Fertelli, and C.J. Donskey. 2013. *Evaluation of a commercial real-time polymerase chain reaction assay for detection of environmental contamination with Clostridium difficile. The Journal of hospital infection.* 85:76–78.

Desvaux, M., M. Hebraud, R. Talon, and I.R. Henderson. 2009. *Secretion and subcellular localizations of bacterial proteins: a semantic awareness issue. Trends Microbiol.* 17:139–145.

Dillon, S.T., E.J. Rubin, M. Yakubovich, C. Pothoulakis, J.T. LaMont, L.A. Feig, and R.J. Gilbert. 1995. Involvement of Ras-related Rho proteins in the mechanisms of action of Clostridium difficile toxin A and toxin B. Infect. Immun. 63:1421–1426.

Dingle, T., S. Wee, G.L. Mulvey, A. Greco, E.N. Kitova, J. Sun, S. Lin, J.S. Klassen, M.M. Palcic, K.K. Ng, and G.D. Armstrong. 2008. Functional properties of the carboxy-terminal host cell-binding domains of the two toxins, TcdA and TcdB, expressed by Clostridium difficile. Glycobiology. 18:698–706.

Doder, R., N. Kovacevic, D. Muncan, A. Potkonjak, B. Tomasev, and M. Ruzic. 2013. [Outcomes of Clostridium difficile enterocolitis after administration of antibiotics along with probiotic supplement]. Med. Pregl. 66:209–213.

Dolwani, S., M. Metzner, J.J. Wassell, A. Yong, and A.B. Hawthorne. 2004. Diagnostic accuracy of faecal calprotectin estimation in prediction of abnormal small bowel radiology. Aliment Pharmacol Ther. 20:615–621.

Dowling, R.H. 1973. The enterohepatic circulation of bile acids as they relate to lipid disorders. J. Clin. Pathol. Suppl. (Assoc. Clin. Pathol). 5:59–67.

Dubberke, E.R., and M.A. Olsen. 2012. Burden of Clostridium difficile on the healthcare system. Clinical infectious diseases : an official publication of the Infectious Diseases Society of America. 55 Suppl 2:S88–92.

DuPont, H.L. 2011. The search for effective treatment of Clostridium difficile infection. The New England journal of medicine. 364:473–475.

Dupuy, B., N. Mani, S. Katayama, and A.L. Sonenshein. 2005. Transcription activation of a UV-inducible Clostridium perfringens bacteriocin gene by a novel sigma factor. Mol. Microbiol. 55:1196–1206.

Eckert, C., B. Coignard, M. Hebert, C. Tarnaud, C. Tessier, A. Lemire, B. Burghoffer, D. Noel, and F. Barbut. 2013. Clinical and microbiological features of Clostridium difficile infections in France: the ICD-RAISIN 2009 national survey. Med Mal Infect. 43:67–74.

Egerer, M., T. Giesemann, T. Jank, K.J. Satchell, and K. Aktories. 2007. Auto-catalytic cleavage of Clostridium difficile toxins A and B depends on cysteine protease activity. J. Biol. Chem. 282:25314–25321.

Elliott, B., B.J. Chang, C.L. Golledge, and T.V. Riley. 2007. Clostridium difficile-associated diarrhoea. Intern Med J. 37:561–568.

Finkelman, F.D., T. Shea-Donohue, S.C. Morris, L. Gildea, R. Strait, K.B. Madden, L. Schopf, and J.F. Urban, Jr. 2004. Interleukin-4- and interleukin-13-mediated host protection against intestinal nematode parasites. Immunol Rev. 201:139–155.

Florin, I., and M. Thelestam. 1983. Internalization of Clostridium difficile cytotoxin into cultured human lung fibroblasts. Biochim. Biophys. Acta. 763:383–392.

Gasteiger E., H.C. Gattiker A., Duvaud S., Wilkins M.R., Appel R.D., Bairoch A. 2005. Protein Identification and Analysis Tools on the ExPASy Server. John M. Walker (ed): The Proteomics Protocols Handbook, Humana Press

Genth, H., S.C. Dreger, J. Huelsenbeck, and I. Just. 2008. *Clostridium difficile* toxins: more than mere inhibitors of Rho proteins. *Int. J. Biochem. Cell Biol.* 40:592–597.

Gerding, D.N., S. Johnson, M. Rupnik, and K. Aktories. 2014. *Clostridium difficile* binary toxin CDT: mechanism, epidemiology, and potential clinical importance. *Gut Microbes.* 5:15–27.

Gerding, D.N., C.A. Muto, and R.C. Owens, Jr. 2008. Measures to control and prevent *Clostridium difficile* infection. *Clinical infectious diseases : an official publication of the Infectious Diseases Society of America.* 46 Suppl 1:S43–49.

Gerhard, R., S. Nottrott, J. Schoentaube, H. Tatge, A. Olling, and I. Just. 2008. Glucosylation of Rho GTPases by *Clostridium difficile* toxin A triggers apoptosis in intestinal epithelial cells. *Journal of medical microbiology.* 57:765–770.

Geric, B., S. Johnson, D.N. Gerding, M. Grabnar, and M. Rupnik. 2003. Frequency of binary toxin genes among *Clostridium difficile* strains that do not produce large Clostridial toxins. *J. Clin. Microbiol.* 41:5227–5232.

Geric, B., M. Rupnik, D.N. Gerding, M. Grabnar, and S. Johnson. 2004. Distribution of *Clostridium difficile* variant toxinotypes and strains with binary toxin genes among clinical isolates in an American hospital. *J. Med. Microbiol.* 53:887–894.

Gonda, D.K., A. Bachmair, I. Wunning, J.W. Tobias, W.S. Lane, and A. Varshavsky. 1989. Universality and structure of the N-end rule. *J. Biol. Chem.* 264:16700–16712.

Gould, C.V., J.R. Edwards, J. Cohen, W.M. Bamberg, L.A. Clark, M.M. Farley, H. Johnston, J. Nadle, L. Winston, D.N. Gerding, L.C. McDonald, and F.C. Lessa. 2013. Effect of Nucleic Acid Amplification Testing on Population-Based Incidence Rates of *Clostridium difficile* Infection. *Clinical infectious diseases : an official publication of the Infectious Diseases Society of America.*

Gouma, D.J., J.C. Coelho, J.D. Fisher, J.F. Schlegel, Y.F. Li, and F.G. Moody. 1986. Endotoxemia after relief of biliary obstruction by internal and external drainage in rats. *Am. J. Surg.* 151:476–479.

Govind, R., and B. Dupuy. 2012. Secretion of *Clostridium difficile* toxins A and B requires the holin-like protein TcdE. *PLoS Pathog.* 8:e1002727.

Grabowski, G.A., S. Gatt, J. Kruse, and R.J. Desnick. 1984. Human lysosomal beta-glucosidase: kinetic characterization of the catalytic, aglycon, and hydrophobic binding sites. *Arch. Biochem. Biophys.* 231:144–157.

Greco, A., J.G. Ho, S.J. Lin, M.M. Palcic, M. Rupnik, and K.K. Ng. 2006. Carbohydrate recognition by *Clostridium difficile* toxin A. *Nat Struct Mol Biol.* 13:460–461.

Guruprasad, K., B.V. Reddy, and M.W. Pandit. 1990. Correlation between stability of a protein and its dipeptide composition: a novel approach for predicting in vivo stability of a protein from its primary sequence. *Protein Eng.* 4:155–161.

Hall, I.C., O'Toole, E. 1935. Intestinal flora in new–born infants with a description of a new pathogenic anaerobe, *Bacillus difficilis*. *Arch Pediatr Adolesc Med.* 49:390–402.

Hammond, G.A., and J.L. Johnson. 1995. The toxigenic element of *Clostridium difficile* strain

VPI 10463. Microb. Pathog. 19:203–213.

Han, S., J.A. Craig, C.D. Putnam, N.B. Carozzi, and J.A. Tainer. 1999. Evolution and mechanism from structures of an ADP-ribosylating toxin and NAD complex. Nat. Struct. Biol. 6:932–936.

Hansen, D., L.D. Pollan, and H. Fernando. 2013. Fulminant Clostridium difficile Colitis: A Complication of Perioperative Antibiotic Prophylaxis. Journal of oral and maxillofacial surgery : official journal of the American Association of Oral and Maxillofacial Surgeons.

Henriques, A.O., and C.P. Moran, Jr. 2007. Structure, assembly, and function of the spore surface layers. Annu Rev Microbiol. 61:555–588.

Heuman, D.M., A.S. Mills, J. McCall, P.B. Hylemon, W.M. Pandak, and Z.R. Vlahcevic. 1991a. Conjugates of ursodeoxycholate protect against cholestasis and hepatocellular necrosis caused by more hydrophobic bile salts. In vivo studies in the rat. Gastroenterology. 100:203–211.

Heuman, D.M., W.M. Pandak, P.B. Hylemon, and Z.R. Vlahcevic. 1991b. Conjugates of ursodeoxycholate protect against cytotoxicity of more hydrophobic bile salts: in vitro studies in rat hepatocytes and human erythrocytes. Hepatology. 14:920–926.

Hilbert, D.W., and P.J. Piggot. 2004. Compartmentalization of gene expression during Bacillus subtilis spore formation. Microbiol Mol Biol Rev. 68:234–262.

Ho, J.G., A. Greco, M. Rupnik, and K.K. Ng. 2005. Crystal structure of receptor-binding C-terminal repeats from Clostridium difficile toxin A. Proc. Natl. Acad. Sci. U. S. A. 102:18373–18378.

Hofmann, F., C. Busch, U. Prepens, I. Just, and K. Aktories. 1997. Localization of the glucosyltransferase activity of Clostridium difficile toxin B to the N-terminal part of the holotoxin. J Biol Chem. 272:11074–11078.

Holleran, W.M., Y. Takagi, G. Imokawa, S. Jackson, J.M. Lee, and P.M. Elias. 1992. beta-Glucocerebrosidase activity in murine epidermis: characterization and localization in relation to differentiation. J. Lipid Res. 33:1201–1209.

Howerton, A., M. Patra, and E. Abel-Santos. 2013. A new strategy for the prevention of Clostridium difficile infection. The Journal of infectious diseases. 207:1498–1504.

Huelsenbeck, S.C., M. May, G. Schmidt, and H. Genth. 2009. Inhibition of cytokinesis by Clostridium difficile toxin B and cytotoxic necrotizing factors – reinforcing the critical role of RhoA in cytokinesis. Cell Motil. Cytoskeleton. 66:967–975.

Hundsberger, T., V. Braun, M. Weidmann, P. Leukel, M. Sauerborn, and C. von Eichel-Streiber. 1997. Transcription analysis of the genes tcdA-E of the pathogenicity locus of Clostridium difficile. Eur. J. Biochem. 244:735–742.

Iwakura, Y., and H. Ishigame. 2006. The IL-23/IL-17 axis in inflammation. J. Clin. Invest. 116:1218–1222.

Jafari, N.V., S.A. Kuehne, C.E. Bryant, M. Elawad, B.W. Wren, N.P. Minton, E. Allan, and M. Bajaj-Elliott. 2013. Clostridium difficile Modulates Host Innate Immunity via Toxin-

Independent and Dependent Mechanism(s). PLoS One. 8:e69846.

Jank, T., and K. Aktories. 2008. *Structure and mode of action of Clostridial glucosylating toxins: the ABCD model. Trends Microbiol. 16:222–229.*

Jank, T., T. Giesemann, and K. Aktories. 2007. *Rho-glucosylating Clostridium difficile toxins A and B: new insights into structure and function. Glycobiology. 17:15R–22R.*

Ji, G., R. Beavis, and R.P. Novick. 1997. *Bacterial interference caused by autoinducing peptide variants. Science. 276:2027–2030.*

Jiang, Z.D., K.W. Garey, M. Price, G. Graham, P. Okhuysen, T. Dao-Tran, M. LaRocco, and H.L. DuPont. 2007. *Association of interleukin-8 polymorphism and immunoglobulin G anti-toxin A in patients with Clostridium difficile-associated diarrhea. Clin Gastroenterol Hepatol. 5:964–968.*

Joshi, S., S.J. Lewis, S. Creanor, and R.M. Ayling. 2010. *Age-related faecal calprotectin, lactoferrin and tumour M2–PK concentrations in healthy volunteers. Ann Clin Biochem. 47:259–263.*

Jump, R.L., M.J. Pultz, and C.J. Donskey. 2007. *Vegetative Clostridium difficile survives in room air on moist surfaces and in gastric contents with reduced acidity: a potential mechanism to explain the association between proton pump inhibitors and C. difficile-associated diarrhea? Antimicrob Agents Chemother. 51:2883–2887.*

Just, I., and R. Gerhard. 2004. *Large clostridial cytotoxins. Rev. Physiol. Biochem. Pharmacol. 152:23–47.*

Just, I., J. Selzer, M. Wilm, C. von Eichel-Streiber, M. Mann, and K. Aktories. 1995a. *Glucosylation of Rho proteins by Clostridium difficile toxin B. Nature. 375:500–503.*

Just, I., M. Wilm, J. Selzer, G. Rex, C. von Eichel-Streiber, M. Mann, and K. Aktories. 1995b. *The enterotoxin from Clostridium difficile (ToxA) monoglucosylates the Rho proteins. J. Biol. Chem. 270:13932–13936.*

Kamiya, S., K. Yamakawa, H. Ogura, and S. Nakamura. 1989. *Recovery of spores of Clostridium difficile altered by heat or alkali. J. Med. Microbiol. 28:217–221.*

Kane, S.V., W.J. Sandborn, P.A. Rufo, A. Zholudev, J. Boone, D. Lyerly, M. Camilleri, and S.B. Hanauer. 2003. *Fecal lactoferrin is a sensitive and specific marker in identifying intestinal inflammation. Am J Gastroenterol. 98:1309–1314.*

Karadsheh, Z., and S. Sule. 2013. *Fecal transplantation for the treatment of recurrent Clostridium difficile infection. North American journal of medical sciences. 5:339–343.*

Karlsson, K.A. 1995. *Microbial recognition of target-cell glycoconjugates. Curr. Opin. Struct. Biol. 5:622–635.*

Karlsson, S., B. Dupuy, K. Mukherjee, E. Norin, L.G. Burman, and T. Akerlund. 2003. *Expression of Clostridium difficile toxins A and B and their sigma factor TcdD is controlled by temperature. Infect. Immun. 71:1784–1793.*

Kelly, C.R., L. de Leon, and N. Jasutkar. 2012. *Fecal microbiota transplantation for relapsing Clostridium difficile infection in 26 patients: methodology and results. J. Clin.*

Gastroenterol. 46:145–149.

Khan, M.S., B.K. Sridhar, and A. Srinatha. 2010. *Development and Evaluation of pH-Dependent Micro Beads for Colon Targeting. Indian J Pharm Sci. 72:18–23.*

Khodaverdian, V., M. Pesho, B. Truitt, L. Bollinger, P. Patel, S. Nithianantham, G. Yu, and M. Shoham. 2013. *Discovery of anti-virulence agents against MRSA. Antimicrob. Agents Chemother.*

Konikoff, M.R., and L.A. Denson. 2006. *Role of fecal calprotectin as a biomarker of intestinal inflammation in inflammatory bowel disease. Inflamm Bowel Dis. 12:524–534.*

Krivan, H.C., G.F. Clark, D.F. Smith, and T.D. Wilkins. 1986. *Cell surface binding site for Clostridium difficile enterotoxin: evidence for a glycoconjugate containing the sequence Gal alpha 1-3Gal beta 1-4GlcNAc. Infect. Immun. 53:573–581.*

Kuehne, S.A., S.T. Cartman, J.T. Heap, M.L. Kelly, A. Cockayne, and N.P. Minton. 2010. *The role of toxin A and toxin B in Clostridium difficile infection. Nature. 467:711–713.*

Kyne, L., M.B. Hamel, R. Polavaram, and C.P. Kelly. 2002. *Health care costs and mortality associated with nosocomial diarrhea due to Clostridium difficile. Clin Infect Dis. 34:346–353.*

Lankford, C.S., and D.M. Frucht. 2003. *A unique role for IL-23 in promoting cellular immunity. J. Leukoc. Biol. 73:49–56.*

Lofland, D., F. Josephat, and S. Partin. 2013. *Fecal transplant for recurrent Clostridium difficile infection. Clinical laboratory science : journal of the American Society for Medical Technology. 26:131–135.*

Longtin, Y., S. Trottier, G. Brochu, B. Paquet-Bolduc, C. Garenc, V. Loungnarath, C. Beaulieu, D. Goulet, and J. Longtin. 2013. *Impact of the type of diagnostic assay on Clostridium difficile infection and complication rates in a mandatory reporting program. Clinical infectious diseases : an official publication of the Infectious Diseases Society of America. 56:67–73.*

Loo, V.G., L. Poirier, M.A. Miller, M. Oughton, M.D. Libman, S. Michaud, A.M. Bourgault, T. Nguyen, C. Frenette, M. Kelly, A. Vibien, P. Brassard, S. Fenn, K. Dewar, T.J. Hudson, R. Horn, P. Rene, Y. Monczak, and A. Dascal. 2005. *A predominantly clonal multi-institutional outbreak of Clostridium difficile-associated diarrhea with high morbidity and mortality. N. Engl. J. Med. 353:2442–2449.*

Lyerly, D.M., H.C. Krivan, and T.D. Wilkins. 1988. *Clostridium difficile: its disease and toxins. Clin. Microbiol. Rev. 1:1–18.*

Lyerly, D.M., K.E. Saum, D.K. MacDonald, and T.D. Wilkins. 1985. *Effects of Clostridium difficile toxins given intragastrically to animals. Infect. Immun. 47:349–352.*

Magill, S.S., J.R. Edwards, W. Bamberg, Z.G. Beldavs, G. Dumyati, M.A. Kainer, R. Lynfield, M. Maloney, L. McAllister-Hollod, J. Nadle, S.M. Ray, D.L. Thompson, L.E. Wilson, and S.K. Fridkin. 2014. *Multistate point-prevalence survey of health care-associated infections. The New England journal of medicine. 370:1198–1208.*

Mani, N., and B. Dupuy. 2001. *Regulation of toxin synthesis in Clostridium difficile by an alternative RNA polymerase sigma factor.* Proc. Natl. Acad. Sci. U. S. A. 98:5844–5849.

Mani, N., D. Lyras, L. Barroso, P. Howarth, T. Wilkins, J.I. Rood, A.L. Sonenshein, and B. Dupuy. 2002. *Environmental response and autoregulation of Clostridium difficile TxeR, a sigma factor for toxin gene expression.* J. Bacteriol. 184:5971–5978.

Matamouros, S., P. England, and B. Dupuy. 2007. *Clostridium difficile toxin expression is inhibited by the novel regulator TcdC.* Mol. Microbiol. 64:1274–1288.

McDonald, L.C., G.E. Killgore, A. Thompson, R.C. Owens, Jr., S.V. Kazakova, S.P. Sambol, S. Johnson, and D.N. Gerding. 2005. *An epidemic, toxin gene-variant strain of Clostridium difficile.* N Engl J Med. 353:2433–2441.

Moncrief, J.S., L.A. Barroso, and T.D. Wilkins. 1997. *Positive regulation of Clostridium difficile toxins.* Infect. Immun. 65:1105–1108.

Montoya, M., and O. Detorres. 2013. *Antimicrobial Selection and Its Impact on the Incidence of Clostridium difficile-Associated Diarrhea.* Journal of pharmacy practice.

Murphy, K.M., and S.L. Reiner. 2002. *The lineage decisions of helper T cells.* Nat Rev Immunol. 2:933–944.

O'Brien, J.A., B.J. Lahue, J.J. Caro, and D.M. Davidson. 2007. *The emerging infectious challenge of Clostridium difficile-associated disease in Massachusetts hospitals: clinical and economic consequences.* Infect. Control Hosp. Epidemiol. 28:1219–1227.

Olling, A., S. Seehase, N.P. Minton, H. Tatge, S. Schroter, S. Kohlscheen, A. Pich, I. Just, and R. Gerhard. 2012. *Release of TcdA and TcdB from Clostridium difficile cdi 630 is not affected by functional inactivation of the tcdE gene.* Microb. Pathog. 52:92–100.

Oppmann, B., R. Lesley, B. Blom, J.C. Timans, Y. Xu, B. Hunte, F. Vega, N. Yu, J. Wang, K. Singh, F. Zonin, E. Vaisberg, T. Churakova, M. Liu, D. Gorman, J. Wagner, S. Zurawski, Y. Liu, J.S. Abrams, K.W. Moore, D. Rennick, R. de Waal-Malefyt, C. Hannum, J.F. Bazan, and R.A. Kastelein. 2000. *Novel p19 protein engages IL-12p40 to form a cytokine, IL-23, with biological activities similar as well as distinct from IL-12.* Immunity. 13:715–725.

Parham, C., M. Chirica, J. Timans, E. Vaisberg, M. Travis, J. Cheung, S. Pflanz, R. Zhang, K.P. Singh, F. Vega, W. To, J. Wagner, A.M. O'Farrell, T. McClanahan, S. Zurawski, C. Hannum, D. Gorman, D.M. Rennick, R.A. Kastelein, R. de Waal Malefyt, and K.W. Moore. 2002. *A receptor for the heterodimeric cytokine IL-23 is composed of IL-12Rbeta1 and a novel cytokine receptor subunit, IL-23R.* J. Immunol. 168:5699–5708.

Perelle, S., M. Gibert, P. Bourlioux, G. Corthier, and M.R. Popoff. 1997. *Production of a complete binary toxin (actin-specific ADP-ribosyltransferase) by Clostridium difficile CD196.* Infect. Immun. 65:1402–1407.

Peters, S.P., P. Coyle, and R.H. Glew. 1976. *Differentiation of beta-glucocerebrosidase from beta-glucosidase in human tissues using sodium taurocholate.* Arch. Biochem. Biophys. 175:569–582.

Pfeifer, G., J. Schirmer, J. Leemhuis, C. Busch, D.K. Meyer, K. Aktories, and H. Barth. 2003.

Cellular uptake of Clostridium difficile toxin B. Translocation of the N-terminal catalytic domain into the cytosol of eukaryotic cells. J. Biol. Chem. 278:44535–44541.

Popoff, M.R., E.J. Rubin, D.M. Gill, and P. Boquet. 1988. *Actin-specific ADP-ribosyltransferase produced by a Clostridium difficile strain. Infect. Immun. 56:2299–2306.*

Pothoulakis, C. 2000. *Effects of Clostridium difficile toxins on epithelial cell barrier. Ann. N. Y. Acad. Sci. 915:347–356.*

Poupon, R.E., B. Balkau, E. Eschwege, and R. Poupon. 1991. *A multicenter, controlled trial of ursodiol for the treatment of primary biliary cirrhosis. UDCA-PBC Study Group. The New England journal of medicine. 324:1548–1554.*

Queneau, P.E., P. Bertault-Peres, E. Mesdjian, A. Durand, and J.C. Montet. 1993. *Diminution of an acute cyclosporin-induced cholestasis by tauroursodeoxycholate in the rat. Transplantation. 56:530–534.*

Raffestin, S., B. Dupuy, J.C. Marvaud, and M.R. Popoff. 2005. *BotR/A and TetR are alternative RNA polymerase sigma factors controlling the expression of the neurotoxin and associated protein genes in Clostridium botulinum type A and Clostridium tetani. Mol. Microbiol. 55:235–249.*

Redelings, M.D., F. Sorvillo, and L. Mascola. 2007. *Increase in Clostridium difficile-related mortality rates, United States, 1999–2004. Emerg Infect Dis. 13:1417–1419.*

Reineke, J., S. Tenzer, M. Rupnik, A. Koschinski, O. Hasselmayer, A. Schrattenholz, H. Schild, and C. von Eichel-Streiber. 2007. *Autocatalytic cleavage of Clostridium difficile toxin B. Nature. 446:415–419.*

Reinert, D.J., T. Jank, K. Aktories, and G.E. Schulz. 2005. *Structural basis for the function of Clostridium difficile toxin B. J. Mol. Biol. 351:973–981.*

Rogers, D.S., S. Kundrupu, V.C. Sunkesula, and C.J. Donskey. 2013. *Comparison of Perirectal versus Rectal Swabs for Detection of Asymptomatic Carriers of Toxigenic Clostridium difficile. J. Clin. Microbiol. 51(10):3421–2.*

Rolfe, R.D., and W. Song. 1993. *Purification of a functional receptor for Clostridium difficile toxin A from intestinal brush border membranes of infant hamsters. Clin. Infect. Dis. 16 Suppl 4:S219–227.*

Rupnik, M., J.S. Brazier, B.I. Duerden, M. Grabnar, and S.L. Stubbs. 2001. *Comparison of toxinotyping and PCR ribotyping of Clostridium difficile strains and description of novel toxinotypes. Microbiology. 147:439–447.*

Rupnik, M., S. Pabst, C. von Eichel-Streiber, H. Urlaub, and H.D. Soling. 2005. *Characterization of the cleavage site and function of resulting cleavage fragments after limited proteolysis of Clostridium difficile toxin B (TcdB) by host cells. Microbiology. 151:199–208.*

Rupnik, M., M.H. Wilcox, and D.N. Gerding. 2009. *Clostridium difficile infection: new developments in epidemiology and pathogenesis. Nat Rev Microbiol. 7:526–536.*

Schutze, G.E., and R.E. Willoughby. 2013. *Clostridium difficile infection in infants and children.*

Pediatrics. 131:196–200.

Setlow, P. 2003. *Spore germination. Curr Opin Microbiol. 6:550–556.*

Shastri, Y.M., D. Bergis, N. Povse, V. Schafer, S. Shastri, M. Weindel, H. Ackermann, and J. Stein. 2008. *Prospective multicenter study evaluating fecal calprotectin in adult acute bacterial diarrhea. Am J Med. 121:1099–1106.*

Shikita, M., J.W. Fahey, T.R. Golden, W.D. Holtzclaw, and P. Talalay. 1999. *An unusual case of 'uncompetitive activation' by ascorbic acid: purification and kinetic properties of a myrosinase from Raphanus sativus seedlings. Biochem. J. 341 (Pt 3):725–732.*

Sorg, J.A., and A.L. Sonenshein. 2010. *Inhibiting the initiation of Clostridium difficile spore germination using analogs of chenodeoxycholic acid, a bile acid. J. Bacteriol. 192:4983–4990.*

Stare, B.G., M. Delmee, and M. Rupnik. 2007. *Variant forms of the binary toxin CDT locus and tcdC gene in Clostridium difficile strains. J. Med. Microbiol. 56:329–335.*

Steiner, T.S., C.A. Flores, T.T. Pizarro, and R.L. Guerrant. 1997. *Fecal lactoferrin, interleukin-1beta, and interleukin-8 are elevated in patients with severe Clostridium difficile colitis. Clin Diagn Lab Immunol. 4:719–722.*

Stubbe, H., J. Berdoz, J.P. Kraehenbuhl, and B. Corthesy. 2000. *Polymeric IgA is superior to monomeric IgA and IgG carrying the same variable domain in preventing Clostridium difficile toxin A damaging of T84 monolayers. J. Immunol. 164:1952–1960.*

Sun, X., T. Savidge, and H. Feng. 2010. *The enterotoxicity of Clostridium difficile toxins. Toxins (Basel). 2:1848–1880.*

Tan, K.S., B.Y. Wee, and K.P. Song. 2001. *Evidence for holin function of tcdE gene in the pathogenicity of Clostridium difficile. J Med Microbiol. 50:613–619.*

Teneberg, S., I. Lonnroth, J.F. Torres Lopez, U. Galili, M.O. Halvarsson, J. Angstrom, and K.A. Karlsson. 1996. *Molecular mimicry in the recognition of glycosphingolipids by Gal alpha 3 Gal beta 4 GlcNAc beta-binding Clostridium difficile toxin A, human natural anti alpha-galactosyl IgG and the monoclonal antibody Gal-13: characterization of a binding-active human glycosphingolipid, non-identical with the animal receptor. Glycobiology. 6:599–609.*

Thelestam, M., and E. Chaves-Olarte. 2000. *Cytotoxic effects of the Clostridium difficile toxins. Curr Top Microbiol Immunol. 250:85–96.*

Tixier, E., F. Lalanne, I. Just, J.P. Galmiche, and M. Neunlist. 2005. *Human mucosa/submucosa interactions during intestinal inflammation: involvement of the enteric nervous system in interleukin-8 secretion. Cell Microbiol. 7:1798–1810.*

Tobias, J.W., T.E. Shrader, G. Rocap, and A. Varshavsky. 1991. *The N-end rule in bacteria. Science. 254:1374–1377.*

Tucker, K.D., and T.D. Wilkins. 1991. *Toxin A of Clostridium difficile binds to the human carbohydrate antigens I, X, and Y. Infect. Immun. 59:73–78.*

Viscidi, R., S. Willey, and J.G. Bartlett. 1981. *Isolation rates and toxigenic potential of Clostridium difficile isolates from various patient populations. Gastroenterology. 81:5–9.*

von Eichel-Streiber, C., P. Boquet, M. Sauerborn, and M. Thelestam. 1996. *Large clostridial cytotoxins – a family of glycosyltransferases modifying small GTP-binding proteins. Trends Microbiol.* 4:375–382.

Voth, D.E., and J.D. Ballard. 2005. *Clostridium difficile toxins: mechanism of action and role in disease. Clin. Microbiol. Rev.* 18:247–263.

Vyas, D., E. L'Esperance H, and A. Vyas. 2013. *Stool therapy may become a preferred treatment of recurrent Clostridium difficile? World journal of gastroenterology : WJG.* 19:4635–4637.

Wang, I.N., D.L. Smith, and R. Young. 2000. *Holins: the protein clocks of bacteriophage infections. Annu. Rev. Microbiol.* 54:799–825.

Warny, M., J. Pepin, A. Fang, G. Killgore, A. Thompson, J. Brazier, E. Frost, and L.C. McDonald. 2005. *Toxin production by an emerging strain of Clostridium difficile associated with outbreaks of severe disease in North America and Europe. Lancet.* 366:1079–1084.

Weese, J.S., H.R. Staempfli, and J.F. Prescott. 2000. *Isolation of environmental Clostridium difficile from a veterinary teaching hospital. J Vet Diagn Invest.* 12:449–452.

Wilkins, T.D., and D.M. Lyerly. 2003. *Clostridium difficile testing: after 20 years, still challenging. J Clin Microbiol.* 41:531–534.

Yen, D., J. Cheung, H. Scheerens, F. Poulet, T. McClanahan, B. McKenzie, M.A. Kleinschek, A. Owyang, J. Mattson, W. Blumenschein, E. Murphy, M. Sathe, D.J. Cua, R.A. Kastelein, and D. Rennick. 2006. *IL-23 is essential for T cell-mediated colitis and promotes inflammation via IL-17 and IL-6. J Clin Invest.* 116:1310–1316.

Young, I., I. Wang, and W.D. Roof. 2000. *Phages will out: strategies of host cell lysis. Trends Microbiol.* 8:120–128.

Zilberberg, M.D., A.F. Shorr, and M.H. Kollef. 2008. *Increase in adult Clostridium difficile-related hospitalizations and case-fatality rate, United States, 2000–2005. Emerg. Infect. Dis.* 14:929–931.

Chapter 12

Purification of PEGylated Proteins

Mina Sepahi[1], Shahin Hadadian[2], Reza Ahangari Cohan[3] and
Dariush Norouzian[3]

1 Introduction

Proteins are biomolecules produced by living cells. They can be of medicinal or industrial interest. Thereby, they need to be appropriately modified chemically in order to increase their stability against mostly proteolysis. This can be achieved by conjugating the targeted proteins to polyethylene glycol reagents. Conjugation of therapeutic proteins through polyethylene glycol technology causes increase in half life circulation of such drug in the body. But the adverse effect could be loss of pharmacokinetic properties of the drug under investigation.

Proteins can be either randomly or selectively PEGylated. However, the PEGylated forms of protein must be separated from the unpegyalted one which can be achieved by size exclusion, ion exchange and reveres phase chromatography methods depending on the strategy employed.

Polyethylene glycol (PEG) is generally regarded as a non-biodegradable polymer that reacts and attaches covalently to particular functional groups present in proteins. Non-biodegradability is not hundred percent accepted and some reports show oxidative degradation by various agents and enzymes, such as alcohol and aldehyde dehydrogenases (Jevsevar et al., 2010; Roberts et al., 2002) furthermore, PEG chains with molecular weight less than 400 Da (Dalton) are in vivo metabolized by alcohol dehydrogenases to toxic metabolites.

[1] Recombinant Biopharmaceuticals Production Department, Production and Research Complex Pasteur Institute of Iran, Iran

[2] Research and Development Department, Production and Research Complex, Pasteur Institute of Iran, Iran

[3] Pilot Nano Biotechnology Department, Pasteur Institute of Iran, Iran

The PEG larger than 400 Da which are used for PEGylation of proteins, are not susceptible to enzymatic dehydrogenation/oxidation to yield such toxic metabolite requiring different mechanisms to clear the toxic substances (Veronese & Pasut, 2005). Such removal mechanism varies with the molecular weight of employed polyethylene glycol. The detoxification /removal of toxic metabolites is brought about through renal filtration system for PEG molecules having a molecular weight of less than 20 kDa (Veronese & Pasut, 2005). There are other cleaning pathways like liver uptake and immune system (Veronese & Pasut, 2005).

2   Types of PEG

However, different lengths, shapes and chemistries of polyethylene glycol (PEG) reagents are available in international market. The most famous brands in PEG market are NOF Corporation (Japan); Creative PEG Works (USA); Chirotech Technology Limited (UK), Dr. Peddy's Lab (India); and JenKem (China) (Jevsevar *et al.*, 2010).

At the beginning of using PEG as a technology, researcher used linear PEG but nowadays new practices employ both linear and branched PEGs with the molecular weight up to 40 kDa with good results and improvement in pharmacokinetic properties (Jevsevar *et al.*, 2010; Veronese & Pasut, 2005; Gaberc-Porekar *et al.*, 2008). New PEG formats such as forked, multi-arm and comb-shaped PEGs show promises for the future. According to PEG reactivity with proteins or non proteinicious drugs, two distinct generations of PEG appeared viz, first and second and third generations.

2.1   First-Generation of PEG

This generation was begun with the alpha or epsilon amino groups of lysine reactivity. By introducing this generation, a wide range of proteins were coupled to commercially available PEG. Due to disadvantages such as small rang of molecular weights, unstable linkages between proteins and PEG, importantly non selective modification and PEG impurities shifted the route to next generation (Jevsevar *et al.*, 2010; Roberts, Bentley & Harris, 2002; Veronese & Pasut, 2005; Ryan, Mantovani, Wang *et al.*, 2008)

2.2   Second –Generation of PEG

This generation created to cover some problem like lack of selectivity in modification and unstable linkages. This generation is also known as site-specific PEGylation. According to PEG site, there are different modified polyethylene glycols such as PEG-propionaldehyde, PEG-acetaldehyde and the well known one is free cysteine PEGylation reagent like malemidyl-PEG (Roberts *et al.*, 2002; Shaunak, *et al.*, 2006; Zhang *et al.*, 2012).

It is important to notice that PEGylation methods described here mostly belong to second generation of PEGylation. It means that researchers exactly predict where the reaction can take place. Bioinformatics is an important tool in second generation PEGylation. Here we describe some methods that cover both generations (Ahangar Cohan *et al.*, 2011). There are different methods to categorize the PEGs, according to length, shape, etc. Each company, brand or book uses a method to explain different derivative of PEG. Here, we explain some example of this subject.

2.2.1   Amine PEGylation

This kind of PEG reacts with amino group present on protein or peptide surface, includes an activated N-hydroxylsuccinimide (NHS) form of polyethylene glycol (NHS-PEG). Nowadays, there are different forms of NHS-PEG like, PEG succinimidyl ester, PEG succinimidyl carbonate with different molecular weights which are commercially available (Roberts *et al.*, 2002).

2.2.2   Thiol PEGylation

A thiol group is a functional group having generally a sulfur atom bonded to hydrogen atom i. E -SH. Site-specific PEGylation at native cysteine residues is seldom carried out because these residues are usually in the form of disulfide bonds or otherwise, are required for biological activity. On the other hand, site- directed engineering needed to be used to introduce a cysteine residue at the surface of engineered protein for thiol PEGylation. The cysteine mutated protein must be accessible to PEG and maintain its biological activity after modification by PEG (Roberts *et al.*, 2002; Shaunak *et al.*, 2006; Ahangar Cohan *et al.*, 2011).

2.2.3   N-terminal PEGylation

N-terminal PEGylation, means using a reductive alkylation step with a PEG- aldehyde reagent and a reducing agent (Roberts, Bentley & Harris, 2002).

2.2.4   Oxidized Carbohydrates or N-terminus PEGylation

Oxidation of carbohydrate sited at N-terminal of serine or threonine is a new method for site-directed PEGylation of proteins. Oxidation of carbohydrate by enzyme or chemical reagent creates aldehyde groups which can react with PEG- hydrazide to build up a hydrazone linkage.

2.3   Third-Generation of PEG

In this generation, the polymers are available in Y, branched or combed shapes and have received growing attention because they show enhanced pharmacokinetic properties as compared to linear PEG conjugation (Jevsevar, Kunstelj & Porekar, 2010; Roberts, Bentley & Harris, 2002; Veronese & Pasut, 2005).

They demonstrate low viscosity and unable to be accumulated in the organs/ tissues (Veronese & Pasut, 2005).

3   Type Techniques Used to Purify PEGylated Proteins

Lower immunogenicity, longer half life due to lower circulation clearance rate and higher resistance to proteolytic degradation has made PEGylated proteins as widely spreading technology in biopharmaceuticals. Biopharmaceuticals bear more complex structure in comparison to chemical therapeutics and amongst these, PEGylated bio-pharmaceutical are more complex due to their structural heterogenicity with aspect to various PEGylation sites, extent of PEGylation (partially or fully PEGylation) and the length of PEG chains attached to the molecule. The most important parameters to be considered in protein-polymer conjugation are: a) protein structure, spatial distances between PEGylation and protein functional sites, the number of linked polymer chains, protein molecular weight and b) polymer composition, polymer molecular weight, shape and its conjugation chemistry (Caliceti, and Veronese, 2003). By keeping the above, the differences in bioactivity of PEGylated protein have been observed as compared to non-PEGylated protein. Such alteration in biological activity could be due to the i) spatial differences between protein functional and PEGylation sites in different isomers ,ii) the steric hindrance on protein caused by PEG molecule (Grace *et al.*, 2005).

Since PEG molecules are relatively inert and neutral hydrophilic polymer, differences in molecular size of protein -PEG conjugates and their native forms (unPEGylated forms) are not relatively small. Methods used to purify PEGylated form of proteins from unPEGyalted form must show good resolution (Veronese, 2009).

However, one of the most challenging tasks in conjugating proteins to PEG reagents is low yield of the conjugated forms of protein. Therefore, to purify the conjugated protein from non conjugated counterpart, it is essential to implement the techniques which can separate the two forms of proteins with high resolution. Some of the techniques which can be used to attain the goals are as follows:

3.1   Separation Based on Size Differences

PEG molecules are more hydrophilic than proteins, so increase in polymer's length increments the stoke radius of PEGylated protein significantly and apparent molecular weight anomalously. For instance, a 5 KDa PEG conjugated to interferon α-2b (23.1 KDa, 21.2 °A) results to a PEG- protein with 73.3 KDa apparent molecular weight (absolute molecular weight 28.1 KDa) and 33.6 °A.

Stokes radius and also linear PEG molecules can cause more increase in molecular weight of conjugated protein as compared to branched type of polyethylene glycol (Grace *et al.*, 2005). The stock or hydrodynamic radius of PEGylated protein can be calculated by Equation 1 (Veronese, 2009):

$$R_{h,\text{PEG prot}} = \frac{A}{6} + \frac{2}{3A} R_{h,PEG}{}^2 + \frac{1}{3} R_{h,PEG},$$
$$A = [108 R_{h,prot}{}^3 + 8 R_{h,PEG}{}^3 + 12(81 R_{h,prot}{}^6 + 12 R_{h,prot}{}^3 R_{h,PEG}{}^3)^{1/2}]^{1/3}. \tag{1}$$

$R_{h,\text{ PEG prot}}$, $R_{h,prot}$ and $R_{h,PEG}$ are hydrodynamic radius of PEGylated protein, protein and

PEG molecule respectively. Two latter are calculated according Equations 2 (Fee & Alstine, 2004) and 3 (Hagel, 1998).

$$R_{h,\,PEG} = 0.1912 M_{r,PEG}^{0.559},\tag{2}$$

$$R_{h,\,PEG} \approx (0.82 \pm 0.02) M_{r,prot}^{1/3},\tag{3}$$

where M_r is the molecular weight.

One should consider that true molecular weight of commercial PEGylating reagents differs from their nominal molecular weight such as 5 KDa commercial PEG is 5589 ± 56 Da (Veronese, 2009). It is an essential to select an appropriate PEG size and a better shielding of the proteins which lead to delayed clearance from kidney ultra filtration and decrease immune system recognition (Caliceti & Veronese, 2003; Caserman, 2009).

The reactivity of PEG molecule and subsequently PEGylation reaction yield can be decreased by increasing PEG molecular weight, PEGylation reaction step will also increase the cost of production because more consumption of PEG (more excess molar ratio of PEG)is required (Zhai, Zhao, Lei *et al.*, 2009). PEGylation of proteins starts with pure sample but there is no reaction with 100% conversion and yield, so separation of PEGylation reaction mixture which means separation of products from reaction feeds (unPEGylated protein and PEG molecules) is the first aim of purification process. High PEGylation may decrease bioactivity and low PEGylation may have no or low half life clearance (Daly, Przybycien & Tilton, 2005). Challenges start when the target protein has different PEGylation sites and the fractionation of positional isoforms is the real adversity. PEGylation extent (the number of PEG adducts on each molecule, N), and positional isomerism (the positions of the PEG adducts on each molecule) should be exactly defined.

Size exclusion chromatography makes the advantages of differences in molecular size which sometimes is related to molecular weight in normal practice during protein separations. But in PEGylated – conjugates separation, elution volume is correlated with molecular size / apparent molecular weight and the stock radius too. Good resolution between high resolution gel filtration fractionation is usually accessible when the two fractions molecular weight differences is more than two fold (Veronese, 2009; Skoog, Holler & Crouch, 2007). For example mono and di PEGylated chicken egg lysozyme (35.5, 56.2 KDa) showed two connected peak which need to lose peak overlapping section to avoid cross contamination of two fractions, but both as mentioned above have a good resolution with unPEGylated form (14.6 KDa) (Daly, Przybycien & Tilton, 2005). Hence size exclusion chromatography (SEC) is a useful technique for separation of PEGylated forms from PEGylation mixture. Therefore heavier PEG molecule will result better fraction resolution in high performance size exclusion chromatography (HPSEC) (Zhai, Zhao, Lei *et al.*, 2009).

For low PEGylation extent, SEC will be effective but the resolution between peaks is expected to be decreased as PEGylation extent is increased (Fee & Alstine, 2006). Considering the PEGylation of protein with a 20 KDa PEG, if the number of PEG adducts on each molecule (N) is more than three, mono PEGylated form could not be separated from the others efficiently (Veronese, 2009). Also, the low flow rates and small amount of sample loading onto the column are obstacles for scaling up (Yu & Ghosh, 2010).

The PEGylated protein peaks overlap at positions where total molecular weight of PEG adducts is equal, regardless of the number of PEG chains used to reach the total the molecular weight (Fee & Alstine, 2006) so this method does not work properly for site specific PEGylation isomers with the same extent of PEGylations (Grace et al., 2005; Knudson, Farkas & McGinley, 2006). Superdex 75 (Yu & Ghosh, 2010), Superdex 200 (Grace et al., 2005; Zhai, Zhao, Lei, Su et al., 2009; Yu & Ghosh, 2010) and Sephacryl S-300 (Daly, Przybycien & Tilton, 2005) are the most high performance size exclusion chromatography media, which have been used for this purpose.

3.2   Separation Based on Electrostatic Charges Differences Using Ion Exchange Chromatography

PEGylation changes the isoelectric point (pI) of a protein because it neutralizes a charged residue such as lysine on the protein surface depending on the size of protein, number of charged residues on the protein and the shape of protein titration curve near its isoelectric point (Veronese, 2009). It is applicable to divide the PEG molecule to two groups from the aspect of protein charge affection. In the first group, PEGylation on N terminal residue does not significantly change the net charge of protein, so PEGylated protein has the same charge of un- PEGylated form. But even in this condition, ion exchange chromatography could resolve PEGylated protein from reaction mixture. Thus shielding of steric effect and weakening the interaction of PEGylated species with the resin, could be the reason (Zhai, Zhao, Lei et al., 2009; Kusterle, Jevševar, and Porekar, 2008). The extent of shielding increases with the degree of PEGylation (Yu & Ghosh, 2010), usually higher PEGylated species including higher number of PEGylation or higher molecular weight of PEG elute at lower ionic strengths (Pabst, Buckley, Rama-subramanyan et al., 2007) and somehow in flow through fraction without binding to the column(Fee & Alstine, 2006). The first mentioned group consists of PEG-aldehyde (labels only the α- amino group), PEG- tresyl or tosyl (not much used because the chemistry leads to a mixture of products), PEG-dichlorotriazine or chlorotriazine (abandoned for therapeutic application because of toxicity) and PEG- epoxide which is slowly reactive and rarely used (Veronese & Pasut, 2005). The second group consists of PEG- carboxilate and PEG- carbonate derivatives which decrease the positive charge of the protein conjugate after bonding to amino group. PEG- carbonates derivatives include PEG-p- nitrophenyl carbonate, PEG- benzotriazolyl carbonate, PEG-2, 3, 5, thrichlorophenyl carbonate and PEG- succinimidyl carbonate yield a urethane linkage with amine and all of them are slowly reactive. The PEG- carboxilate derivatives include derivatives with one or more CH2 groups between PEG and carboxylic group which the kinetic rate of conjugation depends on the numbers and eventual ramification of CH2 group linked to the carboxyl group. PEG- succinimidyl succinate, in which the ester bond between succinate acid and PEG is easily hydrolyzed, is another example of PEG- carboxilates group. The other members are PEG- amino acid- succinimidyl ester and PEG- peptide-succinimidyl ester. Easy quantification of the number of linked PEG chains is possible by NLE or βAla amino acid analysis in PEG- amino acid- succinimidylester family and easily localization of PEGylation site is possible by CNBr treatment of Met- Nle or Met-βAla in the PEG- peptide- succinimidyl ester family (Veronese & Pasut, 2005). Ion exchange chromatography is the most commonly used technique for Purification of PEGylated proteins using different cationic and anionic resin are cited in literatures (Grace *et al.*, 2005; Zhai, Zhao, Lei, Su *et al.*, 2009; Yu & Ghosh, 2010; Abzalimov, Frimpong & Kaltashov, 2012). It is a diffusion limited process and diffusivity decreases adversely by increasing of PEGylation extent (hydrodynamic radius increasing). So restricted flow rate are allowed, a range of 90 cm/hr up to 136 cm/h are reported (Yu & Ghosh, 2010). The other disadvantage is small differences of the strengths of electrostatic interactions between positional isomers which cannot be exploited effectively at the preparative scale (Veronese, 2009). Lower dynamic binding because of the lower diffusivity and access to internal pores in chromatography media is another problem of this technique (Pabst, Buckley, Ramasubramanyan *et al.*, 2007), sometimes adsorption capacity is 10 times lower than is normal for non-PEGylated proteins. Removal of free PEG before loading the sample to the column is a very important parameter in obtaining good resolution (Fee & Alstine, 2006). PEG molecule is not a UV visible substance so does not show a peak in chromatogram and should be detected by SDS- page stained with barium iodine (Zhai, Zhao, Lei *et al.*, 2009) and the UV absorbance of PEGylated isoforms is due to the protein part of them. Its UV absorption but could be detected by Evaporative Light Scattering Detector (ELSD) (Yu *et al.*, 2010). It is possible to use membrane for ion exchange chromatography. In membrane chromatography, porous chromatography media are substituted by the stacks of micro porous membranes. Low back pressure and rapid separation make this method as a effective technique for separation of PEG molecules at large scales. At a operational investigation research, Only a 1 bar backpressure at a 240 cm/h flow rate was seen and by comparing flow rates of 24, 96, 144 and 240 cm/h, the best resolution was reported at the highest one which is in contrary to observed behavior in packed bed column chromatography where both resolution and peak sharpness decrease at high superficial velocities. This can be explained by the enhancement of mass transfer phenomena. In membrane chromatography the convectional transport is dominant to diffusion and diffusion only takes place within the stagnant thin film layer very closed to the pores walls and the thickness of this layer reduces by increasing the velocity which causes better mass transport and resolution consequently (Yu & Ghosh, 2010) .

3.3   Separation Based on Hydrophobicity Differences Using Reverse Phase Chromatography

As mention PEGylation increase the hydrophilic properties of the protein, so cause a reduction in retention time of PEGylated forms in high performance reveres phase chromatography. In this case more PEGylated species elute sooner. Also this phenomena is detectable between different PEG molecule, the more heavy one has less retention time (Zhai, Zhao, Lei *et al.*, 2009) although there are some literature reporting reverse (Lee, Kwon, Kim *et al.*, 2007; Lakshmi & Palaniswamy, 2013; Na & Lee, 2004; Yu *et al.*,

2007). Stationary phase chemistry, temperature, mobile phase gradient and pH are important factor need to be considered and optimized for good resolution in site specific isomers with similar PEGylation extent (Knudson, Farkas & McGinley, 2006). Fee and Alstine have been prepared a detailed list of different chromatography methods for different PEGylated proteins in details (Fee & Alstine, 2006). A research shows that slightly improved resolution between different PEGylated forms can be achieved by increasing temperature in reverse phase chromatography also a C4 column shows a slightly better resolution than C18 but not significant improvement (Knudson, Farkas and McGinley, 2006).

4   Conclusion

Engineering purification of conjugated proteins is often of prime importance in designing the bioseparation strategy. In this chapter, the strategy is built on physicochemical properties of the biomolecule under study. These properties include molecular size, surface charge distribution and relative hydrophobicity for size exclusion, ion exchange and hydrophobic interaction chromatography respectively. Purification of PEGylated proteins involves the separation of unconjugated protein and unreacted PEG from the conjugated proteins. Therefore, it would be an essential to consider the physicochemical properties of the target biomolecule. Furthermore, PEGylation of already purified proteins imposes purification challenges. The challenges involve the separation of PEGylated protein from other reaction products like unreacted PEG and proteins and achievement of high resolution of the PEGylated protein on the basis of their extent of PEGylation. Thus, the purification strategy for separation of PEGylated proteins, extent of PEGylation from unreacted protein and PEG are discussed which seems to be state of arts in purification of PEGylated proteins of medicinal and industrial importance.

References

Abzalimov, R. R., Frimpong, A., & Kaltashov, I. A. (2012). Structural characterization of protein–polymer conjugates. I. Assessing heterogeneity of a small PEGylated protein and mapping conjugation sites using ion exchange chromatography and top-down tandem mass spectrometry. International Journal of Mass Spectrometry, 312: 135–143.

Ahangar Cohan R., Madadkar-Sobhani A., Khanahmad H., Roohv, F., Aghasadeghi M.R., Hedayati M.H., Barghi Z., Shafiee-Ardestani M., Inanlou D.N. & Norouzian D. (2011). Design, modeling, expression, and chemoselective PEGylation of a new nano size cysteine analog of erythropoietin. International Journal of Nanomedicine.

Caliceti, P. & Veronese, F. M. (2003). Pharmacokinetic and biodistribution properties of poly (ethylene glycol)–protein conjugates. Advanced drug delivery reviews, 55(10): 1261–1277.

Caserman, S., Kusterle, M., Kunstelj, M., Milunović, T., Schiefermeier, M., Jevševar, S. & Gaberc Porekar, V. (2009). Correlations between in vitro potency of polyethylene glycol–

protein conjugates and their chromatographic behavior. Analytical biochemistry, 389(1): 27–31.

Daly, S.M., Przybycien, T.M., & Tilton, R.D. (2005). Adsorption of poly (ethylene glycol)-modified lysozyme to silica. Langmuir, 21(4): 1328–1337.

Fee, C.J. & Van Alstine, J.M. (2004). Prediction of the viscosity radius and the size exclusion chromatography behavior of PEGylated proteins. Bioconjugate chemistry, 15(6): 1304–1313.

Fee, C.J. & Van Alstine, J.M. (2006). PEG-proteins: Reaction engineering and separation issues. Chemical engineering science, 61(3): 924–939

Gaberc-Porekar, V., Zore, I., Podobnik, B. & Menart, V. (2008). Obstacles and pitfalls in the PEGylation of therapeutic proteins. Current Opinion in Drug Discovery and Development, 11(2): 242.

Grace, M.J., Lee, S., Bradshaw, S., Chapman, J., Spond, J., Cox, S., DeLorenzo, M., Brassard, D., Wylie, D. & Cannon-Carlson, S. (2005). Site of pegylation and polyethylene glycol molecule size attenuate interferon-α antiviral and antiproliferative activities through the JAK/STAT signaling pathway. Journal of Biological Chemistry, 280(8): 6327–6336.

Hagel, L. (1998). Gel Filtration: in Protein Purification. L. J.-C. Janson & Rydén, Editors., New York: John Wiley & Sons.

Jevsevar, S., Kunstelj M., & Porekar V.G. (2010). PEGylation of therapeutic proteins. Biotechnol J., 5(1): 113–28.

Knudson, V., Farkas, T. & McGinley, M. (2006). Investigations into Improving the Separation of PEGylated Proteins. Insulin, 800(1000): 1200.

Kusterle, M., Jevševar, S., & Porekar, V.G. (2008). Size of Pegylated Protein Conjugates Studied by Various Methods. Acta Chimica Slovenica, 55(3).

Lakshmi, N.S. & Palaniswamy, M.S. (2013). N-Terminal Site-Specific PEGylation and Analytical-Scale Purification of PEG Lysozyme. Agilent Technologies, Inc.

Lee, B.K., Kwon, J.S., Kim, H.J., Yamamoto, S. & Lee, E. (2007). Solid-phase PEGylation of recombinant interferon α-2a for site-specific modification: process performance, characterization, and in vitro bioactivity. Bioconjugate chemistry, 18(6): 1728–1734.

Na, D.H. & Lee, K.C. (2004). Capillary electrophoretic characterization of PEGylated human parathyroid hormone with matrix-assisted laser desorption/ionization time-of-flight mass spectrometry. Analytical biochemistry, 331(2): 322–328.

Pabst, T.M., Buckley, J.J., Ramasubramanyan, N. & Hunter, A.K. (2007). Comparison of strong anion-exchangers for the purification of a PEGylated protein. Journal of Chromatography A, 1147(2): 172–182.

Roberts, M.J., Bentley, M.D. & Harris J.M. (2002). Chemistry for peptide and protein PEGylation. Adv Drug Deliv Rev, 54(4): 459–76.

Ryan, S.M., Mantovani G., Wang X., Haddleton, D.M. & Brayden D.J. (2008). Advances in PEGylation of Important Biotech Molecules: Delivery Aspects. Expert Opinion in Drug Delivery. Apr;5(4): 371–83.

Shaunak, S., Godwin, A., Choi, J.-W., Balan, S., Pedone, E., Vijayarangam, D., Heidelberger, S., Teo, I., Zloh, M. & Brocchini, S. (2006). Site-specific PEGylation of native disulfide bonds in therapeutic proteins. Nature chemical biology, 2(6): 312–313.

Skoog, D.A., Holler, F.J., & Crouch, S.R. (2007). Principles of Instrumental Analysis., Thomson, Brooks/Cole Publishing Company, Pacific Grove: Belmont, CA.

Veronese, F.M. & Pasut, G. (2005). PEGylation, successful approach to drug delivery. Drug discovery today, 10(21): p. 1451–1458.

Veronese, F.M. (2009). PEGylated Protein Drugs: Basic Science and Clinical Applications: Basic Science and Clinical Applications. Springer.

Yu, D. & Ghosh, R. (2010). Purification of PEGylated protein using membrane chromatography. Journal of pharmaceutical sciences, 99(8): 3326–3333.

Yu, P., Qin, G., Qin, D. & Zhang, Z. (2010). A liquid chromatographic method for determination of the modification degree of proteins: PEGylated arginase as an example. Analytical biochemistry, 396(2): p. 325–327.

Yu, P., Zheng, C., Chen, J., Zhang, G., Liu, Y., Suo, X., Zhang, G. & Su, Z. (2007). Investigation on PEGylation strategy of recombinant human interleukin-1 receptor antagonist. Bioorganic & medicinal chemistry, 15(16): 5396–5405.

Zhang, C., Yang, X.-l., Yuan, Y.-h., Pu, J. & Liao, F. (2012). Site-specific PEGylation of therapeutic proteins via optimization of both accessible reactive amino acid residues and PEG derivatives. BioDrugs, 26(4): 209–215.

Zhai, Y., Zhao, Y., Lei, J., Su, Z. & Ma, G. (2009). Enhanced circulation half-life of site-specific PEGylated rhG-CSF: Optimization of PEG molecular weight. Journal of biotechnology, 142(3): 259–266.

www.ingramcontent.com/pod-product-compliance
Lightning Source LLC
Chambersburg PA
CBHW081053220326
41598CB00038B/7083